# STUDY GUIDE & LABORATORY MANUAL

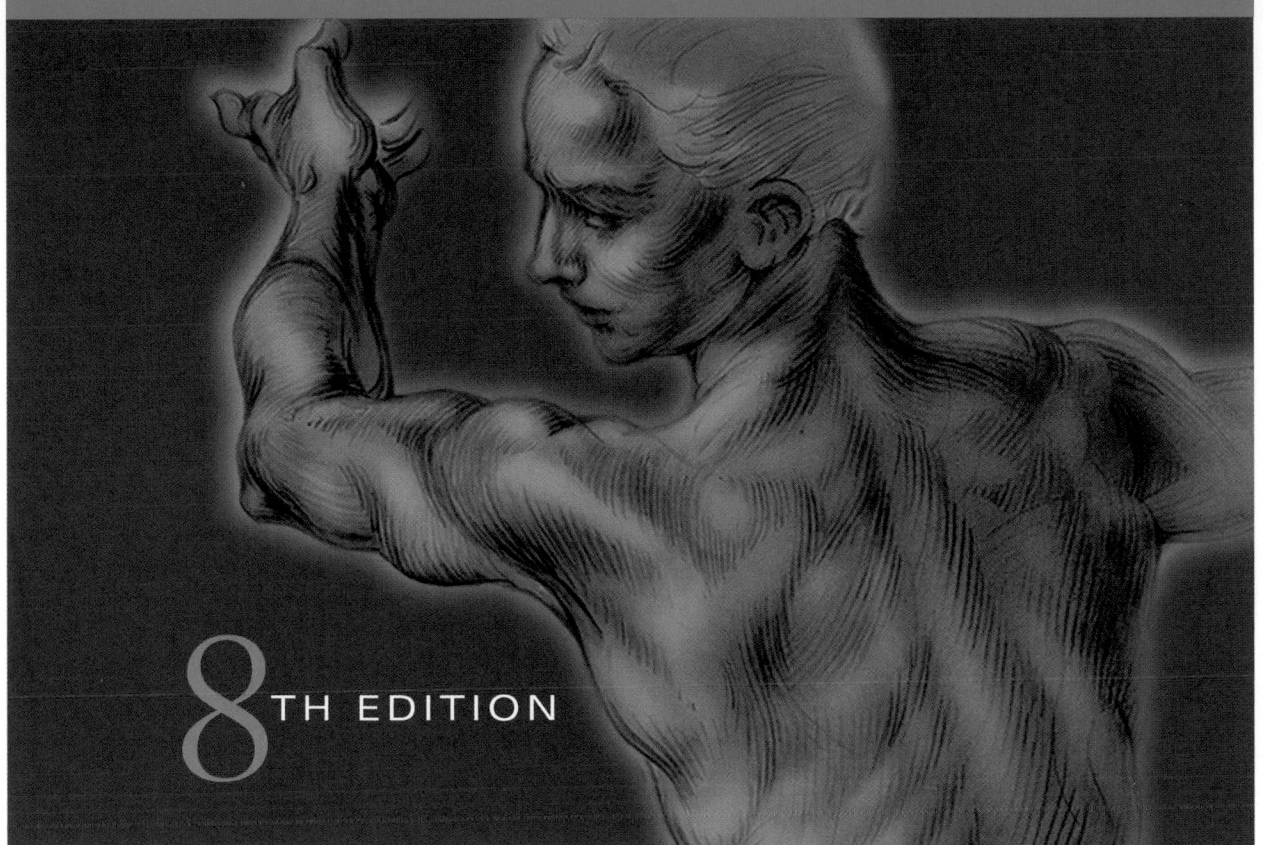

# 8TH EDITION

# Physical Examination & Health Assessment

## CAROLYN JARVIS, PhD, APRN, CNP

Professor of Nursing
Illinois Wesleyan University
Bloomington, Illinois
and
Family Nurse Practitioner
Bloomington, Illinois

## With Ann Eckhardt, PhD, RN

Associate Professor of Nursing
Illinois Wesleyan University
Bloomington, Illinois

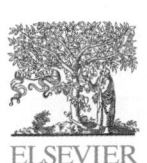

ELSEVIER

STUDY GUIDE & LABORATORY MANUAL FOR
PHYSICAL EXAMINATION & HEALTH
ASSESSMENT, EIGHTH EDITION

ISBN: 978-0-323-53203-7

---

**Notice**

Practitioners and researchers must always rely on their own experience and knowledge in evaluating and using any information, methods, compounds or experiments described herein. Because of rapid advances in the medical sciences, in particular, independent verification of diagnoses and drug dosages should be made. To the fullest extent of the law, no responsibility is assumed by Elsevier, authors, editors or contributors for any injury and/or damage to persons or property as a matter of products liability, negligence or otherwise, or from any use or operation of any methods, products, instructions, or ideas contained in the material herein.

---

Previous editions copyrighted 2016, 2012, 2008, 2004, 2000, 1996, 1993.

**International Standard Book Number: 978-0-323-53203-7**

*Executive Content Strategist:* Lee Henderson
*Senior Content Development Specialist:* Heather Bays
*Publishing Services Manager:* Julie Eddy
*Senior Project Manager:* Jodi M. Willard
*Design Direction:* Brian Salisbury

Printed in Canada

Last digit is the print number:  9  8  7  6  5  4  3

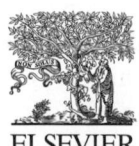

ELSEVIER

3251 Riverport Lane
St. Louis, Missouri 63043

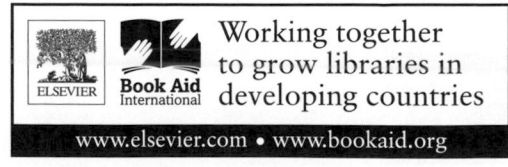

# Contributor/Reviewer

## CONTRIBUTOR

**Lydia Bertschi, DNP, APRN, ACNP-BC**
Assistant Professor
Illinois Wesleyan University
Bloomington, Illinois
*Sections of Chapter 22, Abdomen*

## REVIEWER

**Heidi Monroe MSN, RN-BC, CAPA**
Assistant Professor of Nursing
NCLEX-RN Coordinator
Bellin College
Green Bay, Wisconsin

# Preface

This *Study Guide & Laboratory Manual* is intended to accompany the textbook *Physical Examination & Health Assessment*, 8th edition. You, the student, will use it in two places: in your own study area and in the skills laboratory.

As a *Study Guide*, this workbook highlights and reinforces the content from the text. Each chapter corresponds to a chapter in the textbook and contains exercises and questions in varying formats to synthesize and master content from the text. Fill out the lab manual chapter and answer the questions before coming to the skills laboratory. This will reinforce your lectures, expose any areas in which you have questions for your clinical instructor, and prime you for the skills laboratory/clinical experience.

Once in the skills laboratory, use the *Laboratory Manual* as a direct clinical tool. Each chapter contains assessment forms on perforated, tear-out pages. Usually you will work in pairs and perform the regional physical examinations on each other under the tutelage of your instructor. As you perform the examination on your peer, you can fill out the regional write-up and turn it in to the instructor for feedback.

## FEATURES

Each chapter is divided into two parts—cognitive and clinical—and contains:
- Purpose—A brief summary of the material you are learning in the chapter.
- Reading Assignment—The corresponding chapter and page numbers from the *Physical Examination & Health Assessment* textbook.
- Suggested journal articles—All new for the 8th edition, these are current and choice readings for critical thinking and for interventions.
- Glossary—Important or specialized terms with accompanying definitions.
- Study Guide—Specific short-answer and fill-in questions to help you highlight and learn content from the chapter. New critical thinking questions are included to coordinate the reading and video assignments. Important illustrations of human anatomy, in full color, have been reproduced from the textbook with the labels deleted so you can identify and fill in the names of the structures yourself.
- Review Questions—Multiple-choice questions, matching, and short-answer questions so you can monitor your own mastery of the material. Take the self-exam when you are ready and then check your answers against the answer key provided in the back of the book.
- Critical Thinking Exercises—all new for the 8th edition.
- Clinical Objectives—behavioral objectives that you should achieve during your peer practice in the regional examinations.
- Regional Write-Up Sheets—complete yet succinct physical exam forms that you can use in the skills lab or in the clinical setting. These serve as a memory prompt, listing key history questions and physical examination steps, and as a means of recording data during the patient encounter.
- Narrative Summary Forms—SOAP format, so you can learn to chart narrative accounts of the history and physical exam findings. These forms have accompanying sketches of regional anatomy and are especially useful for those studying advanced practice roles.

Learning the skills of history taking and physical examination requires two types of practice: cognitive and clinical. It is our hope that this manual will help you achieve both of these learning and practice modalities.

CAROLYN JARVIS

ANN ECKHARDT

# Acknowledgments

We are grateful to those on the team at Elsevier who worked on the *Laboratory Manual*. Our thanks extend to Lee Henderson, Executive Content Strategist; Heather Bays, Senior Content Development Specialist; Jodi Willard, Senior Project Manager; Julie Eddy, Publishing Services Manager; and Brian Salisbury, Book Designer. We are dependent on this wonderful team to bring our vision into print and to make it useful for our students.

# Contents

# CHAPTER
# 1

# Evidence-Based Assessment

## PURPOSE

This chapter discusses the characteristics of evidence-based practice, diagnostic reasoning, the nursing process, and critical thinking. This chapter also introduces the concept of health, helps you understand that it is the definition of health that determines the types of factors that are assessed, and shows you that the amount of data gathered during assessment varies with the person's age, developmental state, physical condition, risk factors, and culture.

## READING ASSIGNMENT

Jarvis: *Physical Examination and Health Assessment*, 8th ed., Chapter 1, pp. 1-9.

Suggested reading:
Cunha, B.A. (2017). The master clinician's approach to diagnostic reasoning. *Am J Med, 130*(1), 5-7.

## GLOSSARY

Study the following terms after completing the reading assignment. You should be able to cover the definition on the right and define the term out loud.

**Assessment** . . . . . . . . . . . . . . . . . the collection of data about an individual's health state

**Biomedical model** . . . . . . . . . . the Western European/North American tradition that views health as the absence of disease

**Complete database** . . . . . . . . . . a complete health history and full physical examination

**Critical thinking** . . . . . . . . . . . . simultaneously problem solving while self-improving one's own thinking ability

**Diagnostic reasoning** . . . . . . . . a method of collecting and analyzing clinical information with the following components: (1) attending to initially available cues, (2) formulating diagnostic hypotheses, (3) gathering data relative to the tentative hypotheses, (4) evaluating each hypothesis with the new data collected, and (5) arriving at a final diagnosis

**Emergency database** . . . . . . . . rapid collection of the database, often compiled concurrently with lifesaving measures

**Environment** . . . . . . . . . . . . . . the total of all the conditions and elements that make up the surroundings and influence the development of a person

**Evidence-based practice** . . . . . . a systematic approach emphasizing the best research evidence, the clinician's experience, patient preferences and values, physical examination, and assessment

**Focused database** . . . . . . . . . . used for a limited or short-term problem; concerns mainly one problem, one cue complex, or one body system

**Follow-up database** . . . . . . . . . used in all settings to monitor progress of short-term or chronic health problems

**Holistic health** . . . . . . . . . . . . . the view that the mind, body, and spirit are interdependent and function as a whole within the environment

**Nursing process** . . . . . . . . . . . . a method of collecting and analyzing clinical information with the following components: (1) assessment, (2) diagnosis, (3) outcome identification, (4) planning, (5) implementation, and (6) evaluation

**Objective data** . . . . . . . . . . . . . what the health professional observes by inspecting, palpating, percussing, and auscultating during the physical examination

**Prevention** . . . . . . . . . . . . . . . . any action directed toward promoting health and preventing the occurrence of disease

**Subjective data** . . . . . . . . . . . . . what the person says about himself or herself during history taking

**Wellness** . . . . . . . . . . . . . . . . . . a dynamic process and view of health; a move toward optimal functioning

## STUDY GUIDE

After completing the reading assignment, you should be able to answer the following questions in the spaces provided.

1. The steps of the diagnostic reasoning process are listed below. Consider the clinical example given for "cue recognition," and fill in the remaining diagnostic reasoning steps.

| Stage | Example |
| --- | --- |
| 1.  Cue recognition | 1.  A.J., 62-year-old man, appears pale, diaphoretic, and anxious |
| 2.  Hypothesis formulation | 2. |
| 3.  Data gathering for hypothesis testing | 3. |
| 4.  Hypothesis evaluation | 4. |

2. One of the critical-thinking skills is identifying assumptions. Explain how the following statement contains an assumption. What is a more appropriate response? *"Ellen, you have to break up with your boyfriend. He is too rough with you. He is no good for you."*

3. Another critical-thinking skill involves validation, or checking the accuracy and reliability of data. Describe how you would validate the following data.

   Mr. Quinn tells you his weight this morning was 165 lb.

   The primary counselor tells you Ellen is depressed and angry about being admitted to residential treatment in the clinic.

   When auscultating the heart, you hear a blowing, swooshing sound between the first and second heart sounds.

4. List the barriers to evidence-based practice, both on an individual level and on an organizational level.

5. Differentiate **subjective** data from **objective** data by placing an **S** or an **O** after each of the following: complaint of sore shoulder _____; unconscious _____; blood in the urine _____; family has just moved to a new area _____; dizziness _____; sore throat _____; earache _____; weight gain _____.

6. For the following situations, state the type of data collection you would perform (i.e., *complete* database, *focused* or problem-centered database, *follow-up* database, *emergency* database).
   OxyContin overdose _____; ambulatory, apparently well individual who presents at outpatient clinic with a rash _____; first visit to a health care provider for a checkup _____; recently placed on antihypertensive medication _____.

7. Discuss the impact that racial and cultural diversity of individuals has on the U.S. health care system.

8. List three health care interactions you have experienced with another person from a culture or ethnicity different from your own. Were they positive or negative? What could or should have been done differently?

9. Using one sentence or group of phrases, how would you describe your own health state to someone you are meeting for the first time?

## REVIEW QUESTIONS

This test is for you to check your own mastery of the content. Answers are provided in Appendix A.

1. The concept of health and healing has evolved in recent years. Which is the best description of health?

   a. Health is the absence of disease.
   b. Health is a dynamic process toward optimal functioning.
   c. Health depends on an interaction of mind, body, and spirit within the environment.
   d. Health is the prevention of disease.

2. Which would be included in the database for a new patient admission to a surgical unit?

   a. All subjective and objective data gathered by a health practitioner from a patient
   b. All objective data obtained from a patient through inspection, percussion, palpation, and auscultation
   c. A summary of a patient's record, including laboratory studies
   d. All subjective and objective data, data gathered from a patient, and the results of any laboratory or diagnostic studies completed

3. You are reviewing assessment data of a 45-year-old male patient and note pain of 8 on a scale of 10, labored breathing, and pale skin color on the electronic health record. This documentation is an example of:

    a. Hypothetical reasoning.
    b. Diagnostic reasoning.
    c. Data cluster.
    d. Signs and symptoms.

4. A patient is in the emergency department with nausea and vomiting. Which would you include in the database?

    a. A complete health history and full physical examination
    b. A diet and GI history
    c. Previously identified problems
    d. Start collection of data in conjunction with lifesaving measures

5. A patient has recently received health insurance and would like to know how often he should visit the provider. How do you respond?

    a. "It would be most efficient if you visit on an annual basis."
    b. "There is no recommendation for the frequency of health care visits."
    c. "Your visits may vary, depending on your level of wellness."
    d. "Your visits will be based on your preference."

6. You are reviewing concepts related to steps in the nursing process for determining prioritization and developing patient outcomes. To what are these actions attributed?

    a. Planning
    b. Assessment
    c. Implementation
    d. Diagnosis

7. Which best describes evidence-based nursing practice?

    a. Combining clinical expertise with the use of nursing research to provide the best care for patients while considering the patient's values and circumstances
    b. Appraising and looking at the implications of one or two articles as they relate to the culture and ethnicity of the patient
    c. Completing a literature search to find relevant articles that use nursing research to encourage nurses to use good practices
    d. Finding value-based resources to justify nursing actions when working with patients of diverse cultural backgrounds

8. What can be determined when the nurse clusters data as part of the critical-thinking process?

    a. This step identifies problems that may be urgent and require immediate action.
    b. This step involves making assumptions in the data.
    c. The nurse recognizes relevant information among the data.
    d. Risk factors can be determined so the nurse knows how to offer health teaching.

9. A patient says she is very nervous and nauseated, and she feels as if she will vomit. This data would be what type of data?

    a. Objective
    b. Reflective
    c. Subjective
    d. Introspective

10. The expert nurse differs from the novice nurse by acting without consciously thinking about the actions. This is referred to as:

    a. Deductive reasoning.
    b. Intuition.
    c. The nursing process.
    d. Focused assessment.

11. Which would be considered a risk diagnosis?

    a. Identifying existing levels of wellness
    b. Evaluating previous problems and goals
    c. Identifying potential problems the individual may develop
    d. Focusing on strengths and reflecting an individual's transition to higher levels of wellness

12. Which would be included in a holistic model of assessment?

    a. Nursing goals for the patient
    b. Anticipated growth and development patterns
    c. A patient's perception of his or her health status
    d. The nurse's perception of disease related to the patient

13. The nurse uses health promotion activities with a new patient. What would this focus include?

    a. The nurse would try to change the patient's perceptions of disease.
    b. The nurse would search for identification of biomedical model interventions.
    c. The nurse would help to identify negative health acts of the patient.
    d. The nurse would empower the patient to choose a healthier lifestyle.

14. Which is an example of objective data?

    a. Patient's history of allergies
    b. Patient's use of medications at home
    c. Last menstrual period 1 month ago
    d. 2- × 5-cm scar present on the right lower forearm

15. During the evaluation phase of the nursing process, which action would be included?

    a. Validating the nursing diagnosis
    b. Establishing priorities related to patient care
    c. Including the patient and family members
    d. Establishing a timeline for planned outcomes

# Cultural Assessment

## PURPOSE

This chapter reviews the demographic profile of the United States, the National Standards for Culturally and Linguistically Appropriate Services in Health Care, traditional HEALTH/ILLNESS beliefs and practices, and the steps to cultural competency. At the end of the chapter, you will be able to perform a cultural assessment.

## READING ASSIGNMENT

Jarvis: *Physical Examination and Health Assessment,* 8th ed., Chapter 2, pp. 11-22.

Suggested reading:
Centers for Disease Control and Prevention. (2015). CDC Health Disparities & Inequalities Report. https://www.cdc.gov/minorityhealth/chdireport.html.

## GLOSSARY

Study the following terms after completing the reading assignment. You should be able to cover the definition on the right and define the term out loud.

**Acculturation** . . . . . . . . . . . . . . process of social and psychological exchanges with encounters between persons of different cultures, resulting in changes in either group

**Cultural and linguistic competence** . . . . . . . . . . . . . . . a set of congruent behaviors, attitudes, and policies that come together in a system among professionals that enables work in cross-cultural situations

**Cultural care** . . . . . . . . . . . . . . . professional health care that is culturally sensitive, appropriate, and competent

**Culture** . . . . . . . . . . . . . . . . . . . the nonphysical attributes of a person—the thoughts, communications, actions, beliefs, values, and institutions of racial, ethnic, religious, or social groups

**Ethnicity** . . . . . . . . . . . . . . . . . a social group within the social system that claims to possess variable traits such as a common geographic origin, migratory status, and religion

**Ethnocentrism** . . . . . . . . . . . . . tendency to view your own way of life as the most desirable, acceptable, or best and to act superior to another culture's way of life

**Folk healer** . . . . . . . . . . . . . . . . lay healer in the person's culture apart from the biomedical or scientific health care system

**Health or illness** . . . . . . . . . . . . the balance or imbalance of the person, both within one's being (physical, mental, and/or spiritual) and in the outside world (natural, communal, and/or metaphysical)

**Religion** . . . . . . . . . . . . . . . . . . . an organized system of beliefs concerning the cause, nature, and purpose of the universe, as well as attendance at regular services

**Socialization** . . . . . . . . . . . . . . . the process of being raised within a culture and acquiring the characteristics of that group

**Spirituality** . . . . . . . . . . . . . . . . a broad term focused on a connection to something larger than oneself, and a belief in transcendence

**Title VI of the Civil**
**Rights Act of 1964** . . . . . . . . . . a federal law that mandates that when people with limited English proficiency (LEP) seek health care in health care settings such as hospitals, nursing homes, clinics, daycare centers, and mental health centers, services cannot be denied to them

**Values** . . . . . . . . . . . . . . . . . . . . . a desirable or undesirable state of affairs and a universal feature of all cultures

## STUDY GUIDE

After completing the reading assignment, you should be able to answer the following questions in the spaces provided.

1. Describe the provisions of Title VI of the Civil Rights Act of 1964.

2. Describe the rationale for providing culturally competent care.

3. List the basic characteristics of culture.

4. List and describe factors related to socialization.

5. List and define 3 major theories about how people view the causes of illness.

6. Define the *yin yang theory* of health and illness, and relate this to different types of foods.

7. Define the *hot and cold theory* of health and illness, and relate this to different types of foods and illnesses.

8. List at least 5 names for various folk healers and the culture they represent.

9. Describe 5 methods of complementary interventions.

## REVIEW QUESTIONS

This test is for you to check your own mastery of the content. Answers are provided in Appendix A.

1. Which statement best describes religion?

   a. An organized system of beliefs concerning the cause, nature, and purpose of the universe
   b. Belief in a divine or superhuman spirit to be obeyed and worshiped
   c. Affiliation with one of the 1200 recognized religions in the United States
   d. The following of established rituals, especially in conjunction with health-seeking behaviors

2. The major factor contributing to the need for cultural care nursing is:

   a. An increasing birth rate.
   b. Limited access to health care services.
   c. Demographic change.
   d. A decreasing rate of immigration.

3. The term *culturally competent* implies that the nurse:

   a. Is prepared in nursing.
   b. Possesses knowledge of the traditions of diverse peoples.
   c. Applies underlying knowledge to providing nursing care.
   d. Understands the cultural context of the patient's situation.

4. You are the triage nurse in the emergency department and perform the initial intake assessment on a patient who does not speak English. Based on your understanding of linguistic competence, which action would present as a barrier to effective communication?

   a. Maintaining a professional respectful demeanor
   b. Allowing for additional time to complete the process
   c. Providing the patient with a paper and pencil so he or she can write down the answers to the questions that you are going to ask
   d. Seeing if there are any family members present who may assist with the interview process

5. Which culture would describe illness as hot and cold imbalance?

   a. Asian-American heritage
   b. African-American heritage
   c. Hispanic-American heritage
   d. American Indian heritage

6. Of what does the patient believe the amulet is protective?

   a. The evil eye
   b. Being kidnapped
   c. Exposure to bacterial infections
   d. An unexpected fall

7. Which statement best illustrates the difference between religion and spirituality?

   a. Religion reflects an individual's reaction to life events whereas spirituality is based on whether the individual attends religious services.
   b. Religion is characterized by identification of a higher being shaping one's destiny, whereas spirituality reflects an individual's perception of one's life having worth or meaning.
   c. Religion is the expression of spiritual awakening whereas spirituality is based on belief in divine right.
   d. Religion is the active interpretation of one's spirituality.

8. The first step to cultural competency by a nurse is to:

   a. Identify the meaning of health to the patient.
   b. Understand how a health care delivery system works.
   c. Develop a frame of reference to traditional health care practices.
   d. Understand your own heritage and its basis in cultural values.

9. Which statement is true in regard to pain?

   a. Nurses' attitudes toward their patients' pain are unrelated to their own experiences with pain.
   b. The cultural background of a patient is important in a nurse's assessment of that patient's pain.
   c. A nurse's area of clinical practice is most likely to determine his or her assessment of a patient's pain.
   d. A nurse's years of clinical experience and current position are a strong indicator of his or her response to patient pain.

10. Which factor is identified as a *priority* influence on a patient's health status?

    a. Poverty
    b. Lifestyle factors
    c. Legislative action
    d. Occupational status

11. Which statement is most appropriate to use when initiating an assessment of cultural beliefs with an older American Indian patient?

    a. "Are you of the Christian faith?"
    b. "Do you want to see a medicine man?"
    c. "How often do you seek help from medical providers?"
    d. What cultural or spiritual beliefs are important to you?"

12. Which statement best describes ethnocentrism?

    a. The government's description of various cultures
    b. A central belief that accepts all cultures as one's own
    c. The tendency to view your own way of life as the most desirable
    d. The tendency to impose your beliefs, values, and patterns of behaviors on an individual from another culture

13. Which category is appropriate in a cultural assessment?

    a. Family history
    b. Chief complaint
    c. Past medical history
    d. Health-related beliefs

14. Which health belief practice is associated with patients who are of American Indian heritage?

    a. Wearing bangle bracelets to ward off evil spirits
    b. Believing that forces of nature must be kept in natural balance
    c. Using swamp root as a traditional home remedy
    d. Believing in a shaman as a traditional healer

15. Which statement best reflects the Magicoreligious causation of illness?

    a. Each being is but a part of a larger structure in the world of nature as it relates to health and illness.
    b. Causality relationship exists, leading to expression of illness.
    c. Belief in the struggle between good and evil is reflected in the regulation of health and illness.
    d. Illness occurs as a result of disturbances between hot and cold reactions.

## CRITICAL THINKING EXERCISE 1

Consider the following clinical examples. What is your reaction to each example? How would you handle the situation if you were a part of the conversation or overheard either conversation?

- **Situation 1:** You receive report on a new admission who is coming in with pancreatitis. During report, you are told that the woman's primary language is Spanish. After you share this information with the admitting physician, the physician states, "Oh, great! I sure hope she has somebody with her who can speak English. You KNOW what a pain it is to set up and use the translator system. What am I saying?! She is sure to have SOMEONE with her who speaks English. Those people ALWAYS come in packs."
- **Situation 2:** You are at the nurses' station and overhear the following conversation:
  **Person 1:** "I need to know which patient is going home so that I can write discharge orders."
  **Person 2:** "The Indian family."
  **Person 1 (laughing):** "Indian how? Red dot or red feather?"

## CRITICAL THINKING EXERCISE 2

With a partner or a small group, discuss common stereotypes you have heard, seen, or believe. Be open and honest in your discussion. Where do the stereotypes come from? How might a negative stereotype impact the care you provide a patient? How will being aware of stereotypes potentially enhance patient care?

## SKILLS LABORATORY AND CLINICAL SETTING

You are now ready for the clinical component of this chapter. The purpose of the clinical component is to collect data for a heritage assessment on a peer in the skills laboratory or on a patient in the clinical setting. Although you may not yet have been assigned chapters on the health history, the questions in the heritage assessment tool are clearly defined and should pose no problem. The best experience would be for you to pair up with a peer from a cultural heritage *different* from your own. If this is not possible, you still will gain insight and sensitivity into the cultural dimensions of health and will gain mastery of the assessment tool.

# BOX 2-1    SPECTOR'S HERITAGE ASSESSMENT

1. Where were you born? _____

2. Where were your parents and grandparents born?

   a. Mother: _____
   b. Father: _____
   c. Mother's mother: _____
   d. Mother's father: _____
   e. Father's mother: _____
   f. Father's father: _____

3. How many brothers _____ and sisters _____ do you have?

4. In what setting did you grow up? Urban _____ Rural _____ Suburban _____

   Where? _____

5. In what country did your parents and grandparents grow up?

   a. Mother: _____
   b. Father: _____
   c. Mother's mother: _____
   d. Mother's father: _____
   e. Father's mother: _____
   f. Father's father: _____

6. How old were you when you came to the United States? _____

7. How old were your parents and grandparents when they came to the United States?

   a. Mother: _____
   b. Father: _____
   c. Mother's mother: _____
   d. Mother's father: _____
   e. Father's mother: _____
   f. Father's father: _____

8. When you were growing up, who lived with you? _____

9. Have you maintained contact with:

   a. Aunts, uncles, cousins? _____ Yes _____ No
   b. Brothers and sisters? _____ Yes _____ No
   c. Parents? _____ Yes _____ No
   d. Grandparents? _____ Yes _____ No

10. Does most of your family live near you? _____ Yes _____ No

11. Approximately how often do (did) you visit your family members who live(d) outside your home?

    _____ Daily _____ Weekly _____ Monthly _____ Less than once a year _____ Never

12. Was your original family name changed? _____ Yes _____ No

_____

Reprinted by permission of Pearson Education, Inc., New York, New York.

13. What is your religious preference? _____ Catholic _____ Jewish

    _____ Protestant (denomination): _____ Other _____ None

14. Is your significant other of the same religion? _____ Yes _____ No

15. Is your significant other of the same ethnic background as you? _____ Yes _____ No

16. What kind of school did you attend? _____ Public _____ Private _____ Parochial

17. As an adult, do you live in a neighborhood where the neighbors are the same religion and ethnic

    background as you? _____ Yes _____ No

18. Do you belong to a religious institution? _____ Yes _____ No

19. Would you describe yourself as an active member? _____ Yes _____ No

20. How often do you attend your religious institution? _____ More than once a week _____ Weekly

    _____ Monthly _____ Special holidays only _____ Never

21. Do you practice your religion or other spiritual practices in your home? _____ Yes _____ No

    If yes, please specify: _____ Praying _____ Bible reading _____ Diet _____ Celebrating

    religious holidays _____ Meditating _____ Other

22. Do you prepare foods of your ethnic background? _____ Yes _____ No

23. Do you participate in ethnic activities? _____ Yes _____ No

    If yes, specify: _____ Singing _____ Holiday celebrations _____ Dancing _____ Costumes

    _____ Festivals _____ Other

24. Are your friends from the same religious background? _____ Yes _____ No

25. Are your friends of the same ethnic background as you? _____ Yes _____ No

26. What is your native (non-English) language? _____

    Do you speak this language? _____ Prefer _____ Occasionally _____ Rarely

27. Do you read in your native language? _____ Prefer _____ Occasionally _____ Rarely

(You may score this assessment by giving 1 point to each positive answer from the yes/no questions 9 through 27. An exception is that if a person's name was not changed, he or she gets the point. The higher the score, the more likely the person is to use health practices relevant to his or her traditional heritage.)

From Spector, R.E. (2013). *Cultural diversity in health and illness* (8th ed., pp. 376-378). Upper Saddle River, NJ: Prentice Hall.

## HEALTH AND ILLNESS BELIEFS AND PRACTICES DETERMINATION

The next set of questions relates to *your own* personal health and illness beliefs and practices.

1. How do you define health?

2. How do you rate your health? *(Circle 1)*

    a. Excellent
    b. Good
    c. Fair
    d. Poor

3. How do you describe illness?

4. What do you believe causes illness? *(Circle all that apply.)*

    a. Environmental change
    b. Evil eye
    c. Exposure to drafts
    d. God's punishment
    e. Grief and loss
    f. Hexes and spells
    g. Incorrect food combinations
    h. Not enough work
    i. Overwork
    j. Poor eating habits
    k. Viruses, bacteria
    l. Witchcraft
    m. Other

5. What did your family do to maintain and protect your health?

6. How do you maintain and protect your health?

Jarvis, Carolyn: PHYSICAL EXAMINATION AND HEALTH ASSESSMENT: Study Guide and Laboratory Manual, Eighth Edition.

7. What home remedies did your family use to restore health?

8. What home remedies do you use?

9. Healing and curing are the same. _____ Yes _____ No

10. What do you believe brings healing?

# CHAPTER 3

# The Interview

## PURPOSE

This chapter discusses the process of communication; presents the techniques of interviewing, including open-ended versus closed questions, the 9 types of examiner responses, the 10 "traps" of interviewing, and nonverbal skills; and considers variations in technique that are necessary for individuals of different ages, for those with special needs, and for culturally diverse people.

## READING ASSIGNMENT

Jarvis: *Physical Examination and Health Assessment,* 8th ed., Chapter 3, pp. 23-44.

Suggested reading:
Foronda, C., MacWilliams, B., & McArthur, E. (2016). Interprofessional communication in healthcare: An integrative review. *Nurse Educ Pract, 19,* 36-40.

## GLOSSARY

Study the following terms after completing the reading assignment. You should be able to cover the definition on the right and define the term out loud.

| | |
|---|---|
| **Ad hoc interpreter** | using a patient's family member, friend, or child as interpreter for a patient with limited English proficiency (LEP) |
| **Animism** | imagining that inanimate objects (e.g., a blood pressure cuff) come alive and have human characteristics |
| **Avoidance language** | the use of euphemisms to avoid reality or to hide feelings |
| **Clarification** | examiner's response used when the patient's word choice is ambiguous or confusing |
| **Closed questions** | questions that ask for specific information and elicit a short, one- or two-word answer, a "yes" or "no," or a forced choice |
| **Confrontation** | response in which examiner gives honest feedback about what he or she has seen or felt after observing a certain patient action, feeling, or statement |
| **Distancing** | the use of impersonal speech to put space between one's self and a threat |

**Elderspeak** . . . . . . . . . . . . . . . . infantilizing and demeaning language used by a health professional when speaking to an older adult

**Electronic health recording** . . . direct computer entry of a patient's health record while in the patient's presence

**Empathy** . . . . . . . . . . . . . . . . . viewing the world from the other person's inner frame of reference while remaining yourself; recognizing and accepting the other person's feelings without criticism

**Ethnocentrism** . . . . . . . . . . . . . the tendency to view your own way of life as the most desirable, acceptable, or best and to act in a superior manner to another culture's way of life

**Explanation** . . . . . . . . . . . . . . . examiner's statements that inform the patient; examiner shares factual and objective information

**Facilitation** . . . . . . . . . . . . . . . examiner's response that encourages the patient to say more, to continue with the story

**Geographic privacy** . . . . . . . . . private room or space with only the examiner and patient present

**Interpretation** . . . . . . . . . . . . . examiner's statement that is not based on direct observation, but is based on examiner's inference or conclusion; links events, makes associations, or implies cause

**Interview** . . . . . . . . . . . . . . . . . meeting between the examiner and patient with the goal of gathering a complete health history

**Jargon** . . . . . . . . . . . . . . . . . . . medical vocabulary used with a patient in an exclusionary and paternalistic way

**Leading question** . . . . . . . . . . . a question that implies that one answer would be better than another

**Nonverbal communication** . . . message conveyed through body language—posture, gestures, facial expression, eye contact, touch, and even where one places the chairs

**Open-ended question** . . . . . . . asks for longer narrative information; unbiased; leaves the person free to answer in any way

**Reflection** . . . . . . . . . . . . . . . . examiner response that echoes the patient's words; repeats part of what the patient has just said

**Summary** . . . . . . . . . . . . . . . . . final review of what examiner understands patient has said; condenses facts and presents a survey of how the examiner perceives the health problem or need

**Telegraphic speech** . . . . . . . . . speech used by age 3 or 4 years in which three- or four-word sentences contain only the essential words

**Verbal communication** . . . . . . . messages sent through spoken words, vocalizations, or tone of voice

Jarvis, Carolyn: PHYSICAL EXAMINATION AND HEALTH ASSESSMENT: Study Guide and Laboratory Manual, Eighth Edition.
Copyright © 2020, 2016, 2012, 2008, 2004, 2000, 1996 by Elsevier Inc. All rights reserved.

## STUDY GUIDE

After completing the reading assignment, you should be able to answer the following questions in the spaces provided.

1.  List 8 items of information that should be communicated to the client concerning the terms or expectations of the interview.

2.  Describe the points to consider in preparing the physical setting for the interview.

3.  List the pros and cons of note-taking during the interview.

4.  Contrast open-ended versus closed questions, and explain the purpose of each during the interview.

5.  List the 9 types of examiner responses that could be used during the interview, and give a short example of each.

6.  List the 10 traps of interviewing, and give a short example of each.

7.  State at least 7 types of nonverbal behaviors that an interviewer could make.

8.  State a useful phrase to use as a closing when ending the interview.

9. Discuss special considerations when interviewing an older adult.

10. How would you modify your interviewing technique when working with a hearing-impaired person?

11. Formulate a response you would make to a client who has spoken in a sexually aggressive way.

12. List at least 5 points to consider when using an interpreter during an interview.

## REVIEW QUESTIONS

This test is for you to check your own mastery of the content. Answers are provided in Appendix A.

1. The practitioner, entering the examining room to meet a patient for the first time, states: "Hello, I'm M.M., and I'm here to gather some information from you and to perform your examination. This will take about 30 minutes. D.D. is a student working with me. If it's all right with you, she will remain during the examination." Which of the following must be added to cover all aspects of the interview contract?

   a. A statement regarding confidentiality, patient costs, and the expectations of each person
   b. The purpose of the interview and the role of the interviewer
   c. Time and place of the interview and a confidentiality statement
   d. An explicit purpose of the interview and a description of the physical examination, including diagnostic studies

2. _____is exhibiting an accurate understanding of the other person's feelings within a communication context.

   a. Empathy
   b. Liking others
   c. Facilitation
   d. A nonverbal listening technique

3. You conduct an admission interview. Because you are expecting a phone call, you stand near the door. Which would be a more appropriate approach?

   a. Arrange to have someone page you so you can sit on the side of the bed.
   b. Have someone else answer the phone so you can give the patient your full attention.
   c. Use this approach given the circumstances.
   d. Arrange for a time free of interruptions after the initial physical examination is complete.

4. A patient asks the nurse, "May I ask you a question?" This is an example of:

    a. An open-ended question.
    b. A reflective question.
    c. A closed question.
    d. A double-barreled question.

5. Which statement best describes interpretation as a communication technique?

    a. Interpretation is the same as clarification.
    b. Interpretation is a summary of a statement made by a patient.
    c. Interpretation is used to focus on a particular aspect of what the patient has just said.
    d. Interpretation is based on the interviewer's inference from the data that have been presented.

6. Which demonstrates a good understanding of the interview process?

    a. The nurse stops the patient each time something is said that is not understood.
    b. The nurse spends more time listening to the patient than talking.
    c. The nurse is consistently thinking of his or her next response so the patient will know he or she is understood.
    d. The nurse uses "why" questions to seek clarification of unusual symptoms or behavior.

7. During an interview, a patient denies having any anxiety. The patient frequently changes position in the chair, holds his arms folded tight against his chest, and has little eye contact with the interviewer. The interviewer should:

    a. Use confrontation to bring the discrepancy between verbal and nonverbal behavior to the patient's attention.
    b. Proceed with the interview. Patients usually are truthful with a health care practitioner.
    c. Make a mental note to discuss the behavior after the physical examination is completed.
    d. Proceed with the interview and examination as outlined on the agency assessment form. The patient's behavior is appropriate for the circumstances.

8. For what or with whom should touch be used during the interview?

    a. Only with individuals from a Western culture
    b. As a routine way of establishing contact with the person and communicating empathy
    c. Only with patients of the same gender
    d. Only if the interviewer knows the person well

9. Children usually come for health care with a caregiver. At about what age should the interviewer begin to question the child himself or herself regarding presenting symptoms?

    a. 5 years
    b. 7 years
    c. 9 years
    d. 11 years

10. Because of adolescents' developmental level, not all interviewing techniques can be used with them. Which techniques should be avoided?

    a. Facilitation and clarification
    b. Confrontation and explanation
    c. Empathy and interpretations
    d. Silence and reflection

11. Knowledge of the use of personal space is helpful for the health care provider. Personal distance is generally considered to be:

    a. 0 to 1½ feet.
    b. 1½ to 4 feet.
    c. 4 to 12 feet.
    d. 12 or more feet.

12. Mr. B. tells you, "Everyone here ignores me." You respond, "Ignores you?" This technique is best described as:

    a. Clarification.
    b. Selective listening.
    c. Reflecting.
    d. Validation.

13. What does active listening NOT include?

    a. Taking detailed notes during the interview
    b. Watching for clues in body language
    c. Repeating statements back to the person to make sure you have understood
    d. Asking open-ended questions to explore the person's perspective

14. When interviewing a patient who does not speak English, the examiner should:

    a. Take advantage of family members who are readily available and willing to assist.
    b. Use a qualified medical interpreter who is culturally literate.
    c. Seek as much information as possible and then continue with the physical examination.
    d. Wait until a qualified medical interpreter is available before starting the interview.

15. With older adults, how should the examiner proceed with the interview?

    a. Proceed in a more organized and concise manner.
    b. Consider the fatigue of the older person and break the interview into shorter segments.
    c. Ask a family member to complete some of the records while moving ahead with the interview.
    d. Raise your voice if the patient does not appear to hear you.

## CRITICAL THINKING EXERCISE 1

Practice is an important part of developing communication skills. With a partner, record a patient/nurse interaction. Have your partner pretend to be a patient seeking health care at a local clinic. The partner should create a character, such as a single mother describing vague symptoms in an attempt to get a prescription for her uninsured children, an older woman who focuses the interview on the student nurse's personal life instead of answering the questions, or a young man who thinks he has a sexually transmitted infection but does not want to discuss his symptoms. You can choose your own character, but it should be someone who poses a communication challenge. You may want to ask your instructor for potential vignettes. Entering the interview, you will not know the reason for the visit but must rely on therapeutic communication skills to figure out how to effectively communicate with the patient. The interviews should last no more than 10 minutes and will likely be shorter. Once you have been the nurse, pick a new scenario and switch roles. After completing the interactions, analyze the recording with special attention to:
- Therapeutic communication techniques, verbal and nonverbal
- Nontherapeutic communication techniques, verbal and nonverbal
- Areas for improvement
- Skills at which you excelled

A video recording of this exercise is ideal. Although you may be nervous to record yourself, a recording provides the best opportunity to analyze your skills and will help you in your future interactions with patients. What you say to the patient is not as important as your analysis of the interaction.

## CRITICAL THINKING EXERCISE 2

Below is a list of medical terms. Think about different ways to explain them to people with low health literacy, children, and older adults. Likely your explanations will be different depending on your audience. Take time to discuss your descriptions with a partner or in a group.

Hypertension
Diabetes
Cardiac catheterization
Urinary tract infection
Incontinence
Diarrhea
Nausea
Lymphedema
Glaucoma
Disease
Anticoagulation

## CRITICAL THINKING EXERCISE 3

Techniques for appropriate communication are important, but knowing yourself is equally important—your beliefs, your culture, your biases. Patients have to quickly establish rapport with you as a health care professional, and you need to make sure that you can adequately meet their needs in a nonjudgmental way. Negative facial expression or other negative nonverbal messages can break communication and shatter the rapport you have established. By knowing yourself and your personal biases, you may be able to control your nonverbal expressions. Most people have beliefs about subjects like teen pregnancy, alcohol or illicit drug use, and homosexuality. Awareness of personal prejudices can help you maintain neutrality when faced with difficult patient situations. Answer the following questions or complete the following statements openly and honestly without editing your thoughts in an effort to get to know yourself better.

1. What do I believe about gender roles?
2. What is my definition of health?
3. When I take care of a person from a different religion, I feel …
4. When I meet someone new, I make the following assumptions …
5. I am most fearful of working with …
6. When I see a same-sex couple, I feel …
7. I have the following assumptions/stereotypes about people who are
    a. Homeless
    b. Unemployed
    c. Teen mothers
    d. Drug addicts
    e. Catholic
    f. Muslim
    g. Christian
    h. Jewish

## SKILLS LABORATORY AND CLINICAL SETTING

Note that the clinical component of this chapter is the gathering of the complete health history. The history forms are included in Chapter 4.

# The Complete Health History

## PURPOSE

This chapter helps you learn the elements of a complete health history, interview a patient to gather the data for a complete health history, analyze the patient data, and record the history accurately.

## READING ASSIGNMENT

Jarvis: *Physical Examination and Health Assessment,* 8th ed., Chapter 4, pp. 45-62.

Suggested reading:
Klein, D. A., Goldenring, J. M., & Adelman, W. P. (2014). HEEADSSS 3.0: The psychosocial interview for adolescents updated for a new century fueled by media. *Contemp Pediatr, 31*(1), 16-28.

## STUDY GUIDE

After completing the reading assignment, you should be able to answer the following questions in the spaces provided.

1. State the purpose of the complete health history.

2. List and define the critical characteristics used to explore each symptom the patient identifies.

3. Define the elements of the health history: reason for seeking care; present health state or present illness; past history, family history; review of systems; functional patterns of living.

4. Discuss the rationale for obtaining a family history.

5. Define a pedigree or genogram.

6. Discuss the rationale for obtaining a systems review.

7. Describe the items included in a functional assessment.

## REVIEW QUESTIONS

This test is for you to check your own mastery of the content. Answers are provided in Appendix A.

1. When reading a medical record, you see the following notation: Patient states, "I have had a cold for about a week, and now I am having difficulty breathing." This is an example of:

   a. A past health history.
   b. A review of systems.
   c. A functional assessment.
   d. A reason for seeking care.

2. You have reason to question the reliability of the information being provided by a patient. One way to verify the reliability within the context of the interview is to:

   a. Rephrase the same questions later in the interview.
   b. Review the patient's previous medical records.
   c. Call the person identified as the emergency contact to verify the data provided.
   d. Provide the patient with a printed history to complete and then compare the data provided.

3. The statement "Reason for seeking care" has replaced the "chief complaint." This change is significant because:

   a. The "chief complaint" is really a diagnostic statement.
   b. The newer term allows another individual to supply the necessary information.
   c. The newer term incorporates wellness needs.
   d. The "reason for seeking care" can incorporate the history of the present illness.

4. During an initial interview, the examiner says, "Mrs. J., tell me what you do when your headaches occur?" This is an example of which type of information?

   a. The patient's perception of the problem
   b. Aggravating or relieving factors
   c. The frequency of the problem
   d. The severity of the problem

5. Which is an appropriate recording of a patient's reason for seeking health care?

   a. Angina pectoris, duration 2 hours
   b. Substernal pain radiating to left axilla, 1 hour duration
   c. "Grabbing" chest pain for 2 hours
   d. Pleurisy, 2 days' duration

6. A genogram is used for which reasons?

   a. Past history
   b. Past health history, specifically hospitalizations
   c. Family history
   d. The 8 characteristics of presenting symptoms

7. What is the best description of "review of systems" as a part of the health history?

   a. The evaluation of the past and present health state of each body system
   b. A documentation of the problem as described by the patient
   c. The recording of the objective findings of the practitioner
   d. A statement that describes the overall health state of the patient

8. Which finding is considered to be subjective?

   a. Temperature of 101.2° F
   b. Pulse rate of 96 beats/min
   c. Measured weight loss of 20 pounds since the previous measurement
   d. Pain lasting 2 hours

9. When taking a health history for a child, what information, in addition to that for an adult, is usually obtained?

   a. Coping and stress management
   b. A review of immunizations received
   c. Environmental hazards
   d. Hospitalization history

10. Functional assessment measures how a person manages day-to-day activities. The impact of adoption on the daily activities of a child is referred to as:

    a. Developmental history.
    b. Instrumental activities of daily living.
    c. Reason for seeking care.
    d. Interpersonal relationship assessment.

11. Which two sections of the child's health history become separate sections because of their importance to the child's current health status?

    a. Play activities and rest patterns
    b. Prenatal and postnatal status
    c. Developmental and nutritional history
    d. Accidents, injuries, and immunizations

12. Which statement best describes the purpose of a health history?

    a. To provide an opportunity for interaction between the patient and examiner
    b. To provide a form for obtaining the patient's biographic information
    c. To document the normal and abnormal findings of a physical assessment
    d. To provide a database of subjective information about the patient's past and present health

13. While assessing a man for allergies, he states he is allergic to penicillin. Which response is best?

    a. "Are you allergic to any other drugs?"
    b. "How often have you received penicillin?"
    c. "I'll write your allergy on your chart so you won't receive any."
    d. "Please describe what happens to you when you take penicillin."

## CRITICAL THINKING EXERCISE

Visit *https://familyhistory.hhs.gov*, and complete a "My Family Health Portrait." After completion, consider the following questions:

1. How difficult was it for you to obtain the information necessary to complete the health portrait?
2. Were there questions that you could not answer even after consulting with other family members? How did that make you feel?
3. Did you identify unknown health risks through completion of your personal genogram?
4. How will completing your genogram impact the way in which you describe the importance of family history when interacting with patients?

## SKILLS LABORATORY AND CLINICAL SETTING

The purpose of the clinical component is to practice conducting a complete health history on a peer in the skills laboratory and to achieve the following.

### Clinical Objectives

1. Demonstrate knowledge of interviewing skills by: arranging a private, quiet, comfortable setting; introducing yourself and stating your goals for the interview; posing open-ended and direct questions appropriately; listening to the patient in an attentive, nonjudgmental manner; and choosing appropriate vocabulary the patient understands.

2. Demonstrate knowledge of the components of a health history by: recording the reason for seeking care in the person's own words; eliciting all the critical characteristics to describe the patient's symptom(s); gathering pertinent data for the past history, family history, and systems review; identifying self-care behaviors and risk factors from the functional assessment.

3. Record the history data accurately and as a reflection of what the patient believes the true health state to be.

### Instructions

Work in pairs and obtain a complete health history from a peer. Although you already know each other as student colleagues, play your role straight as examiner or patient for the best learning experience. Be aware that some of the history questions cover personal content. When you are acting as the patient, you have the right to withhold an answer if you do not feel comfortable with the amount of material you will be asked to divulge. Your own rights to privacy must coexist with the goals of the learning experience.

Familiarize yourself with the following history form and practice phrasing your questions ahead of time. Note that the language on this form is intended as a prompt for the examiner and must be translated into clear and appropriate phrases for the patient. As a beginning examiner, you will need to use one copy of the form as a worksheet during the actual interview and use a fresh copy of the form for your rewritten formal record.

## WRITE-UP—HEALTH HISTORY

**Date** _____

**Examiner** _____

### 1. Biographic Data

Name _____ Phone _____

Address _____

Birthdate _____ Birthplace _____

Age _____ Gender _____ Marital Status _____ Occupation _____

Race/ethnic origin _____ Employer _____

### 2. Source and Reliability

### 3. Reason for Seeking Care

### 4. Present Health or History of Present Illness

### 5. Past Health

Describe general health _____

Childhood illnesses _____

Accidents or injuries (include age) _____

Serious or chronic illnesses (include age) _____

Hospitalizations (what for? location?) _____

Operations (name procedure, age) _____

Obstetric history: Gravida _____ Term _____ Preterm _____
                          (# Pregnancies)        (# Term pregnancies)    (# Preterm pregnancies)

                  Ab/incomplete _____ Children living _____
                  (# Abortions or miscarriages)

Course of pregnancy_____
(Date delivery, length of pregnancy, length of labor, baby's weight and sex, vaginal delivery or cesarean section, complications, baby's condition)

Immunizations_____

Last examination date: Physical _____ Dental _____ Vision _____

Allergies _____ Reaction _____

Current medications _____

_____

6. **Family History—Specify Which Relative(s)**

Heart disease_____  Allergies_____
High blood pressure_____  Asthma_____
Stroke_____  Obesity_____
Diabetes_____  Alcoholism or drug addiction _____
Blood disorders_____  Mental illness _____
Breast or ovarian cancer_____  Suicide _____
Cancer (other)_____  Seizure disorder _____
Sickle cell_____  Kidney disease _____
Arthritis_____  Tuberculosis _____

Construct genogram below.

7. **Review of Systems**
   (Circle both past health problems that have been resolved and current problems, including date of onset.) | Describe circled items.

   **General Overall Health State:** Present weight (gain or loss, period of time, by diet or other factors), fatigue, weakness or malaise, fever, chills, sweats or night sweats

   **Skin:** History of skin disease (eczema, psoriasis, hives), pigment or color change, change in mole, excessive dryness or moisture, pruritus, excessive bruising, rash or lesion

   **Hair:** Recent loss, change in texture

   **Nails:** Change in shape, color, or brittleness
   **Health Promotion:** Amount of sun exposure, method of self-care for skin and hair

   **Head:** Any unusually frequent or severe headache, any head injury, dizziness (syncope), or vertigo

   **Eyes:** Difficulty with vision (decreased acuity, blurring, blind spots), eye pain, diplopia (double vision), redness or swelling, watering or discharge, glaucoma or cataracts
   **Health Promotion:** Wears glasses or contacts, last vision check or glaucoma test, how coping with loss of vision, if any

   **Ears:** Earaches, infections, discharge and its characteristics, tinnitus, or vertigo
   **Health Promotion:** Hearing loss, hearing aid use, how loss affects daily life, any exposure to environmental noise, method of cleaning ears

   **Nose and Sinuses:** Discharge and its characteristics, any unusually frequent or severe colds, sinus pain, nasal obstruction, nosebleeds, allergies or hay fever, or change in sense of smell

   **Mouth and Throat:** Mouth pain, frequent sore throat, bleeding gums, toothache, lesion in mouth or tongue, dysphagia, hoarseness or voice change, tonsillectomy, altered taste
   **Health Promotion:** Pattern of daily dental care, use of prostheses (dentures, bridge), and last dental checkup

   **Neck:** Pain, limitation of motion, lumps or swelling, enlarged or tender nodes, goiter

   **Breast:** Pain, lump, nipple discharge, rash, history of breast disease, any surgery on breasts
   **Axilla:** Tenderness, lump or swelling, rash
   **Health Promotion:** Performs breast self-examination, including frequency and method used, last mammogram and results

(Circle if present.)                                          Describe circled items.

**Respiratory System:** History of lung disease (asthma, emphysema, bronchitis, pneumonia, tuberculosis), chest pain with breathing, wheezing or noisy breathing, shortness of breath, how much activity produces shortness of breath, cough, sputum (color, amount), hemoptysis, toxin or pollution exposure
    **Health Promotion:** Last chest x-ray examination

**Cardiovascular System:** Precordial or retrosternal pain, palpitation, cyanosis, dyspnea on exertion (specify amount of exertion it takes to produce dyspnea), orthopnea, paroxysmal nocturnal dyspnea, nocturia, edema, history of heart murmur, hypertension, coronary artery disease, anemia
    **Health Promotion:** Date of last ECG or other heart tests and results

**Peripheral Vascular System:** Coldness, numbness and tingling, swelling of legs (time of day, activity), discoloration in hands or feet (bluish red, pallor, mottling, associated with position, especially around feet and ankles), varicose veins or complications, intermittent claudication, thrombophlebitis, ulcers
    **Health Promotion:** If work involves long-term sitting or standing, avoid crossing legs at the knees; wear support hose.

**Gastrointestinal System:** Appetite, food intolerance, dysphagia, heartburn, indigestion, pain (associated with eating), other abdominal pain, pyrosis (esophageal and stomach burning sensation with sour eructation), nausea and vomiting (character), vomiting blood, history of abdominal disease (ulcer, liver or gallbladder, jaundice, appendicitis, colitis), flatulence, frequency of bowel movement, any recent change, stool characteristics, constipation or diarrhea, black stools, rectal bleeding, rectal conditions, hemorrhoids, fistula)
    **Health Promotion:** Use of antacids or laxatives

**Urinary System:** Frequency, urgency, nocturia (the number of times awakens at night to urinate, recent change), dysuria, polyuria or oliguria, hesitancy or straining, narrowed stream, urine color (cloudy or presence of hematuria), incontinence, history of urinary disease (kidney disease, kidney stones, urinary tract infections, prostate); pain in flank, groin, suprapubic region, or low back
    **Health Promotion:** Measures to avoid or treat urinary tract infections, use of Kegel exercises

**Male Genital System:** Penis or testicular pain, sores or lesions, penile discharge, lumps, hernia
    **Health Promotion:** Perform testicular self-examination? How frequently?

**Female Genital System:** Menstrual history (age at menarche, last menstrual period, cycle and duration, any amenorrhea or menorrhagia, premenstrual pain or dysmenorrhea, intermenstrual spotting), vaginal itching, discharge and its characteristics, age at menopause, menopausal signs or symptoms, postmenopausal bleeding.
    **Health Promotion:** Last gynecologic checkup, last Pap test and results

(Circle if present.)                                             | Describe circled items.

**Sexual Health:** Presently in a relationship involving intercourse? Are aspects of sex satisfactory to you and partner, any dyspareunia (for female), any changes in erection or ejaculation (for male), use of contraceptive, is contraceptive method satisfactory? Use of condoms, how frequently? Aware of any contact with partner who has sexually transmitted infection (gonorrhea, herpes, chlamydia, venereal warts, HIV/AIDS, syphilis)?

**Musculoskeletal System:** History of arthritis or gout. In the joints: pain, stiffness, swelling (location, migratory nature), deformity, limitation of motion, noise with joint motion. In the muscles: any pain, cramps, weakness, gait problems or problems with coordinated activities. In the back: any pain (location and radiation to extremities), stiffness, limitation of motion, or history of back pain or disk disease.
　　**Health Promotion:** How much walking per day? What is the effect of limited range of motion on daily activities, such as on grooming, feeding, toileting, dressing? Any mobility aids used?

**Neurologic System:** History of seizure disorder, stroke, fainting, blackouts. In motor function: weakness, tic or tremor, paralysis, coordination problems. In sensory function: numbness and tingling (paresthesia). In cognitive function: memory disorder (recent or distant, disorientation). In mental status: any nervousness, mood change, depression, or any history of mental health dysfunction or hallucinations.

**Hematologic System:** Bleeding tendency of skin or mucous membranes, excessive bruising, lymph node swelling, exposure to toxic agents or radiation, blood transfusion and reactions.

**Endocrine System:** History of diabetes or diabetic symptoms (polyuria, polydipsia, polyphagia), history of thyroid disease, intolerance to heat or cold, change in skin pigmentation or texture, excessive sweating, relationship between appetite and weight, abnormal hair distribution, nervousness, tremors, need for hormone therapy.

## Functional Assessment (Including Activities of Daily Living)

**Self-Esteem, Self-Concept:** Education (last grade completed, other significant training) _____

_____

Financial status (income adequate for lifestyle and/or health concerns) _____

_____

Value-belief system (religious practices and perception of personal strengths) _____

_____

Self-care behaviors_____

_____

**Activity and Exercise:** Daily profile, usual pattern of a typical day _____

_____

Independent or needs assistance with ADLs, feeding, bathing, hygiene, dressing, toileting, bed-to-chair

transfer, walking, standing, climbing stairs _____

_____

Leisure activities_____

Exercise pattern (type, amount per day or week, method of warm-up session, method of monitoring

body's response to exercise) _____

_____

Other self-care behaviors_____

**Sleep and Rest:** Sleep patterns, daytime naps, any sleep aids used_____

_____

Other self-care behavior _____

**Nutrition and Elimination:** Record 24-hour diet recall. _____

_____

Is this menu pattern typical of most days? _____

Who buys food? _____ Who prepares food? _____

Finances adequate for food?_____

Who is present at mealtimes? _____

Other self-care behaviors _____

**Interpersonal Relationships and Resources:** Describe own role in family _____

How getting along with family, friends, co-workers, classmates _____

_____

Get support with a problem from _____

How much daily time spent alone? _____

Is this pleasurable or isolating? _____

Other self-care behaviors _____

**Coping and Stress Management:** Describe stresses in life now _____

_____

Change(s) in past year _____

Methods used to relieve stress _____

Are these methods helpful? _____

**Personal Habits:** Daily intake caffeine (coffee, tea, colas) _____

Smoke cigarettes? _____ Number packs per day _____

Daily use for how many years _____ Age started _____

Ever tried to quit? _____ How did it go? _____

Drink alcohol?_____ Date of last alcohol use _____

Amount of alcohol that episode _____

Out of last 30 days, on how many days had alcohol? _____

Ever told had a drinking problem? _____

Any use of street drugs? _____

Marijuana? _____ Cocaine? _____

Crack cocaine? _____ Amphetamines? _____

Heroin? _____ Prescription painkillers? _____

Barbiturates? _____ LSD? _____

Ever been in treatment for drugs or alcohol? _____

**Environment and Hazards:** Housing and neighborhood (type of structure, live alone, know neighbors) _____

_____

Safety of area _____

Adequate heat and utilities _____

Access to transportation _____

Involvement in community services _____

Hazards at workplace or home _____

Use of seatbelts _____

Travel to or residence in other countries _____

Military service in other countries _____

Self-care behaviors _____

**Intimate Partner Violence:** How are things at home? Do you feel safe? _____

_____

Ever been emotionally or physically abused by your partner or someone important to you? _____

Ever been hit, slapped, kicked, pushed, or shoved or otherwise physically hurt by your partner or ex-partner?

_____

Partner ever force you into having sex? _____

Are you afraid of your partner or ex-partner? _____

**Occupational Health:** Please describe your job. _____

Work with any health hazards (e.g., asbestos, inhalants, chemicals, repetitive motion)? _____

_____

Any equipment at work designed to reduce your exposure? _____

Any work programs designed to monitor your exposure? _____

Any health problems that you think are related to your job? _____

What do you like or dislike about your job? _____

**Perception of Own Health:** How do you define health? _____

View of own health now _____

What are your concerns? _____

What do you expect will happen to your health in future? _____

_____

Your health goals _____

Your expectations of nurses, physicians _____

# Mental Status Assessment

## PURPOSE

This chapter helps you learn the components of the mental status examination, including assessing a person's appearance, behavior, cognitive functions, and thought processes and perceptions; understanding the rationale and methods of examination of mental status; and recording the assessment accurately.

## READING ASSIGNMENT

Jarvis: *Physical Examination and Health Assessment,* 8th ed., Chapter 5, pp. 63-83.

Suggested reading:
Bennett, C. (2017). Identifying delirium in older adults with pre-existing mental illness. *Nurse Pract, 42*(6), 39-44.

## GLOSSARY

Study the following terms after completing the reading assignment. You should be able to cover the definition on the right and define the term out loud.

**Abstract reasoning** . . . . . . . . . . pondering a deeper meaning beyond the concrete and literal

**Attention** . . . . . . . . . . . . . . . . . . concentration, ability to focus on one specific thing

**Bereavement** . . . . . . . . . . . . . . . state of loss, sorrow, and/or grief due to the death of a loved one, decline in personal or a loved one's health, or the end of an important relationship

**Consciousness** . . . . . . . . . . . . . being aware of one's own existence, feelings, and thoughts and being aware of the environment

**Delirium** . . . . . . . . . . . . . . . . . . . an acute confusional change or loss of consciousness and perceptual disturbance that may accompany acute illness; usually resolves when the underlying cause is treated

**Dementia** . . . . . . . . . . . . . . . . . a gradual progressive process, causing decreased cognitive function even though the person is fully conscious and awake; not reversible

**Executive function** . . . . . . . . . . high-level cognitive skills, including organizational and regulatory ability

**Language** . . . . . . . . . . . . . . . . . . using the voice to communicate one's thoughts and feelings

**Memory** . . . . . . . . . . . . . . . . . . . ability to lay down and store experiences and perceptions for later recall

**Mood** . . . . . . . . . . . . . . . . . . . . prolonged display of a person's feelings

**Orientation** . . . . . . . . . . . . . . . . awareness of the objective world in relation to the self

**Perceptions** . . . . . . . . . . . . . . . awareness of objects through any of the five senses

**Thought content** . . . . . . . . . . . . *what* the person thinks—specific ideas, beliefs, the use of words

**Thought process** . . . . . . . . . . . the *way* a person thinks, the logical train of thought

**Visuospatial** . . . . . . . . . . . . . . ability to process visual information and perceive relationships between objects in space

## STUDY GUIDE

After completing the reading assignment, you should be able to answer the following questions in the spaces provided.

1. Define the term *mental disorder*.

2. Differentiate *organic brain disorder* from *psychiatric mental disorder*.

3. List 4 situations in which it would be necessary to perform a complete mental status examination.

4. Explain 4 factors that could affect a patient's response to the mental status examination but have nothing to do with mental disorders.

5. State convenient ways to assess a person's recent memory within the context of the initial health history.

6. Which mental function is the Four Unrelated Words Test intended to test?

7. List at least 4 questions you could ask a patient that would screen for suicide ideation.

8. Describe the patient response level of consciousness that would be graded as:

Lethargic or somnolent _____

Obtunded _____

Stupor or semicoma _____

Coma _____

Delirium _____

## CRITICAL THINKING EXERCISE

Utilize the Montreal Cognitive Assessment (MoCA) on the next page to complete a cognitive screen on a partner. Switch partners and complete the Mini-Cog (http://mini-cog.com/mini-cog-instrument/standardized-mini-cog-instrument/) on a different partner. Compare and contrast the differences between the screening tools. Which seemed more appropriate for use in an outpatient clinic? The hospital? Were you comfortable providing instructions and scoring each instrument? What questions do you have about scoring?

Next, use the MoCA and Mini-Cog in a clinical setting. Complete the MoCA and Mini-Cog on different older adults (>65 years). Did you have to change your delivery with an older person? Discuss the experience with classmates to identify differences found with different patients and in different settings.

## REVIEW QUESTIONS

This test is for you to check your own mastery of the content. Answers are provided in Appendix A.

1. Although a full mental status examination may not be required, you must be aware of the 4 main headings of the assessment while performing the interview and physical examination. These headings are:

   a. Mood, affect, consciousness, and orientation.
   b. Memory, attention, thought content, and perceptions.
   c. Language, orientation, attention, and abstract reasoning.
   d. Appearance, behavior, cognition, and thought process.

2. Select the finding that most accurately describes appearance of a patient.

   a. Tense posture and restless activity. Clothing clean but not appropriate for season (e.g., patient wearing T-shirt and shorts in cold weather).
   b. Oriented × 3. Affect appropriate for circumstances.
   c. Alert and responds to verbal stimuli. Tearful when diagnosis discussed.
   d. Laughing inappropriately, oriented × 3.

3. You are assessing short-term cognitive function. Which assessment shows the ability to lay down new memories?

   a. Noting whether the patient completes a thought without wandering
   b. A test of general knowledge
   c. A description of past medical history
   d. Use of the Four Unrelated Words Test

# MONTREAL COGNITIVE ASSESSMENT (MOCA)
Version 7.1 Original Version

NAME :
Education :　　　　Date of birth :
Sex :　　　　DATE :

| VISUOSPATIAL / EXECUTIVE | | | POINTS |
|---|---|---|---|

Copy cube

Draw CLOCK (Ten past eleven)
( 3 points )

(E) End　(A)

(5)　(B)　(2)

(1) Begin

(D)　(4)　(3)

(C)

[ ]　　　　[ ]

[ ] Contour　[ ] Numbers　[ ] Hands　__/5

## NAMING

[ ]　　　　[ ]　　　　[ ]　__/3

## MEMORY

Read list of words, subject must repeat them. Do 2 trials, even if 1st trial is successful. Do a recall after 5 minutes.

| | | FACE | VELVET | CHURCH | DAISY | RED | |
|---|---|---|---|---|---|---|---|
| | 1st trial | | | | | | No points |
| | 2nd trial | | | | | | |

## ATTENTION

| Read list of digits (1 digit/ sec.). | Subject has to repeat them in the forward order | [ ] 2 1 8 5 4 | |
|---|---|---|---|
| | Subject has to repeat them in the backward order | [ ] 7 4 2 | __/2 |

Read list of letters. The subject must tap with his hand at each letter A. No points if ≥ 2 errors

[ ] F B A C M N A A J K L B A F A K D E A A A J A M O F A A B　__/1

Serial 7 subtraction starting at 100　[ ] 93　[ ] 86　[ ] 79　[ ] 72　[ ] 65

4 or 5 correct subtractions: **3 pts**, 2 or 3 correct: **2 pts**, 1 correct: **1 pt**, 0 correct: **0 pt**　__/3

## LANGUAGE

Repeat : I only know that John is the one to help today. [ ]
The cat always hid under the couch when dogs were in the room. [ ]　__/2

Fluency / Name maximum number of words in one minute that begin with the letter F　[ ] _____ (N ≥ 11 words)　__/1

## ABSTRACTION

Similarity between e.g. banana - orange = fruit　[ ] train – bicycle　[ ] watch - ruler　__/2

## DELAYED RECALL

| Has to recall words WITH NO CUE | FACE [ ] | VELVET [ ] | CHURCH [ ] | DAISY [ ] | RED [ ] | Points for UNCUED recall only | __/5 |
|---|---|---|---|---|---|---|---|
| **Optional** Category cue | | | | | | | |
| Multiple choice cue | | | | | | | |

## ORIENTATION

[ ] Date　[ ] Month　[ ] Year　[ ] Day　[ ] Place　[ ] City　__/6

© Z.Nasreddine MD　　www.mocatest.org　　Normal ≥ 26 / 30　TOTAL　__/30

Administered by: _____

Add 1 point if ≤ 12 yr edu

4. You are preparing the discharge plan for a patient with aphasia. What assessment should you include in the plan?

   a. Ask the patient to calculate serial 7s.
   b. Ask the patient to name his or her grandchildren and their birthdays.
   c. Ask the patient to demonstrate word comprehension by naming articles in the room or on the body as you point to them.
   d. Ask the patient to interpret a proverb.

5. During an interview with a patient diagnosed with a seizure disorder, the patient states, "I plan to be an airline pilot." If the patient continues to have this as a career goal after teaching regarding seizure disorders has been provided, you might question the patient's:

   a. Thought processes.
   b. Judgment.
   c. Attention span.
   d. Recent memory.

6. On a patient's second day in an acute care hospital, the patient complains about the "bugs" on the bed. The bed is clean. This would be an example of altered:

   a. Thought processes.
   b. Orientation.
   c. Perception.
   d. Higher intellectual function.

7. One way to assess cognitive function and to screen dementia is with:

   a. The Proverb Interpretation Test.
   b. The Mini-Cog.
   c. The Denver II.
   d. The Older Adult Behavioral Checklist.

8. A major characteristic of dementia is:

   a. Impairment of short- and long-term memory.
   b. Hallucinations.
   c. Sudden onset of symptoms.
   d. Substance-induced.

9. What statement is an example of a patient with dysarthria?

   a. When asked a question, the patient responds fluently but uses words incorrectly or makes up words so that speech may be incomprehensible.
   b. The word choice and grammar are appropriate, but the sounds are distorted so speech is unintelligible.
   c. The pitch and volume of words are difficult and the voice may be hoarse, but language is intact.
   d. Comprehension is intact but there is difficulty in expressing thoughts, with nouns and verbs being the dominant word choices.

10. You are leading a discussion of the planned activities for the day at an adult living center and state, "We will be having snacks at 9:30 and lunch will be at noon." One of the participants responds in a very monotone manner, "Snacks at 9:30, lunch at noon, snacks at 9:30, lunch at noon." This patient is exhibiting signs of:

   a. Echolalia.
   b. Confabulation.
   c. Flight of ideas.
   d. Neologisms.

11. You are performing a mental status examination. Which assessments would be most appropriate?

   a. Examining the patient's EEG
   b. Observing the patient as he or she takes an IQ test
   c. Observing the patient and inferring health or dysfunction
   d. Examining the patient's response to a specific set of questions

12. What is a priority assessment for aging adults?

   a. Phobias
   b. General intelligence
   c. Irrational thinking patterns
   d. Sensory perceptive abilities

13. You are assessing a 75-year-old man. What is an expected finding?

    a. He will have no decrease in any of his abilities, including response time.
    b. He will have difficulty on tests of remote memory because this typically decreases with age.
    c. It may take him a little longer to respond but his general knowledge and abilities should not have declined.
    d. He will have had a decrease in his response time due to language loss and a decrease in general knowledge.

14. When assessing mental status in children, what statement is true?

    a. All aspects of mental status in children are interrelated.
    b. Children are highly labile and unstable until the age of 2.
    c. Children's mental status is largely a function of their parents' level of functioning until the age of 7.
    d. A child's mental status is impossible to assess until the child develops the ability to concentrate.

Match column B to column A.

**Column A—Definition**

15. _____ Lack of emotional response
16. _____ Loss of identity
17. _____ Excessive well-being
18. _____ Apprehensive from the anticipation of a danger whose source is unknown
19. _____ Annoyed, easily provoked
20. _____ Loss of control
21. _____ Sad, gloomy, dejected
22. _____ Rapid shift of emotions
23. _____ Worried about known external danger

**Column B—Type of Mood and Affect**

a. Depression
b. Anxiety
c. Flat affect
d. Euphoria
e. Lability
f. Rage
g. Irritability
h. Fear
i. Depersonalization

24. Write a narrative account of a mental status assessment with normal findings.

## SKILLS LABORATORY AND CLINICAL SETTING

The purpose of the clinical component is to achieve beginning competency with the administration of the mental status examination. You will also screen your patient for anxiety (GAD-7) and depression (PHQ-9). The GAD-7 and PHQ-9 are available in your textbook.

Practice steps of the full mental status examination, screening for anxiety and screening for depression on a peer or patient in the clinical setting. Give appropriate instructions throughout the examination. Use the regional write-up sheet that follows to record your findings.

# REGIONAL WRITE-UP—MENTAL STATUS EXAMINATION

Date _____

Examiner _____

**Patient** _____  Age _____  Gender _____

**Occupation** _____

## Mental Status

(Before testing, tell the person the four words you want him or her to remember and recall in a few minutes for the Four Unrelated Words Test.)

1. **Appearance**

   Posture _____
   Body movements _____
   Dress _____
   Grooming and hygiene _____

2. **Behavior**

   Level of consciousness _____
   Facial expression _____
   Speech:
      Quality _____
      Pace _____
      Word choice _____
   Mood and affect _____

3. **Cognitive Functions**

   Orientation:
      Time _____ Place_____ Person_____
   Attention span _____
   Recent memory _____
   Remote memory _____
   New learning—Four Unrelated Words Test _____
   Additional testing for aphasia:
      Word comprehension _____
      Reading _____
      Writing _____
   Judgment _____

4. **Thought Processes and Perceptions**
   Thought processes _____
   Thought content _____
   Perceptions _____
   Suicidal thoughts _____

**NOTES**

# Substance Use Assessment

## PURPOSE

This chapter presents the scope of the problem regarding primary care and hospital patients who drink excessive alcohol and use illicit drugs. Screening tools and interview approaches are presented.

## READING ASSIGNMENT

Jarvis: *Physical Examination and Health Assessment*, 8th ed., Chapter 6, pp. 85-97.

Suggested reading:
DiBartolo, M. C., & Jarosinski, J. M. (2017). Alcohol use disorder in older adults. *Issues Ment Health Nurs*, *38*(1), 25-32.

## GLOSSARY

Study the following terms after completing the reading assignment. You should be able to cover the definition on the right and define the term out loud.

**Alcohol abuse** . . . . . . . . . . . . . . one or more of the following events in a year: recurrent use resulting in failure to fulfill major role obligations; recurrent use in hazardous situations; recurrent alcohol-related legal problems (e.g., DUI); continued use despite social or interpersonal problems caused or exacerbated by alcohol

**Alcohol use disorder** . . . . . . . . two or more of the following events in a year: tolerance (increased amounts to achieve effect; diminished effect from same amount); withdrawal; a great deal of time spent obtaining alcohol, using it, or recovering from its effect; important activities given up or reduced because of alcohol; drinking more or longer than intended; persistent desire or unsuccessful efforts to cut down or control alcohol use; use continued despite knowledge of having a psychological problem caused or exacerbated by alcohol

**Binge drinking** . . . . . . . . . . . . . . on one occasion: 5 or more standard alcohol drinks for men; 4 or more standard alcohol drinks for women

**Heavy alcohol use** . . . . . . . . . . . binge drinking on 5 or more days in the past month (SAMHSA). Or for men, 15 or more drinks per week; for women, 8 or more drinks per week (CDC)

**Standard alcohol drink**. . . . . . . 14 grams of pure alcohol as found in one 12-ounce beer (5% alcohol); one 8-ounce malt liquor (7% alcohol); one 5-ounce glass of wine (12% alcohol); or 1.5 ounces of spirits (gin, vodka, whiskey, rum) (40% alcohol)

# STUDY GUIDE

After completing the reading assignment, you should be able to answer the following questions in the space provided.

1. What proportion of Americans ages 12 and older report being current alcohol drinkers? And report being binge drinkers (≥5 drinks/occasion)?

2. List the effects of alcohol on 4 traumatic or disease conditions.

3. Define the use of prescription opioid pain relievers for a nonmedical use.

4. Discuss the extra risk alcohol drinking poses to the aging adult.

5. Contrast the use and settings for the following alcohol screening tools: AUDIT; AUDIT-C; CAGE questionnaire.

6. State 3 clinical laboratory findings that are used to detect or monitor alcohol use.

# CRITICAL THINKING EXERCISES

1. Read your daily newspaper for 4 days, making a list of all news stories (e.g., auto accidents, drowning, personal injury) that are or possibly could be alcohol-related.

2. In a group of three or four students, interview a primary care physician, emergency department physician, and intensive care unit physician. Ask each one for clinical examples of alcohol-related cases in their units.

3. Attend one open meeting of Alcoholics Anonymous. Enter your zip code in the AA website (www.aa.org) to find locations. Be fully aware of the anonymous tradition of these meetings, and do not repeat any personal information.

4. Look up your school or university alcohol policy in your student handbook. The ideal handbook statement might be different from the actual situation on your campus. How is this different?

## REVIEW QUESTIONS

This test is for you to check your own mastery of the content. Answers are provided in Appendix A.

1. The phase of addiction characterized by tolerance, increasing time spent in substance-related activities, unsuccessful attempts to quit, and continued use despite known harm is:

   a. Relief.
   b. Withdrawal.
   c. Dependency.
   d. Preoccupation.

2. The unpleasant effect that occurs when use of a drug is stopped is called:

   a. Potency.
   b. Withdrawal.
   c. Metabolism.
   d. Threshold.

3. The need for increasingly larger doses of a substance to achieve the same effect that was initially experienced from using is called:

   a. Tolerance.
   b. Addiction.
   c. Abuse.
   d. Dependence.

4. Which health issue is NOT a result of prolonged heavy drinking?

   a. Kidney and liver damage
   b. Increased risk for oral cancer
   c. Increased resistance to pneumonia and other infectious diseases
   d. Damage to the brain and peripheral nervous system

5. How many drinks does a man consume in one sitting for it to be considered binge drinking?

   a. 3
   b. 5
   c. 7
   d. 8

6. A pregnant woman explains that she does not intend to stop drinking because her friends continued to drink during pregnancy, and "nothing happened to them or their kids." How should the clinician respond to this statement?

   a. "While it's true that there is no scientific evidence that alcohol harms the fetus, abstinence is recommended because of the physical effects on your body."
   b. "No amount of alcohol has been determined to be safe for a pregnant woman so I would ask you to stop drinking alcohol completely."
   c. "Maybe you could cut back on your alcohol intake, at least until you're in the third trimester, when the effects on the fetus are minimal."
   d. "If you can limit yourself to only one drink per day, you will be helping yourself and your baby."

7. Which is the most commonly used laboratory test to identify chronic alcohol drinking?

   a. Blood urea nitrogen
   b. Liver enzyme panel
   c. Gamma-glutamyl transferase (GGT)
   d. Mean corpuscular volume (MCV)

8. The CAGE screening tool is used to assess:

   a. Sexual activity.
   b. Depression.
   c. Problem alcohol use.
   d. Decreased mental status.

9. While assessing a man during a physical examination for work, you suspect alcohol use. Which assessment tool is appropriate in this situation?

   a. AUDIT screening tool
   b. Rapid eye test
   c. Mental status examination
   d. Holmes Social Readjustment Rating Scale

10. You are screening patients for excessive alcohol consumption. Which patient would be considered over the recommended limit?

    a. The man who reports drinking 2 beers each day
    b. The woman who reports drinking 2 vodka martinis each day
    c. The older adult man who reports drinking 1 glass of sherry before going to bed each night
    d. The woman who reports drinking 1 glass of wine with dinner each day

11. You are performing a sports physical on a 16-year-old girl. Which question would most likely yield an accurate substance use assessment?

    a. "Many teenagers have tried street drugs. Have you tried these drugs? "
    b. "Tell me which street drugs your friends have offered to you?"
    c. "Do most of your friends drink alcohol or do street drugs?"
    d. "Your high school has a reputation for drug use. Do you use drugs?"

12. During the assessment, you will observe for which problems in addition to alcohol withdrawal syndrome?

    a. Renal insufficiency
    b. Hypertension
    c. Irritable bowel syndrome
    d. Impaired glucose tolerance

13. You are assessing a patient's cardiac risk factors secondary to chronic alcohol use. Which condition might this patient exhibit?

    a. Bradycardia
    b. Ventral fibrillation
    c. Hypertension
    d. Hypotension

14. You are assessing a male patient's alcohol consumption. Which statement would alert you to investigate further?

    a. "I drink at wedding and holidays."
    b. "I enjoy a few beers on the weekend."
    c. "No matter how much I drink I don't get drunk."
    d. "I drink a beer with dinner every day."

## SKILLS LABORATORY AND CLINICAL SETTING

Pair up with a classmate and interview each other using the AUDIT questionnaire. Keep your answers confidential and share the questionnaire after use—this is not to turn in to the instructor. Note that questions 1 to 3 cover alcohol consumption, questions 4 to 6 cover drinking behavior, and questions 7 to 10 cover adverse consequences from alcohol. Record the score at the end of each line and total; the maximum total is 400%. A cutpoint of 8 or more for men or 4 or more for women, adolescents, and persons older than 60 years indicates hazardous alcohol consumption.

Now role-play, and one of you take the role of the nurse and the other take the role of the hospitalized person in possible alcohol withdrawal. Proceed through the CIWA assessment guide. A complete assessment takes about 5 minutes. Note the points at which medication by protocol is recommended as needed or is ordered.

# THE ALCOHOL USE DISORDERS IDENTIFICATION TEST—AUDIT*

| Questions | 0 | 1 | 2 | 3 | 4 |
|---|---|---|---|---|---|
| 1. How often do you have a drink containing alcohol? | Never | Monthly or less | 2 to 4 times a month | 2 to 3 times a week | 4 or more times a week |
| 2. How many drinks containing alcohol do you have on a typical day when you are drinking? | 1 or 2 | 3 or 4 | 5 or 6 | 7 to 9 | 10 or more |
| 3. How often do you have five or more drinks on one occasion? | Never | Less than monthly | Monthly | Weekly | Daily or almost daily |
| 4. How often during the last year have you found that you were not able to stop drinking once you had started? | Never | Less than monthly | Monthly | Weekly | Daily or almost daily |
| 5. How often during the last year have you failed to do what was normally expected of you because of drinking? | Never | Less than monthly | Monthly | Weekly | Daily or almost daily |
| 6. How often during the last year have you needed a first drink in the morning to get yourself going after a heavy drinking session? | Never | Less than monthly | Monthly | Weekly | Daily or almost daily |
| 7. How often during the last year have you had a feeling of guilt or remorse after drinking? | Never | Less than monthly | Monthly | Weekly | Daily or almost daily |
| 8. How often during the last year have you been unable to remember what happened the night before because of your drinking? | Never | Less than monthly | Monthly | Weekly | Daily or almost daily |
| 9. Have you or someone else been injured because of your drinking? | No | | Yes, but not in the last year | | Yes, during the last year |
| 10. Has a relative, friend, doctor, or other health care worker been concerned about your drinking or suggested you cut down? | No | | Yes, but not in the last year | | Yes, during the last year |
| | | | | | **Total** |

*Note:** This questionnaire (the AUDIT) is reprinted with permission from the World Health Organization. To reflect standard drink sizes in the United States, the number of drinks in question 3 was changed from six to five. A free AUDIT manual with guidelines for use in primary care settings is available online at www.who.org.

## Alcohol Withdrawal Assessment Scoring Guidelines (CIWA - Ar)

**Nausea/Vomiting** - Rate on scale 0-7.
0 - None
1 - Mild nausea with no vomiting
2
3
4 - Intermittent nausea
5
6
7 - Constant nausea and frequent dry heaves and vomiting

**Tremors -** Have patient extend arms and spread fingers. Rate on scale 0-7.
0 - No tremor
1 - Not visible, but can be felt fingertip to fingertip
2
3
4 - Moderate, with patient's arms extended
5
6
7 - Severe, even w/arms not extended

**Anxiety** - Rate on scale 0-7.
0 - No anxiety, patient at ease
1- Mildly anxious
2
3
4 - Moderately anxious or guarded, so anxiety is inferred
5
6
7 - Equivalent to acute panic states seen in severe delirium or acute schizophrenic reactions

**Agitation** - Rate on scale 0-7.
0 - Normal activity
1 - Somewhat normal activity
2
3
4 - Moderately fidgety and restless
5
6
7 - Paces back and forth, or constantly thrashes about

**Paroxysmal Sweats** - Rate on scale 0-7.
0 - No sweats
1 - Barely perceptible sweating, palms moist
2
3
4 - Beads of sweat obvious on forehead
5
6
7 - Drenching sweats

**Orientation and Clouding of Sensorium** - Ask, "What day is this? Where are you? Who am I?" Rate on scale 0-4.
0 - Oriented
1 - Cannot do serial additions or is uncertain about date
2 - Disoriented to date by no more than 2 calendar days
3 - Disoriented to date by more than 2 calendar days
4 - Disoriented to place and/or person

**Tactile Disturbances** - Ask, "Have you experienced any itching, pins and needles sensation, burning or numbness, or a feeling of bugs crawling on or under your skin?"
Rate on scale 0-7.
0 - None
1 - Very mild itching, pins and needles, burning, or numbness
2 - Mild itching, pins and needles, burning, or numbness
3 - Moderate itching, pins and needles, burning, or numbness
4 - Moderate hallucinations
5 - Severe hallucinations
6 - Extremely severe hallucinations
7 - Continuous hallucinations

**Auditory Disturbances** - Ask, "Are you more aware of sounds around you? Are they harsh? Do they startle you? Do you hear anything that disturbs you or that you know isn't there?"
Rate on scale 0-7.
0 - Not present
1 - Very mild harshness or ability to startle
2 - Mild harshness or ability to startle
3 - Moderate harshness or ability to startle
4 - Moderate hallucinations
5 - Severe hallucinations
6 - Extremely severe hallucinations
7 - Continuous hallucinations

**Visual Disturbances** - Ask, "Does the light appear to be too bright? Is its color different than normal? Does it hurt your eyes? Are you seeing anything that disturbs you or that you know isn't there?" Rate on scale 0-7.
0 - Not present
1 - Very mild sensitivity
2 - Mild sensitivity
3 - Moderate sensitivity
4 - Moderate hallucinations
5 - Severe hallucinations
6 - Extremely severe hallucinations
7 - Continuous hallucinations

**Headache** - Ask, "Does your head feel different than usual? Does it feel like there is a band around your head?" Do not rate dizziness or lightheadedness. Rate on scale 0-7.
0 - Not present
1 - Very mild
2 - Mild
3 - Moderate
4 - Moderately severe
5 - Severe
6 - Very severe
7 - Extremely severe

Procedure:
1. Assess and rate each of the 10 criteria of the CIWA scale. Each criterion is rated on a scale from 0 to 7, except for "Orientation and clouding of sensorium," which is rated on a scale from 0 to 4. Add up the scores for all ten criteria. This is the total CIWA-Ar score for the patient at that time. Document vitals and CIWA-Ar assessment on the Withdrawal Assessment Sheet. Document administration of PRN medications on the assessment sheet as well.
2. The CIWA-Ar scale is the most sensitive tool for assessment of the patient experiencing alcohol withdrawal. Nursing assessment is vitally important. Early intervention for a CIWA-Ar score of 8 or greater provides the best means to prevent the progression of withdrawal.

| Assessment Protocol | | Date | | | | | | | | | | | |
|---|---|---|---|---|---|---|---|---|---|---|---|---|---|
| a. Vitals, Assessment Now. | | Time | | | | | | | | | | | |
| b. If initial score ≥ 8 repeat q1h x 8 hrs, then if stable q2h x 8 hrs, then if stable q4h. | | Pulse | | | | | | | | | | | |
| | | RR | | | | | | | | | | | |
| c. If initial score < 8, assess q4h x 72 hrs. If score < 8 for 72 hrs, d/c assessment. If score ≥ 8 at any time, go to (b) above. | | O₂ sat | | | | | | | | | | | |
| d. If indicated (see indications below), administer PRN medications as ordered and record on MAR and below. | | BP | | | | | | | | | | | |

**Assess and rate each of the following (CIWA-Ar Scale):** Refer to reverse for detailed instructions in use of the CIWA-Ar scale.

| | | | | | | | | | | | | |
|---|---|---|---|---|---|---|---|---|---|---|---|---|
| **Nausea/Vomiting** (0-7) 0 - none; 1 - mild nausea, no vomiting; 4 - intermittent nausea; 7 - constant nausea, frequent dry heaves & vomiting. | | | | | | | | | | | | |
| **Tremors** (0-7) 0 - no tremor; 1 - not visible but can be felt; 4 - moderate w/ arms extended; 7 - severe, even w/ arms not extended. | | | | | | | | | | | | |
| **Anxiety** (0-7) 0 - none, at ease; 1 - mildly anxious; 4 - moderately anxious or guarded; 7 - equivalent to acute panic state. | | | | | | | | | | | | |
| **Agitation** (0-7) 0 - normal activity; 1 - somewhat normal activity; 4 - moderately fidgety/restless; 7 - paces or constantly thrashes about. | | | | | | | | | | | | |
| **Paroxysmal Sweats** (0-7) 0 - no sweats; 1 - barely perceptible sweating, palms moist; 4 - beads of sweat obvious on forehead; 7 - drenching sweat. | | | | | | | | | | | | |
| **Orientation** (0-4) 0 - oriented; 1 - uncertain about date; 2 - disoriented to date by no more than 2 days; 3 - disoriented to date by > 2 days; 4 - disoriented to place and / or person. | | | | | | | | | | | | |
| **Tactile Disturbances** (0-7) 0 - none; 1 - very mild itch, P&N, numbness; 2-mild itch, P&N, burning, numbness; 3 - moderate itch, P&N, burning, numbness; 4 - moderate hallucinations; 5 - severe hallucinations; 6 – extremely severe hallucinations; 7 - continuous hallucinations. | | | | | | | | | | | | |
| **Auditory Disturbances** (0-7) 0 - not present; 1 - very mild harshness/ability to startle; 2 - mild harshness, ability to startle; 3 - moderate harshness, ability to startle; 4 - moderate hallucinations; 5 - severe hallucinations; 6 - extremely severe hallucinations; 7 - continuous hallucinations. | | | | | | | | | | | | |
| **Visual Disturbances** (0-7) 0 - not present; 1 - very mild sensitivity; 2 - mild sensitivity; 3 - moderate sensitivity; 4 - moderate hallucinations; 5 - severe hallucinations; 6 - extremely severe hallucinations; 7 - continuous hallucinations. | | | | | | | | | | | | |
| **Headache** (0-7) 0 - not present; 1 - very mild; 2 - mild; 3 - moderate; 4 - moderately severe; 5 - severe; 6 - very severe; 7 - extremely severe. | | | | | | | | | | | | |
| Total CIWA-Ar score: | | | | | | | | | | | | |

| PRN med: (circle one) Diazepam Lorazepam | Dose given (mg): Route: | | | | | | | | | | | | |
|---|---|---|---|---|---|---|---|---|---|---|---|---|---|
| **Time** of PRN medication administration: | | | | | | | | | | | | | |
| Assessment of response (CIWA-Ar score 30-60 minutes after medication administered) | | | | | | | | | | | | | |
| RN Initials | | | | | | | | | | | | | |

**Scale for Scoring:**
Total Score =
  0-9: absent or minimal withdrawal
  10-19: mild to moderate withdrawal
  More than 20: severe withdrawal

**Indications for PRN medication:**
a. Total CIWA-Ar score 8 or higher if ordered PRN only (symptom-triggered method).
b. Total CIWA-Ar score 15 or higher if on scheduled medication (scheduled + PRN method).
Consider transfer to ICU for any of the following: Total score above 35, q1h assess. x more than 8 hrs required, more than 4 mg/hr lorazepam x 3 hr **or** 20 mg/hr diazepam x 3 hr required, or resp. distress.

Patient Identification (Addressograph)

| Signature/Title | Initials | Signature/Title | Initials |
|---|---|---|---|
| | | | |
| | | | |
| | | | |
| | | | |

This scale is not copyrighted and may be used freely.
Adapted from Sullivan, J. T., Sykora, K., Schneiderman, J., Naranjo, C. A., Sellers, E. M. (1989). Assessment of alcohol withdrawal: The revised Clinical Institute Withdrawal Assessment for Alcohol scale (CIWA-Ar). *Br J Addict 84*:1353-1357. Reprinted from www.ihs.gov, revised 2003.

# Domestic and Family Violence Assessment

## PURPOSE

This chapter helps you learn about intimate partner violence, elder abuse, and child abuse. The content includes how to assess the extent of the abuse, how to assess the extent of physical and psychological harm, and how to document appropriately.

## READING ASSIGNMENT

Jarvis: *Physical Examination and Health Assessment*, 8th ed., Chapter 7, pp. 99-111.

Suggested readings:
Killion, C. M. (2017). Cultural healing practices that mimic child abuse. *Ann Forensic Res Anal*, 4(2).

## GLOSSARY

Study the following terms after completing the reading assignment. You should be able to cover the definition on the right and define the term out loud.

**Child emotional abuse** . . . . . . any pattern of behavior that harms a child's emotional development or sense of self-worth. It includes frequent belittling, rejection, threats, and withholding love and support

**Child neglect** . . . . . . . . . . . . . . failure to provide for a child's basic needs (physical, educational, medical, and emotional)

**Child physical abuse** . . . . . . . . physical injury resulting from punching, beating, kicking, biting, burning, shaking, or otherwise harming a child. Even if the parent or caregiver did not intend to harm the child, such acts are considered abuse when done purposefully

**Child sexual abuse** . . . . . . . . . includes fondling a child's genitals, incest, penetration, rape, sodomy, indecent exposure, and commercial exploitation through prostitution or the production of pornographic materials

**Elder abuse** . . . . . . . . . . . . . . . . willful infliction of force that results in bodily harm, pain, and/or impairment on a person age 65 years or older. Examples include pushing, slapping, hitting, shaking, burning, and rough handling

**Elder neglect (physical)** . . . . . . physical harm (actual or potential) to a person age 65 years or older because of failure to provide for the person's well-being. Examples include inadequate feeding and hydration, unsanitary living conditions, and poor personal hygiene

**Intimate partner violence (IPV)** . . . . . . . . . . . . . physical and/or sexual violence (use of physical force) or threat of such violence; also psychological or emotional abuse and/or coercive tactics when there has been prior physical and/or sexual violence between spouses or non-marital partners (dating, boyfriend-girlfriend) or former spouses or non-marital partners

**Mandatory reporter** . . . . . . . . a specified group of people (e.g., health care providers) is required by law to report abuse (of a specified nature against specified people) to a governmental agency (e.g., protective services, the police)

**Psychological abuse** . . . . . . . . infliction of emotional and/or mental anguish by humiliation, coercion, and threats and/or lack of social stimulation. Examples include yelling, threats of harm, threats of withholding basic medical and/or personal care, and leaving the person alone for long periods

**Routine universal screening for intimate partner violence** . . . . . . . . . . . . asking all adult patients each time they are in the health care system, no matter what their problem or concern, whether they have experienced IPV

## STUDY GUIDE

After completing the reading assignment, you should be able to answer the following questions in the spaces provided.

1. Identify the most common physical health problems that result from intimate partner violence.

2. Identify the most common mental health problems that result from intimate partner violence.

3. Differentiate abuse from neglect.

4. Identify commonly used screening tools for intimate partner violence.

5. Identify commonly used screening questions for older adult abuse.

6. Identify important elements of assessment for an abused person.

7. Discuss bruising in children and how it relates to their development level.

8. Identify some of the important elements of the child's medical history when assessing for suspected child maltreatment.

9. Discuss some of the long-term consequences of child maltreatment.

10. Identify risk factors that may contribute to child maltreatment.

## CRITICAL THINKING EXERCISES

1. Review laws in your state and at least 1 other state related to intimate partner violence, elder abuse, and child maltreatment. Do the laws between the states differ? Were you surprised by any of the laws or mandatory reporting regulations? Talk with at least 1 classmate and compare notes.
2. Identify community resources that help victims of intimate partner violence, elder abuse, and child maltreatment. Create a list of resources and identify any gaps. For example, your community may have a shelter for abused women and children yet lack adequate community resources for male or elderly victims of abuse.

3. During your clinical, screen at least 1 adult patient for intimate partner violence using a screening tool recommended by the U.S. Preventive Services Task Force. How did the interaction make you feel? Was the client willing to answer the questions? What therapeutic communication techniques did you use during the encounter?

## REVIEW QUESTIONS

This test is for you to check your own mastery of the content. Answers are provided in Appendix A.

1. Which scenario is an example of intimate partner violence?

   a. An ex-boyfriend stalks his ex-girlfriend
   b. Marital rape
   c. Hitting a date
   d. All of the above

2. Routine universal screening for domestic violence includes:

   a. Asking everyone each time they come to the health care system if they are abused.
   b. Asking everyone who has injuries if they are abused.
   c. Asking everyone who has symptoms of depression and PTSD if they are abused.
   d. Asking everyone ages 18 to 30 years if they are abused.

3. Patients are at high risk for which mental health problem associated with intimate partner violence?

   a. Hallucinations
   b. Suicidality
   c. Schizophrenia
   d. Attention-deficit/hyperactivity disorder (ADHD)

4. Which gynecologic problem is *not* usually associated with intimate partner violence?

   a. Pelvic pain
   b. Ovarian cysts
   c. STIs
   d. Vaginal tearing

5. Risk factors for intimate partner homicide include:

   a. Abuse during pregnancy.
   b. Victim substance abuse.
   c. Victim unemployment.
   d. History of victim childhood sexual assault.

6. Elder abuse and neglect assessments include:

   a. Willful infliction of force.
   b. Withholding prescription medications without medical orders.
   c. Not replacing broken eyeglasses.
   d. Threatening to place someone in a nursing home.
   e. All of the above.

7. When assessing an injury on a child, which should be considered?

   a. The child's developmental level
   b. The child's medical and medication history
   c. The history of how the injury occurred
   d. All of the above

8. What is a known risk factor for child maltreatment?

   a. Substance abuse
   b. Intimate partner violence
   c. Physical disability and/or mental retardation in the child
   d. All of the above

9. Bruising on a nonwalking or noncruising child:

   a. Is a common finding from normal infant activity.
   b. Needs to be further evaluated for either an abusive or medical explanation.
   c. Is commonly seen on the buttocks.
   d. Cannot be reported until after a full medical evaluation.

10. Which is a forensic term that is related to "purpura" but is not related to blunt force trauma?

    a. Wound
    b. Incision
    c. Ecchymosis
    d. Bruise

11. Which should be routinely included in evaluating a case of elder abuse?

    a. Corroborative interview from caregiver
    b. Baseline laboratory tests
    c. Testing for STIs
    d. TB testing

12. During an examination, you notice a patterned injury on a patient's back. Which is most likely?

    a. A blunt force trauma
    b. A friction rub
    c. A stabbing
    d. A welt from a leather belt

13. During an interview, a woman has answered "yes" to 3 of the Abuse Assessment Screen questions. How should you proceed?

    a. Ask the patient if she has filed a restraining order.
    b. Proceed by asking more questions about the items she answered "yes."
    c. Respond by confirming that the patient was abused.
    d. Interview the woman's partner and compare notes.

14. Which clinical situation would require the examiner to report to the proper authorities?

    a. Statements from the victim
    b. Statements from witnesses
    c. Proof of abuse and/or neglect
    d. Suspicion of elder abuse and/or neglect

15. Which would you include on the chart of the patient who has been the victim of abuse?

    a. Photographic documentation of injuries
    b. A summary of the abused patient's statements
    c. Verbatim documentation of every statement made
    d. A general description of injuries in the progress notes

# NOTES

# CHAPTER 8

# Assessment Techniques and Safety in the Clinical Setting

## PURPOSE

This chapter helps you learn the assessment techniques of inspection, palpation, percussion, and auscultation; learn the items of equipment needed for a complete physical examination; and consider age-specific modifications you would make for the examination of individuals throughout the life cycle.

## READING ASSIGNMENT

Jarvis: *Physical Examination and Health Assessment*, 8th ed., Chapter 8, pp. 113-124.

Suggested reading:
Miller, S., Owens, L., & Silverman, E. (2015). Physical examination of the adult patient with chronic respiratory disease. *Medsurg Nurs 24*(3), 195-198.

## GLOSSARY

Study the following terms after completing the reading assignment. You should be able to cover the definition on the right and define the term out loud.

**Amplitude** . . . . . . . . . . . . . . . . (or intensity) how loud or soft a sound is

**Duration** . . . . . . . . . . . . . . . . . the length of time a note lingers

**Ophthalmoscope** . . . . . . . . . . . an instrument that illuminates the internal eye structures, enabling the examiner to look through the pupil at the fundus (background) of the eye

**Otoscope** . . . . . . . . . . . . . . . . . an instrument that illuminates the ear canal, enabling the examiner to look at the ear canal and tympanic membrane

**Pitch** . . . . . . . . . . . . . . . . . . . . (or frequency) the number of vibrations (or cycles) per second of a note

**Quality** . . . . . . . . . . . . . . . . . . (or timbre) a subjective difference in a sound as a result of the sound's distinctive overtones

## STUDY GUIDE

After completing the reading assignment, you should be able to answer the following questions in the spaces provided.

1. Define and describe the technique of the 4 physical examination skills:

   Inspection _____

   Palpation_____

   Percussion_____

   Auscultation _____

2. Define the characteristics of the following percussion notes:

|  | Pitch | Amplitude | Quality | Duration |
|---|---|---|---|---|
| Resonance |  |  |  |  |
| Hyperresonance |  |  |  |  |
| Tympany |  |  |  |  |
| Dull |  |  |  |  |
| Flat |  |  |  |  |

3. Differentiate among light, deep, and bimanual palpation.

4. List the two endpieces of the stethoscope and the conditions for which each is best suited.

5. Describe the environmental conditions to consider in preparing the examination setting.

6. List 4 situations in which you clean your hands promptly and thoroughly.

7. Describe your own preparation as you encounter the patient for examination: your own dress, your demeanor, safety/Universal Precautions, sequence of examination steps, instructions to patient.

8. What age-specific considerations would you make for the examination of the:

Infant? _____

Toddler? _____

Preschooler? _____

School-age child? _____

Adolescent? _____

Older adult? _____

Acutely ill person? _____

## REVIEW QUESTIONS

This test is for you to check your own mastery of the content. Answers are provided in Appendix A.

1. During the assessment, which part of the hand is best for detecting vibration?

   a. Fingertips
   b. Index finger and thumb in opposition
   c. Dorsum of the hand
   d. Ulnar surface of the hand

2. When performing indirect percussion, the stationary finger is struck:

   a. At the ulnar surface.
   b. At the middle joint.
   c. At the distal interphalangeal joint.
   d. Wherever it is in contact with the skin.

3. The best description of the pitch of a sound wave obtained by percussion is:

   a. The intensity of the sound.
   b. The number of vibrations per second.
   c. The length of time the note lingers.
   d. The overtones of the note.

4. The bell of the stethoscope is used:

   a. For soft, low-pitched sounds.
   b. For high-pitched sounds.
   c. To hold firmly against the skin.
   d. To magnify sound.

5. The ophthalmoscope has 5 apertures. Which aperture is used to assess the eyes of a patient with undilated pupils?

   a. Grid
   b. Slit
   c. Small
   d. Large

6. At the conclusion of the patient examination, the examiner should:

   a. Document findings after leaving the examining room.
   b. Have findings confirmed by another practitioner.
   c. Relate objective findings to the subjective findings for accuracy.
   d. Summarize findings to the patient.

7. When the examiner enters the examining room, the infant patient is asleep. Which assessment should the examiner perform next?

    a. Height and weight
    b. Blood pressure
    c. Heart, lung, and abdomen
    d. Temperature

8. The sequence of an examination changes from beginning with the thorax to that of head to toe when the patient is in what age category?

    a. The infant
    b. The preschool child
    c. The school-age child
    d. The adolescent

9. When inspecting the ear canal of a patient, the examiner chooses which speculum for the otoscope?

    a. A short, broad one
    b. The narrowest for a child
    c. The longest for an adult
    d. The largest that will fit

10. For a health assessment, which assessment technique will you use first?

    a. Palpation
    b. Inspection
    c. Percussion
    d. Auscultation

11. To assess a patient's abdomen by palpation, how should the nurse proceed?

    a. Avoid palpation of reported "tender" areas because this may cause the patient pain.
    b. Quickly palpate a tender area to avoid any discomfort that the patient may experience.
    c. Begin the assessment with deep palpation, encouraging the patient to relax and take deep breaths.
    d. Start with light palpation to detect surface characteristics and to accustom the patient to being touched.

# CHAPTER 9

# General Survey and Measurement

## PURPOSE

This chapter helps you learn the method of gathering data for a general survey on a patient and the techniques for measuring height and weight and for calculating body mass index.

## READING ASSIGNMENT

Jarvis: *Physical Examination and Health Assessment*, 8th ed., Chapter 9, pp. 125-138.

Suggested readings:
Cottrell, D. B., & Williams, J. (2016). Eating disorders in men. *Nurse Pract, 41*(9):49-56.

## STUDY GUIDE

After completing the reading assignment, write or draw the answer in the spaces provided.

1. List the significant information considered in each of the 4 areas of a general survey—physical appearance, body structure, mobility, and behavior.

2. Describe the normal posture, body build, and proportions.

3. Note aspects of normal gait.

4. Describe the clinical appearance of the following variations in stature:

   Hypopituitary dwarfism _____

   Gigantism _____

   Acromegaly _____

   Achondroplastic dwarfism _____

   Marfan syndrome_____

   Endogenous obesity (Cushing syndrome) _____

   Anorexia nervosa _____

5. State the body mass index for a male weighing 190 lb who is 5′10″ tall _____ and for a female weighing 136 lb who is 5′4″ tall _____.

6. For serial weight measurements, what time of day would you instruct the person to have his or her weight measured?

7. Describe the technique for measuring head circumference and chest circumference on an infant.

8. What changes in height and in weight distribution would you expect for an adult in his or her 70s and 80s?

# REVIEW QUESTIONS

This test is for you to check your own mastery of the content. Answers are provided in Appendix A.

1. The 4 areas to consider during the general survey include:

   a. Ethnicity, gender, age, and socioeconomic status
   b. Physical appearance, gender, ethnicity, and affect
   c. Dress, affect, nonverbal behavior, and mobility
   d. Physical appearance, body structure, mobility, and behavior

2. You are assessing a patient's gait. What do you expect to find?

    a. Gait is varied, depending on the height of the person.
    b. Gait is equal to the length of the arm.
    c. Gait is as wide as the shoulder width.
    d. Gait is half the height of the person.

3. An 18-month-old child is brought into the clinic for a health screening visit. To assess the height of the child:

    a. Use a tape measure.
    b. Use a horizontal measuring board.
    c. Have the child stand on the upright scale.
    d. Measure arm span to estimate height.

4. Which changes in head circumference measurements in relation to chest measurements will occur from infancy through early childhood?

    a. A newborn's head should be approximately 5 cm larger than the chest circumference, but by age 2, they should be equal.
    b. The chest grows at a faster rate than the cranium, but at age 1, the measurements will be the same, and after age 2, the chest should be approximately 5 cm larger.
    c. The newborn's head will be approximately 2 cm larger than the chest circumference, but between 6 months and 2 years, they will be about the same.
    d. The head and chest circumferences should be very similar, but between 6 months and 2 years, the chest size will increase and remain that way.

5. Which changes regarding height and weight occur during a person's 80s and 90s?

    a. Both increase.
    b. Weight increases, and height decreases.
    c. Both decrease.
    d. Both remain the same as during the 70s.

## CRITICAL THINKING EXERCISES

1. Your next patient is a 55-year-old man who has experienced shortness of breath for the past 2 days. When you walk into the room you hear audible, labored breathing. Based on the picture below, write a general survey.

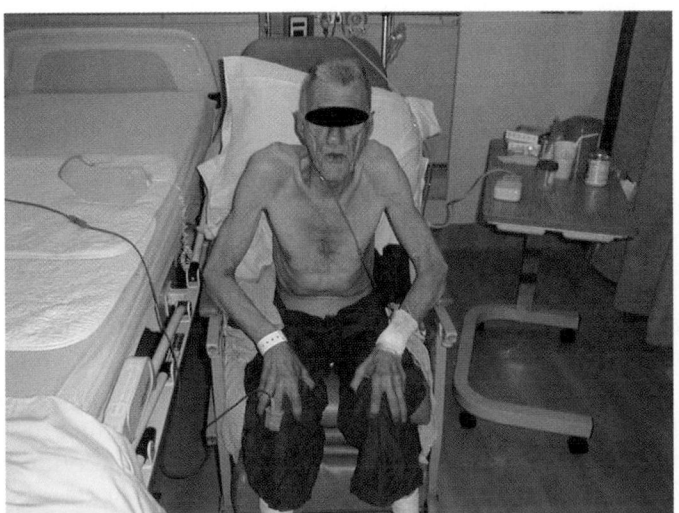

From Goldman, L. & Schafer, A.I. (2012). *Goldman's Cecil medicine* (24 ed.). Philadelphia: Saunders.

2. H.Y. is at your clinic with her mother for a well-child appointment. She is new to your clinic and you have no history other than that she recently turned 1 year old. Based on the picture below, write a general survey.

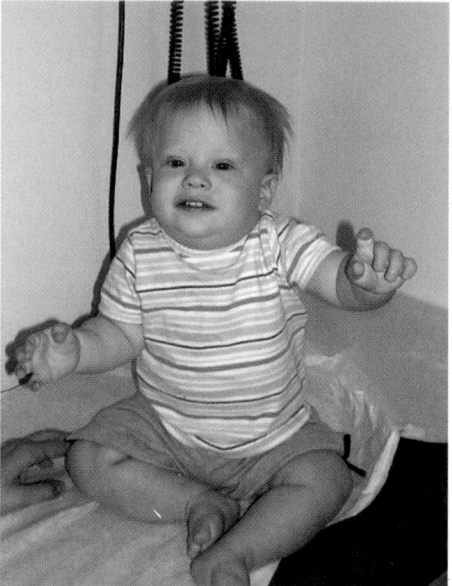

From Zitelli, B.J., McIntire, S.C., & Nowalk, A.J. (2012). *Atlas of pediatric physical diagnosis* (ed. 6). Philadelphia, Saunders.

## SKILLS LABORATORY AND CLINICAL SETTING

You are now ready for the clinical component of Chapters 8 and 9. The purpose of the clinical component is to observe and describe the regional examination on a peer in the skills laboratory and to achieve the following:

### Clinical Objectives

1. Observe and describe the significant characteristics of a general survey.

2. Measure height and weight, and determine if findings are within normal range.

3. Record the physical examination findings accurately.

### Instructions

Set up your section of the skills laboratory for a complete physical examination, attending to proper lighting, tables, and linen. Gather all equipment you will need for a complete physical examination, and make sure you are familiar with its mechanical operation. You will not use all the equipment today, but you will use it during the course of the semester, and this is the time to have it checked out.

Practice the steps of gathering data for a general survey and for height and weight on a peer. Record your findings using the regional write-up sheet that follows. The first section of the sheet is intended as a worksheet. It includes points for you to note that add up to the general survey. The bottom of the sheet has instructions for you to write the general survey statement; this is the topic sentence that will serve as an introduction for the complete physical examination write-up.

# REGIONAL WRITE-UP—GENERAL SURVEY, VITAL SIGNS

Date _____

Examiner _____

Patient _____ Age _____ Gender _____

Occupation _____

## I. Physical Examination

A. General survey
  1. Physical appearance
     Gender_____
     Level of consciousness _____
     Skin color _____
     Facial features _____
  2. Body structure
     Stature _____
     Nutrition _____
     Symmetry_____
     Posture_____
     Position _____
     Body build, contour _____
     Any physical deformity _____
  3. Mobility
     Gait _____
     Range of motion _____
  4. Behavior
     Facial expression _____
     Mood and affect _____
     Speech _____
     Dress _____
     Personal hygiene _____
B. Measurement
  1. Height: _____ cm; _____ ft/inches    3. Body mass index _____
  2. Weight: _____ kg; _____ lb            4. Waist circumference _____ inches

## II. Summary

Write a summary of the general survey, including height and weight. This will serve as an introduction for the complete physical examination write-up.

## Table 9-1 Body Mass Index

| | NORMAL | | | | | | OVERWEIGHT | | | | | | OBESE | | | | | | |
|---|---|---|---|---|---|---|---|---|---|---|---|---|---|---|---|---|---|---|---|---|
| BMI | 19 | 20 | 21 | 22 | 23 | 24 | 25 | 26 | 27 | 28 | 29 | 30 | 31 | 32 | 33 | 34 | 35 | 36 | 37 | 38 | 39 |
| HEIGHT (INCHES) | BODY WEIGHT (POUNDS) | | | | | | | | | | | | | | | | | | | | |
| 58 | 91 | 96 | 100 | 105 | 110 | 115 | 119 | 124 | 129 | 134 | 138 | 143 | 148 | 153 | 158 | 162 | 167 | 172 | 177 | 181 | 186 |
| 59 | 94 | 99 | 104 | 109 | 114 | 119 | 124 | 128 | 133 | 138 | 143 | 148 | 153 | 158 | 163 | 168 | 173 | 178 | 183 | 188 | 193 |
| 60 | 97 | 102 | 107 | 112 | 118 | 123 | 128 | 133 | 138 | 143 | 148 | 153 | 158 | 163 | 168 | 174 | 179 | 184 | 189 | 194 | 199 |
| 61 | 100 | 106 | 111 | 116 | 122 | 127 | 132 | 137 | 143 | 148 | 153 | 158 | 164 | 169 | 174 | 180 | 185 | 190 | 195 | 201 | 206 |
| 62 | 104 | 109 | 115 | 120 | 126 | 131 | 136 | 142 | 147 | 153 | 158 | 164 | 169 | 175 | 180 | 186 | 191 | 196 | 202 | 207 | 213 |
| 63 | 107 | 113 | 118 | 124 | 130 | 135 | 141 | 146 | 152 | 158 | 163 | 169 | 175 | 180 | 186 | 191 | 197 | 203 | 208 | 214 | 220 |
| 64 | 110 | 116 | 122 | 128 | 134 | 140 | 145 | 151 | 157 | 163 | 169 | 174 | 180 | 186 | 192 | 197 | 204 | 209 | 215 | 221 | 227 |
| 65 | 114 | 120 | 126 | 132 | 138 | 144 | 150 | 156 | 162 | 168 | 174 | 180 | 186 | 192 | 198 | 204 | 210 | 216 | 222 | 228 | 234 |
| 66 | 118 | 124 | 130 | 136 | 142 | 148 | 155 | 161 | 167 | 173 | 179 | 186 | 192 | 198 | 204 | 210 | 216 | 223 | 229 | 235 | 241 |
| 67 | 121 | 127 | 134 | 140 | 146 | 153 | 159 | 166 | 172 | 178 | 185 | 191 | 198 | 204 | 211 | 217 | 223 | 230 | 236 | 242 | 249 |
| 68 | 125 | 131 | 138 | 144 | 151 | 158 | 164 | 171 | 177 | 184 | 190 | 197 | 203 | 210 | 216 | 223 | 230 | 236 | 243 | 249 | 256 |
| 69 | 128 | 135 | 142 | 149 | 155 | 162 | 169 | 176 | 182 | 189 | 196 | 203 | 209 | 216 | 223 | 230 | 236 | 243 | 250 | 257 | 263 |
| 70 | 132 | 139 | 146 | 153 | 160 | 167 | 174 | 181 | 188 | 195 | 202 | 209 | 216 | 222 | 229 | 236 | 243 | 250 | 257 | 264 | 271 |
| 71 | 136 | 143 | 150 | 157 | 165 | 172 | 179 | 186 | 193 | 200 | 208 | 215 | 222 | 229 | 236 | 243 | 250 | 257 | 265 | 272 | 279 |
| 72 | 140 | 147 | 154 | 162 | 169 | 177 | 184 | 191 | 199 | 206 | 213 | 221 | 228 | 235 | 242 | 250 | 258 | 265 | 272 | 279 | 287 |
| 73 | 144 | 151 | 159 | 166 | 174 | 182 | 189 | 197 | 204 | 212 | 219 | 227 | 235 | 242 | 250 | 257 | 265 | 272 | 280 | 288 | 295 |
| 74 | 148 | 155 | 163 | 171 | 179 | 186 | 194 | 202 | 210 | 218 | 225 | 233 | 241 | 249 | 256 | 264 | 272 | 280 | 287 | 295 | 303 |
| 75 | 152 | 160 | 168 | 176 | 184 | 192 | 200 | 208 | 216 | 224 | 232 | 240 | 248 | 256 | 264 | 272 | 279 | 287 | 295 | 303 | 311 |
| 76 | 156 | 164 | 172 | 180 | 189 | 197 | 205 | 213 | 221 | 230 | 238 | 246 | 254 | 263 | 271 | 279 | 287 | 295 | 304 | 312 | 320 |

| | EXTREME OBESITY | | | | | | | | | | | | | | |
|---|---|---|---|---|---|---|---|---|---|---|---|---|---|---|---|
| BMI | 40 | 41 | 42 | 43 | 44 | 45 | 46 | 47 | 48 | 49 | 50 | 51 | 52 | 53 | 54 |
| HEIGHT (INCHES) | BODY WEIGHT (POUNDS) | | | | | | | | | | | | | | |
| 58 | 191 | 196 | 201 | 205 | 210 | 215 | 220 | 224 | 229 | 234 | 239 | 244 | 248 | 253 | 258 |
| 59 | 198 | 203 | 208 | 212 | 217 | 222 | 227 | 232 | 237 | 242 | 247 | 252 | 257 | 262 | 267 |
| 60 | 204 | 209 | 215 | 220 | 225 | 230 | 235 | 240 | 245 | 250 | 255 | 261 | 266 | 271 | 276 |
| 61 | 211 | 217 | 222 | 227 | 232 | 238 | 243 | 248 | 254 | 259 | 264 | 269 | 275 | 280 | 285 |
| 62 | 218 | 224 | 229 | 235 | 240 | 246 | 251 | 256 | 262 | 267 | 273 | 278 | 284 | 289 | 295 |
| 63 | 225 | 231 | 237 | 242 | 248 | 254 | 259 | 265 | 270 | 278 | 282 | 287 | 293 | 299 | 304 |
| 64 | 232 | 238 | 244 | 250 | 256 | 262 | 267 | 273 | 279 | 285 | 291 | 296 | 302 | 308 | 314 |
| 65 | 240 | 246 | 252 | 258 | 264 | 270 | 276 | 282 | 288 | 294 | 300 | 306 | 312 | 318 | 324 |
| 66 | 247 | 253 | 260 | 266 | 272 | 278 | 284 | 291 | 297 | 303 | 309 | 315 | 322 | 328 | 334 |
| 67 | 255 | 261 | 268 | 274 | 280 | 287 | 293 | 299 | 306 | 312 | 319 | 325 | 331 | 338 | 344 |
| 68 | 262 | 269 | 276 | 282 | 289 | 295 | 302 | 308 | 315 | 322 | 328 | 335 | 341 | 348 | 354 |
| 69 | 270 | 277 | 284 | 291 | 297 | 304 | 311 | 318 | 324 | 331 | 338 | 345 | 351 | 358 | 365 |
| 70 | 278 | 285 | 292 | 299 | 306 | 313 | 320 | 327 | 334 | 341 | 348 | 355 | 362 | 369 | 376 |
| 71 | 286 | 293 | 301 | 308 | 315 | 322 | 329 | 338 | 343 | 351 | 358 | 365 | 372 | 379 | 386 |
| 72 | 294 | 302 | 309 | 316 | 324 | 331 | 338 | 346 | 353 | 361 | 368 | 375 | 383 | 390 | 397 |
| 73 | 302 | 310 | 318 | 325 | 333 | 340 | 348 | 355 | 363 | 371 | 378 | 386 | 393 | 401 | 408 |
| 74 | 311 | 319 | 326 | 334 | 342 | 350 | 358 | 365 | 373 | 381 | 389 | 396 | 404 | 412 | 420 |
| 75 | 319 | 327 | 335 | 343 | 351 | 359 | 367 | 375 | 383 | 391 | 399 | 407 | 415 | 423 | 431 |
| 76 | 328 | 336 | 344 | 353 | 361 | 369 | 377 | 385 | 394 | 402 | 410 | 418 | 426 | 435 | 443 |

Modified from Clinical guidelines on the identification, evaluation, and treatment of overweight and obesity in adults: The evidence report. June 2009. http://www.nhlbi.nih.gov/guidelines/obesity/bmi_tbl.pdf.

# CHAPTER
# 10
## Vital Signs

## PURPOSE

This chapter helps you learn how to measure and interpret vital signs.

## READING ASSIGNMENT

Jarvis: *Physical Examination and Health Assessment,* 8th ed., Chapter 10, pp. 136-160.

Suggested readings:
Jungquist, C. R., Smith, K., Wiltse Nicely, K. L. et al. (2017). Monitoring hospitalized adult patients for opioid-induced sedation and respiratory depression. *Am J Nurs, 117*(3), S27-S35.

## GLOSSARY

Study the following terms after completing the reading assignment. You should be able to cover the definition on the right and define the term out loud.

**Auscultatory gap** . . . . . . . . . . . . a brief period when Korotkoff sounds disappear during auscultation of blood pressure; may occur with hypertension

**Bradycardia** . . . . . . . . . . . . . . . heart rate fewer than 50 or 60 beats per minute in the adult (depending on agency)

**Sphygmomanometer** . . . . . . . . instrument for measuring arterial blood pressure

**Stroke volume** . . . . . . . . . . . . . amount of blood pumped out of the heart with each heartbeat

**Tachycardia** . . . . . . . . . . . . . . . heart rate greater than 95 beats per minute in the adult

## STUDY GUIDE

After completing the reading assignment, write or draw the answer in the spaces provided.

1. Describe the tympanic membrane and temporal artery thermometers, and compare their use with other forms of temperature measurement.

2. Describe 3 qualities to consider when assessing the pulse.

3. Relate the qualities of normal respirations to the appropriate approach for counting them.

4. Define and describe the relationships among the terms *blood pressure, systolic pressure, diastolic pressure, pulse pressure,* and *mean arterial pressure.*

5. List factors that affect blood pressure.

6. Relate the use of the wrong size blood pressure cuff to the possible findings that might be obtained.

7. Explain the significance of phase I, phase IV, and phase V Korotkoff sounds during blood pressure measurement.

8. Given an apparently healthy 20-year-old adult, state the expected range for oral temperature, pulse, respirations, and blood pressure.

## REVIEW QUESTIONS

This test is for you to check your own mastery of the content. Answers are provided in Appendix A.

1. During an initial home visit, the patient's temperature is noted to be 97.4° F. How would you interpret this?

    a. It cannot be evaluated without knowledge of the person's age.
    b. It is below normal. The person should be assessed for possible hypothermia.
    c. It should be retaken by the rectal route, because this best reflects core body temperature.
    d. It should be reevaluated at the next visit before a decision is made.

2. Select the best description of an accurate assessment of a patient's pulse.

    a. Count for 15 seconds if the pulse is regular.
    b. Begin counting with zero; count for 30 seconds.
    c. Count for 30 seconds and multiply by 2 for all cases.
    d. Count for 1 full minute; begin counting with zero.

3. After assessing the patient's pulse, the practitioner determines it to be "normal." This would be recorded as:

    a. 3+.
    b. 2+.
    c. 1+.
    d. 0.

4. Select the best description of an accurate assessment of a patients' respirations.

    a. Count for a full minute before taking the pulse.
    b. Count for 15 seconds and multiply by 4.
    c. Count after informing the patient where you are in the assessment process.
    d. Count for 30 seconds after pulse assessment.

5. Pulse pressure is described as:

    a. The difference between the systolic and diastolic pressure.
    b. A reflection of the viscosity of the blood.
    c. Another way to express the systolic pressure.
    d. A measure of vasoconstriction.

6. The examiner suspects a patient has coarctation of the aorta. Which assessment finding supports this suspicion?

    a. The thigh pressure is higher than in the arm.
    b. The thigh pressure is equal to that in the arm.
    c. The thigh pressure is unrelated to the arm pressure. There is no constant relationship; findings are highly individual.
    d. The thigh pressure is lower than in the arm.

7. Mean arterial pressure is:

    a. The arithmetic average of systolic and diastolic pressures.
    b. The driving force of blood during systole.
    c. Diastolic pressure plus one third of the pulse pressure.
    d. Corresponding to phase III Korotkoff.

8. Why is it important to match the appropriate size of blood pressure cuff to the person's arm and shape and not to the person's age?

    a. Using a cuff that is too narrow will give a false reading that is high.
    b. Using a cuff that is too wide will give a false reading that is low.
    c. Using a cuff that is too narrow will give a false reading that is low.
    d. Using a cuff that is too wide will give a false reading that is high.

9. A patient is being seen in the clinic for complaints of "fainting episodes that started last week." How should you proceed with the examination?

   a. Take the blood pressure in both arms and thighs.
   b. Ask the person to walk a few paces and then take the blood pressure.
   c. Record the blood pressure in the lying, sitting, and standing positions.
   d. Record the blood pressure in the lying and sitting positions and average these numbers to obtain a mean blood pressure.

10. The nurse is conducting a health fair for older adults. Which statement is true regarding vital sign measurements in aging adults?

    a. The pulse is more difficult to palpate because of the stiffness of the blood vessels.
    b. An increased respiratory rate and a shallower inspiratory phase are possible findings.
    c. A decreased pulse pressure occurs from changes in systolic and diastolic blood pressures.
    d. Changes in the body's temperature regulatory mechanism leave the older adult more likely to develop a fever.

## CRITICAL THINKING EXERCISE

1. Analyze the following vital sign values. Make sure to note any additional information you need to fully analyze the values:

   55-year-old woman: T 37°C, R 18 breaths/min, P 160 bpm, BP 90/60 mm Hg

   2-year-old boy: T 37°C, R 18 breaths/min, P 130 bpm

   89-year-old woman: T 36°C, R 12 breaths/min, P 55 bpm, BP 140/98 mm Hg

   25-year-old man: T 39°C, R 26 breaths/min, P 113 bpm, BP 100/60 mm Hg

## SKILLS LABORATORY AND CLINICAL SETTING

You are now ready for the clinical component of Chapter 10. The purpose of the clinical component is to perform vital signs measurements to achieve the following:

### Clinical Objectives

1. Demonstrate temperature measurement using oral, tympanic, and temporal artery thermometers.

2. Correctly take a radial pulse and describe associated characteristics.

3. Measure blood pressure.

4. Record the vital sign findings accurately.

### Instructions

Practice taking a full set if vital signs on at least 5 peers in the laboratory setting. For each person note the following:
1. Temperature _____
2. Pulse
   a. Rate _____
   b. Rhythm _____
   c. Force _____
3. Respiratory rate _____; description _____
4. Blood pressure _____ R arm; _____ L arm

# CHAPTER 11

# Pain Assessment

## PURPOSE

This chapter helps you learn the structure and function of pain pathways, understand the process of nociception, understand the rationale and methods of pain assessment, and accurately record the findings.

## READING ASSIGNMENT

Jarvis: *Physical Examination and Health Assessment*, 8th ed., Chapter 11, pp. 161-178.

Suggested readings:
Jungquist, C. R., Vallerand, A. H., Sicoutris, C., et al. (2017). Assessing and managing acute pain: A call to action. *Am J Nurs, 117*(3), S4-S11.
Robinson-Lane, S. G., & Booker, S. Q. (2017). Culturally responsive pain management for Black older adults. *J Gerontol Nurs, 43*(8), 33-41.

## GLOSSARY

Study the following terms after completing the reading assignment. You should be able to cover the definition on the right and define the term out loud.

| | |
|---|---|
| **Acute pain** | short-term, self-limiting, often predictable trajectory; stops after injury heals |
| **Allodynia** | experience of pain after a normally nonpainful tactile (e.g., from clothing) or thermal stimulus |
| **Breakthrough pain** | pain restarts or escalates before next scheduled analgesic dose |
| **Chronic (persistent) pain** | pain continues for 6 months or longer after initial injury |
| **Cutaneous pain** | pain originating from skin surface or subcutaneous structures |
| **Incident pain** | occurs predictably after specific movements |
| **Modulation** | pain message inhibited during this last phase of nociception |
| **Neuropathic pain** | abnormal processing of pain message; burning, shooting in nature |
| **Nociception** | process whereby noxious stimuli are perceived as pain; central and peripheral nervous systems intact |
| **Nociceptors** | specialized nerve endings that detect painful sensations |

**Pain** . . . . . . . . . . . . . . . . . . . . . . "An unpleasant sensory and emotional experience associated with actual or potential tissue damage, or described in terms of such damage. Pain is always subjective." (American Pain Society)

**Perception**. . . . . . . . . . . . . . . . . conscious awareness of painful sensation

**Referred pain** . . . . . . . . . . . . . . pain felt at a particular site but originates from another location

**Somatic pain**. . . . . . . . . . . . . . originating from muscle, bone, joints, tendons, or blood vessels

**Transduction** . . . . . . . . . . . . . . first phase of nociception whereby the painful stimulus is changed into an action potential

**Transmission** . . . . . . . . . . . . . . second phase of nociception whereby the pain impulse moves from the spinal cord to the brain

**Visceral pain**. . . . . . . . . . . . . . . originating from internal organs such as the gallbladder or stomach

## STUDY GUIDE

After completing the reading assignment, write or draw the answers in the spaces provided.

1. Describe the process of nociception using the four phases of:

    Transduction _____

    Transmission _____

    Perception _____

    Modulation _____

2. Identify the differences between nociceptive and neuropathic pain. Which words will people use to describe nociceptive and neuropathic pain?

3. List various sources of pain.

4. Explain how acute and chronic pain differ in terms of nonverbal behaviors.

5. Identify the most reliable indicator of a person's pain.

6. What does the mnemonic *PQRST* stand for, and how can it be used to guide pain assessment?

7. Describe physical examination findings that might indicate pain.

## CRITICAL THINKING EXERCISES

1. What conditions are more likely to produce pain in the aging adult?

2. How would you modify your examination when the patient reports having abdominal pain?

3. How would you assess for pain in an individual with dementia?

4. What would you say to someone who tells you that infants do not remember pain and that they are too little for the pain to have any damaging effect?

5. What would you say to a colleague who remarks that the individual with Alzheimer disease does not feel pain and therefore does not require an analgesic?

Fill in the labels indicated on the following illustration:

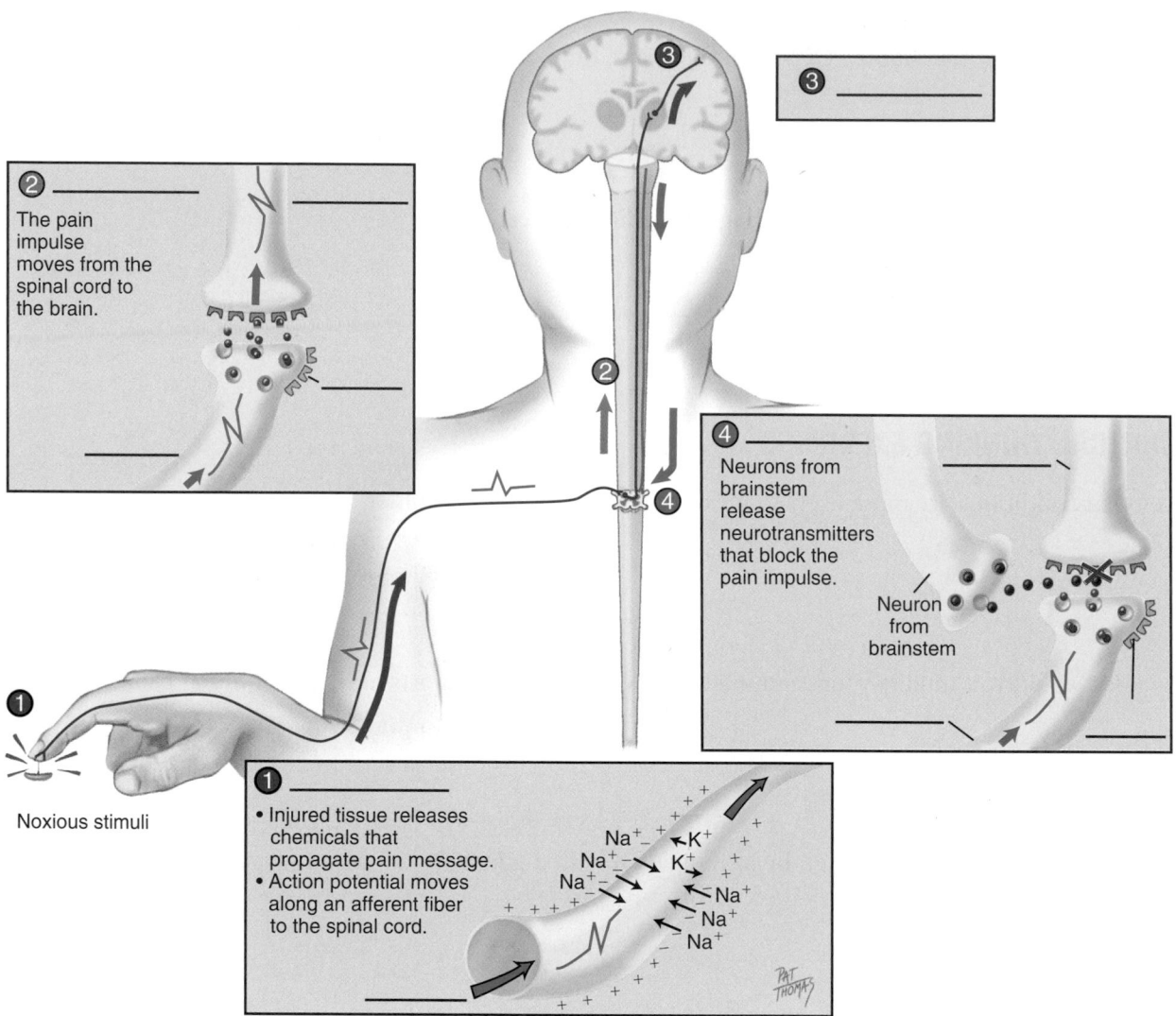

② _____ _____

The pain impulse moves from the spinal cord to the brain.

③ _____

④ _____

Neurons from brainstem release neurotransmitters that block the pain impulse.

Neuron from brainstem

① _____

Noxious stimuli

① _____

• Injured tissue releases chemicals that propagate pain message.
• Action potential moves along an afferent fiber to the spinal cord.

Na⁺ K⁺
Na⁺ K⁺
Na⁺ Na⁺
Na⁺
Na⁺

## REVIEW QUESTIONS

This test is for you to check your own mastery of the content. Answers are provided in Appendix A.

1. At which phase does the individual become aware of a painful sensation?

   a. Modulation
   b. Transduction
   c. Perception
   d. Transmission

2. While taking a history, the patient describes a burning, painful sensation that moves around the toes and bottoms of the feet. These symptoms suggest:

   a. Nociceptive pain.
   b. Neuropathic pain.
   c. Visceral pain.
   d. Muscular pain.

3. During the physical examination, your patient is diaphoretic and pale and complains of dull pain in the LUQ of the abdomen. This is what type of pain?

   a. Cutaneous pain
   b. Somatic pain
   c. Visceral pain
   d. Psychogenic pain

4. While caring for a preterm infant, you are aware that:

   a. Inhibitory neurotransmitters are in sufficient supply by 15 weeks' gestation.
   b. The fetus has less capacity to feel pain.
   c. Repetitive blood draws have minimal long-term consequences.
   d. The preterm infant is more sensitive to painful stimuli.

5. The most reliable indicator of pain in the adult is:

   a. The degree of physical functioning.
   b. Nonverbal behaviors.
   c. The MRI findings.
   d. The patient's self-report.

6. While examining the broken arm of a 4-year-old boy, select the appropriate assessment tool to evaluate his pain status.

   a. 0 to 10 numeric rating scale
   b. Wong-Baker scale
   c. Simple descriptor scale
   d. 0 to 5 numeric rating scale

7. Normal age-related finding in the lower extremities of an 80-year-old woman would be:

   a. Crepitus.
   b. Joint swelling.
   c. Diminished strength bilaterally.
   d. Unilateral muscle atrophy.

8. A patient presents with acute pain of the abdomen. After the initial examination, how would you proceed?

   a. Withhold analgesic until diagnostic testing is completed.
   b. Give pain medications as ordered.
   c. Withhold analgesic until pain subsides.
   d. Determine what type of pain it is and proceed accordingly.

9. For older adult postoperative patients, poorly controlled acute pain places them at higher risk for:

   a. Atelectasis.
   b. Increased myocardial oxygen demand.
   c. Impaired wound healing.
   d. All of the above.

10. A 30-year-old woman reports having persistent intense pain in her right arm related to trauma sustained from a car accident 5 months ago. She states that the slightest touch or clothing can exacerbate the pain. This report is suggestive of:

    a. Referred pain.
    b. Psychogenic pain.
    c. Complex regional pain I.
    d. Cutaneous pain.

11. CRIES is an appropriate pain assessment tool for:

    a. Cognitively impaired older adults.
    b. Children ages 2 to 8 years.
    c. Infants and children.
    d. Preterm and term neonates.

12. Pain issues should be anticipated in a cognitively impaired older adult with a history of:

    a. Constipation.
    b. Peripheral vascular disease.
    c. COPD.
    d. Parkinson disease.

13. Pain in the aging adult is considered to be:

    a. Part of the normal degenerative process.
    b. Perceived to a lesser degree.
    c. An expected finding.
    d. Unrelated to the aging process.

14. Which is considered a common physiologic change that occurs with pain?

    a. Polyuria
    b. Hyperventilation
    c. Hyperactive bowel sounds
    d. Tachycardia

15. A patient is requesting pain medication and expresses a pain level of 9/10; however, the patient is up and smiling. How should you proceed?

    a. Complete a full physical examination.
    b. Reposition patient but withhold pain medication based on behavior.
    c. Call the provider and suggest a substance abuse consult.
    d. Use therapeutic communication techniques to determine the patient's pain scale goal and history of chronic pain.

# SKILLS LABORATORY AND CLINICAL SETTING

The purpose of the clinical component is to practice pain assessment in the clinical setting and to achieve the following:

## Clinical objectives

1. Assess pain in patients using objective and subjective indicators of pain.
2. Use the Faces Pain Scale—Revised to assess pain in at least 1 patient.
3. Use the Brief Pain Inventory to assess pain in at least 1 patient.
4. Use the numeric pain scale (0-10) to assess pain in at least 1 patient.

## Instructions

Use the Faces Pain Scale—Revised, Brief Pain Inventory, and numeric pain scale (0-10) to assess pain in at least 1 patient. If possible, use each tool on multiple patients to assure understanding of how to use each assessment tool. Discuss your findings with your laboratory faculty member and classmates.

**Faces Pain Scale — Revised  (FPS-R)**
In the following instructions, say "hurt" or "pain," whichever seems right for a particular child.
**"These faces show how much something can hurt.  This face** [point to left-most face] **shows no pain. The faces show more and more pain** [point to each from left to right] **up to this one** [point to right-most face] **— it shows very much pain. Point to the face that shows how much you hurt** [right now]."

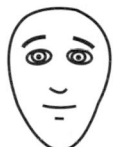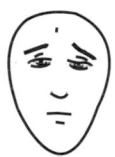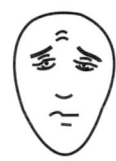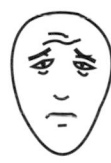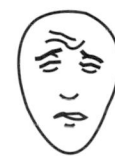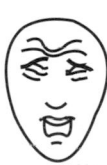

Score the chosen face 0, 2, 4, 6, 8, or 10, counting left to right, so '0' = 'no pain' and '10' = 'very much pain.'  Do not use words like 'happy' and 'sad.'  This scale is intended to measure how children feel inside, not how their face looks.
**Permission for use.** Copyright in the FPS-R is held by the International Association for the Study of Pain (IASP) © 2001.  This material may be photocopied for non-commercial clinical and research use. To request permission from IASP to reproduce the FPS-R in a publication, or for any commercial use, please e-mail **iaspdesk@iasp-pain.org**. For all other information regarding the FPS-R contact **Tiina.Jaaniste@sesiahs.health.nsw.gov.au** (Pain Medicine Unit, Sydney Children's Hospital, Randwick, NSW 2031, Australia).
**Sources.** Hicks, C. L., von Baeyer, C. L., Spafford, P. van Korlaar, I., Goodenough, B. The Faces Pain Scale—Revised: toward a common metric in pediatric pain measurement. *Pain, 93,* 173-183. Bieri, D., Reeve, R., Champion, G. D. et al. The Faces Pain Scale for the self-assessment of the severity of pain experienced by children: development, initial validation and preliminary investigation for ratio scale properties. *Pain, 41,* 139-150.

From Hicks, C. L., von Baeyer, C. L., Spafford, P. A., et al. (2001). The Faces Pain Scale—Revised: toward a common metric in pediatric pain measurement. *Pain, 93,* 173-183. © 2001, International Association for the Study of Pain (IASP).

**Brief Pain Inventory**

Date:___/___/___          Time: _____
Name:_____
        Last          First          Middle initial

1. Throughout our lives, most of us have had pain from time to time (such as minor headaches, sprains, and tooth-aches). Have you had pain other than these everyday kinds of pain today?
   1. Yes    2. No

2. On the diagram, shade in the areas where you feel pain. Put an X on the area that hurts the most.

Right          Left          Left          Right

3. Please rate your pain by circling the one number that best describes your pain at its **worst** in the past 24 hours.

   0   1   2   3   4   5   6   7   8   9   10
   No                              Pain as bad as
   pain                            you can imagine

4. Please rate your pain by circling the one number that best describes your pain at its **least** in the past 24 hours.

   0   1   2   3   4   5   6   7   8   9   10
   No                              Pain as bad as
   pain                            you can imagine

5. Please rate your pain by circling the one number that best describes your pain on the **average**.

   0   1   2   3   4   5   6   7   8   9   10
   No                              Pain as bad as
   pain                            you can imagine

6. Please rate your pain by circling the one number that tells how much pain you have **right now**.

   0   1   2   3   4   5   6   7   8   9   10
   No                              Pain as bad as
   pain                            you can imagine

7. What treatments or medications are you receiving for your pain?

   _____
   _____

8. In the past 24 hours, how much **relief** have pain treatments or medications provided? Please circle the one percentage that most shows how much relief you have received.

   0%  10  20  30  40  50  60  70  80  90  100%
   No                                    Complete
   relief                                relief

9. Circle the one number that describes how, during the past 24 hours, pain has **interfered** with your:
   A: General activity

   0   1   2   3   4   5   6   7   8   9   10
   Does not                        Completely
   interfere                       interferes

   B: Mood

   0   1   2   3   4   5   6   7   8   9   10
   Does not                        Completely
   interfere                       interferes

   C: Walking ability

   0   1   2   3   4   5   6   7   8   9   10
   Does not                        Completely
   interfere                       interferes

   D: Normal work (includes both work outside the home and housework)

   0   1   2   3   4   5   6   7   8   9   10
   Does not                        Completely
   interfere                       interferes

   E: Relations with other people

   0   1   2   3   4   5   6   7   8   9   10
   Does not                        Completely
   interfere                       interferes

   F: Sleep

   0   1   2   3   4   5   6   7   8   9   10
   Does not                        Completely
   interfere                       interferes

   G: Enjoyment of life

   0   1   2   3   4   5   6   7   8   9   10
   Does not                        Completely
   interfere                       interferes

(Copyright © Charles S. Cleeland, 1991.)

# Nutrition Assessment

## PURPOSE

This chapter helps you learn the components of nutritional assessment, including the assessment of dietary intake and nutritional status of individuals; identify the possible occurrence, nature, and extent of impaired nutritional status (ranging from undernutrition to overnutrition); and record the assessment accurately.

## READING ASSIGNMENT

Jarvis: *Physical Examination and Health Assessment*, 8th ed., Chapter 12, pp. 179-195.

Suggested reading:
Mangels, A. R. (2018). Malnutrition in older adults: An evidence-based review of risk factors, assessment, and intervention. *Am J Nurs, 118*(3): 34-42.

## GLOSSARY

Study the following terms after completing the reading assignment. You should be able to cover the definition on the right and define the term out loud.

**Android obesity** . . . . . . . . . . . . . excess body fat that is placed predominantly within the abdomen and upper body, as opposed to the hips and thighs

**Anthropometry** . . . . . . . . . . . . . measurement of the body (e.g., height, weight, circumferences, skinfold thickness)

**Body mass index** . . . . . . . . . . . weight in kilograms divided by height in meters squared (W/H$^2$); value of 30 or more is indicative of obesity; value of less than 18.5 is indicative of undernutrition.

**Diet history** . . . . . . . . . . . . . . . . a detailed record of dietary intake obtainable from 24-hour recalls, food frequency questionnaires, food diaries, and similar sources

**Kwashiorkor** . . . . . . . . . . . . . . . primarily a protein deficiency characterized by edema, growth failure, and muscle wasting

**Malnutrition** . . . . . . . . . . . . . . . may mean any nutrition disorder but usually refers to long-term nutritional inadequacies or excesses

**Marasmic kwashiorkor** . . . . . . . combination of chronic energy deficit and chronic or acute protein deficiency

**Marasmus** . . . . . . . . . . . . . . . . . results from energy and protein deficiency, manifesting with significant loss of body weight, skeletal muscle, and adipose tissue mass, but with serum protein concentrations relatively intact

**Nutritional monitoring** . . . . . . assessment of dietary or nutritional status at intermittent times with the aim of detecting changes in the dietary or nutritional status of a population

**Nutrition screening** . . . . . . . . . a process used to identify individuals at nutritional risk or with nutritional problems

**Obesity** . . . . . . . . . . . . . . . . . . . excessive accumulation of body fat; usually defined as 20% above desirable weight or body mass index of 30.0 to 39.9

**Protein-calorie
malnutrition (PCM)** . . . . . . . . inadequate consumption of protein and energy, resulting in a gradual body wasting and increased susceptibility to infection

**Recommended dietary
allowance (RDA)** . . . . . . . . . . . levels of intake of essential nutrients considered to be adequate to meet the nutritional needs of almost all healthy persons

**Sarcopenic obesity** . . . . . . . . . . combined loss of muscle mass with weight gain occurring in old age

**Skinfold thickness** . . . . . . . . . . double fold of skin and underlying subcutaneous tissue that is measured with skinfold calipers at various body sites

**Waist-to-hip ratio (WHR)** . . . . waist or abdominal circumference divided by the hip or gluteal circumference; method for assessing fat distribution

## STUDY GUIDE

After completing the reading assignment, you should be able to answer the following questions in the spaces provided.

1. Define optimal nutritional status.

2. Describe the unique nutritional needs for various developmental periods throughout the life cycle.

3. Describe the role that cultural heritage and values may play in an individual's nutritional intake.

4. Describe 4 sources of error that may occur when using the 24-hour diet recall.

5. Explain the clinical changes associated with each type of malnutrition:

Obesity _____

Marasmus _____

Kwashiorkor _____

Marasmus-kwashiorkor mix _____

## REVIEW QUESTIONS

This test is for you to check your own mastery of the content. Answers are provided in Appendix A.

1. The balance between nutrient intake and nutrient requirements is described as:

   a. Undernutrition.
   b. Malnutrition.
   c. Nutritional status.
   d. Overnutrition.

2. You are providing health promotion teaching for a newly pregnant woman and recommend which of the following weight gain parameters for a healthy pregnancy?

   a. 25 to 35 pounds
   b. 28 to 40 pounds
   c. 15 to 25 pounds
   d. The recommendation depends on the BMI of the mother at the start of the pregnancy.

3. Which is a normal expected change with aging?

   a. Increase in energy needs
   b. Increase in body water
   c. Decrease in height
   d. Increase in AP diameter of the chest

4. You obtain which data when screening patients for nutritional status?

   a. Temperature, pulse, and respiration
   b. Blood pressure and genogram
   c. Weight and nutrition intake history
   d. Serum creatinine levels

5. A 24-hour recall of dietary intake is used:

   a. As an anthropometric measure of calories consumed.
   b. As a questionnaire or interview of everything eaten within the last 24 hours.
   c. As the same as a food frequency questionnaire.
   d. As a form of food diary.

6. Mary, a 15-year-old, has come for a school physical. During the interview, you learn that menarche has not occurred. The BMI is 17. You suspect:

   a. Nutritional deficiency.
   b. Alcohol intake.
   c. Smoking history.
   d. Possible elevated blood sugar.

7. Which older adult is at lowest risk for alteration in nutritional status?

   a. 80-year-old widow who lives alone
   b. 65-year-old widower who visits a senior center with a meal program 5 days per week
   c. 70-year-old person with poor dentition who lives with a son
   d. 73-year-old couple with low income and no transportation

8. The examiner is completing an initial assessment for a patient admitted to a long-term care facility. The patient is unable to stand for a measurement of height. To obtain this important anthropometric information, the examiner would:

   a. Measure the waist-to-hip circumference.
   b. Estimate the body mass index.
   c. Measure arm span.
   d. Obtain a mid–upper arm muscle circumference to estimate skeletal muscle reserve.

9. Which assessment finding indicates a patient at nutrition risk?

   a. BMI = 24 kg/m$^2$
   b. Waist circumference at 43 inches
   c. Current weight = 200 lb
   d. BMI = 19 kg/m$^2$

10. Marasmus is often characterized by:

    a. Severely depleted visceral proteins.
    b. Elevated triglycerides.
    c. Hyperglycemia.
    d. Low weight for height.

11. Which BMI category in adults is indicative of obesity?

    a. 18.5 to 24.9 kg/m$^2$
    b. 25.0 to 29.9 kg/m$^2$
    c. 30.0 to 39.9 kg/m$^2$
    d. <18.5 kg/m$^2$

12. Why should you ask about the use of medications when assessing a patient's nutritional status?

    a. Medication allergies are on the rise and are a major health concern.
    b. Many drugs can interact with nutrients and impair their digestion, absorption, metabolism, or uptake.
    c. Patients readily discuss their daily use of vitamin and mineral supplements when asked.
    d. The use of anabolic steroids can reduce muscle size and physical performance.

# SKILLS LABORATORY AND CLINICAL SETTING

The purpose of the clinical component is to practice the steps of the assessment on a peer in the skills laboratory and to achieve the following:

## Clinical Objectives

1. Identify persons at risk for developing malnutrition.

2. Develop an appreciation for cultural influences on nutritional status.

3. Use anthropometric measures and laboratory data to assess the nutritional status of an individual.

4. Use nutritional assessment in the provision of health care.

5. Record the assessment findings accurately.

## Instructions

1. Gather nutritional assessment forms and anthropometric equipment. Practice the steps of the *Malnutrition Screening Tool* on a peer in the skills laboratory.
2. Review the questions in the *Mini Nutritional Assessment* with an aging adult. Persons identified as being at risk (MNA score 0-11 points) should undergo a more comprehensive assessment.

---

### MALNUTRITION SCREENING TOOL (MST)

Have you lost weight recently without trying?
| | |
|---|---|
| No | 0 |
| Unsure | 2 |

If yes, how much weight (kilograms) have you lost?
| | |
|---|---|
| 1-5 | 1 |
| 6-10 | 2 |
| 11-15 | 3 |
| >15 | 4 |
| Unsure | 2 |

Have you been eating poorly because of a decreased appetite?
| | |
|---|---|
| No | 0 |
| Yes | 1 |
| Total | |

Score of 2 or more = patient at risk for malnutrition

---

# Mini Nutritional Assessment
## MNA®

**Nestlé**
**NutritionInstitute**

| Last name: | | First name: | | |
|---|---|---|---|---|
| Sex: | Age: | Weight, kg: | Height, cm: | Date: |

Complete the screen by filling in the boxes with the appropriate numbers. Total the numbers for the final screening score.

## Screening

**A  Has food intake declined over the past 3 months due to loss of appetite, digestive problems, chewing or swallowing difficulties?**
0 = severe decrease in food intake
1 = moderate decrease in food intake
2 = no decrease in food intake ☐

**B  Weight loss during the last 3 months**
0 = weight loss greater than 3 kg (6.6 lbs)
1 = does not know
2 = weight loss between 1 and 3 kg (2.2 and 6.6 lbs)
3 = no weight loss ☐

**C  Mobility**
0 = bed or chair bound
1 = able to get out of bed / chair but does not go out
2 = goes out ☐

**D  Has suffered psychological stress or acute disease in the past 3 months?**
0 = yes          2 = no ☐

**E  Neuropsychological problems**
0 = severe dementia or depression
1 = mild dementia
2 = no psychological problems ☐

**F1 Body Mass Index (BMI) (weight in kg) / (height in m)$^2$**
0 = BMI less than 19
1 = BMI 19 to less than 21
2 = BMI 21 to less than 23
3 = BMI 23 or greater ☐

IF BMI IS NOT AVAILABLE, REPLACE QUESTION F1 WITH QUESTION F2.
DO NOT ANSWER QUESTION F2 IF QUESTION F1 IS ALREADY COMPLETED.

**F2 Calf circumference (CC) in cm**
0 = CC less than 31
3 = CC 31 or greater ☐

## Screening score (max. 14 points)

**12 - 14 points:** Normal nutritional status
**8 - 11 points:** At risk of malnutrition
**0 - 7 points:** Malnourished ☐☐

**References**
1. Vellas B, Villars H, Abellan G, *et al.* Overview of the MNA® - Its History and Challenges. *J Nutr Health Aging.* 2006;**10**:456-465.
2. Rubenstein LZ, Harker JO, Salva A, Guigoz Y, Vellas B. Screening for Undernutrition in Geriatric Practice: Developing the Short-Form Mini Nutritional Assessment (MNA-SF). *J. Geront.* 2001; **56A**: M366-377
3. Guigoz Y. The Mini-Nutritional Assessment (MNA®) Review of the Literature - What does it tell us? *J Nutr Health Aging.* 2006; **10**:466-487.
4. Kaiser MJ, Bauer JM, Ramsch C, et al.  Validation of the Mini Nutritional Assessment Short-Form (MNA®-SF): A practical tool for identification of nutritional status.  *J Nutr Health Aging.* 2009; **13**:782-788.
® Société des Produits Nestlé, S.A., Vevey, Switzerland, Trademark Owners © Nestlé, 1994, Revision 2009. N67200 12/99 10M
**For more information: www.mna-elderly.com**

# CHAPTER 13

# Skin, Hair, and Nails

## PURPOSE

This chapter helps you learn the structure and function of the skin and its appendages, understand the rationale for and the methods of inspection and palpation of the skin, and record the assessment accurately.

## READING ASSIGNMENT

Jarvis: *Physical Examination and Health Assessment*, 8th ed., Chapter 13, pp. 197-244.

Suggested readings:

Baranoski, S., LeBlanc, K., & Glockner, M. (2016). Preventing, assessing, and managing skin tears. *Am J Nurs, 116*(11), 24-31.

Kirkland-Kyhn, H., Zaratkicwicz, S., Teleten, O., et al. (2018). Caring for aging skin. *Am J Nurs, 118*(2), 60-63.

## GLOSSARY

Study the following terms after completing the reading assignment. You should be able to cover the definition on the right and define the term out loud.

**Alopecia** . . . . . . . . . . . . . . . . . . baldness; hair loss

**Annular** . . . . . . . . . . . . . . . . . . circular shape to skin lesion

**Bulla** . . . . . . . . . . . . . . . . . . elevated cavity containing free fluid larger than 1 cm in diameter

**Confluent** . . . . . . . . . . . . . . . . skin lesions that run together

**Crust** . . . . . . . . . . . . . . . . . . thick, dried-out exudate left on skin when vesicles or pustules burst or dry up

**Cyanosis** . . . . . . . . . . . . . . . . . . dusky blue color to skin or mucous membranes as a result of increased amount of nonoxygenated hemoglobin

**Erosion** . . . . . . . . . . . . . . . . . . scooped-out, shallow depression in skin

**Erythema** . . . . . . . . . . . . . . . . intense redness of the skin due to excess blood in dilated superficial capillaries, as in fever or inflammation

**Excoriation** . . . . . . . . . . . . . . . . . self-inflicted abrasion on skin due to scratching

**Fissure** . . . . . . . . . . . . . . . . . . . . linear crack in skin extending into dermis

**Furuncle** . . . . . . . . . . . . . . . . . . boil; suppurative inflammatory skin lesion due to infected hair follicle

**Hemangioma** . . . . . . . . . . . . . . skin lesion due to benign proliferation of blood vessels in the dermis

**Iris** . . . . . . . . . . . . . . . . . . . . . . target shape of skin lesion

**Jaundice** . . . . . . . . . . . . . . . . . . yellow color to skin, palate, and sclera due to excess bilirubin in the blood

**Keloid** . . . . . . . . . . . . . . . . . . . . hypertrophic scar, elevated beyond site of original injury

**Lichenification** . . . . . . . . . . . . . tightly packed set of papules that thickens skin; caused by prolonged intense scratching

**Lipoma** . . . . . . . . . . . . . . . . . . . benign fatty tumor

**Maceration** . . . . . . . . . . . . . . . . softening of tissue by soaking

**Macule** . . . . . . . . . . . . . . . . . . . flat skin lesion with only a color change

**Nevus** . . . . . . . . . . . . . . . . . . . . mole; circumscribed skin lesion due to excess melanocytes

**Nodule** . . . . . . . . . . . . . . . . . . . elevated skin lesion larger than 1 cm in diameter

**Pallor** . . . . . . . . . . . . . . . . . . . . excessively pale, whitish-pink color to lightly pigmented skin

**Papule** . . . . . . . . . . . . . . . . . . . palpable skin lesion smaller than 1 cm in diameter

**Plaque** . . . . . . . . . . . . . . . . . . . skin lesion in which papules coalesce or come together

**Pruritus** . . . . . . . . . . . . . . . . . . itching

**Purpura** . . . . . . . . . . . . . . . . . . red-purple skin lesion due to blood in tissues from breaks in blood vessels

**Pustule** . . . . . . . . . . . . . . . . . . . elevated cavity containing thick, turbid fluid

**Scale** . . . . . . . . . . . . . . . . . . . . . compact desiccated flakes of skin from shedding of dead skin cells

**Telangiectasia** . . . . . . . . . . . . . skin lesion due to permanently enlarged and dilated blood vessels that are visible

**Ulcer** . . . . . . . . . . . . . . . . . . . . . sloughing of necrotic inflammatory tissue that causes a deep depression in skin, extending into dermis

**Vesicle** . . . . . . . . . . . . . . . . . . . elevated cavity containing free fluid up to 1 cm in diameter

**Wheal** . . . . . . . . . . . . . . . . . . . . raised red skin lesion due to interstitial fluid

**Zosteriform** . . . . . . . . . . . . . . . linear shape of skin lesion along a nerve route

## STUDY GUIDE

After completing the reading assignment, you should be able to answer the following questions in the spaces provided.

1. List the 3 layers associated with the skin, and describe the contents of each layer.

2. Differentiate among sebaceous, eccrine, and apocrine glands.

3. List at least 5 functions of the skin.

4. Describe the appearance of pallor, erythema, cyanosis, and jaundice in both light-skinned and dark-skinned persons. State common causes of each.

5. List causes of changes in skin temperature, texture, moisture, mobility, and turgor.

6. The white linear markings that normally are visible through the nail and on the pink nail bed are termed _____ _____.

7. Describe the following findings that are common variations on the infant's skin:

   Mongolian spot _____

   Café au lait spot _____

   Erythema toxicum _____

   Cutis marmorata _____

   Physiologic jaundice _____

   Milia _____

8. Describe the following findings that are common variations on the aging adult's skin:

   Lentigines _____

   Seborrheic keratosis _____

   Actinic keratosis _____

   Acrochordons (skin tags) _____

   Sebaceous hyperplasia _____

9. Differentiate among these purpuric lesions: petechiae, bruise, hematoma.

10. Differentiate among the appearance of the skin rash of these childhood illnesses: measles (rubeola), German measles (rubella), chickenpox (varicella).

11. List and describe the 4 stages of pressure injury development.

12. Define and give an example of the following primary skin lesions: macule, papule, plaque, nodule, tumor, wheal, vesicle, pustule.

13. Define and give an example of these secondary lesions: crust, scale, fissure, erosion, ulcer.

Fill in the labels indicated on the following illustrations:

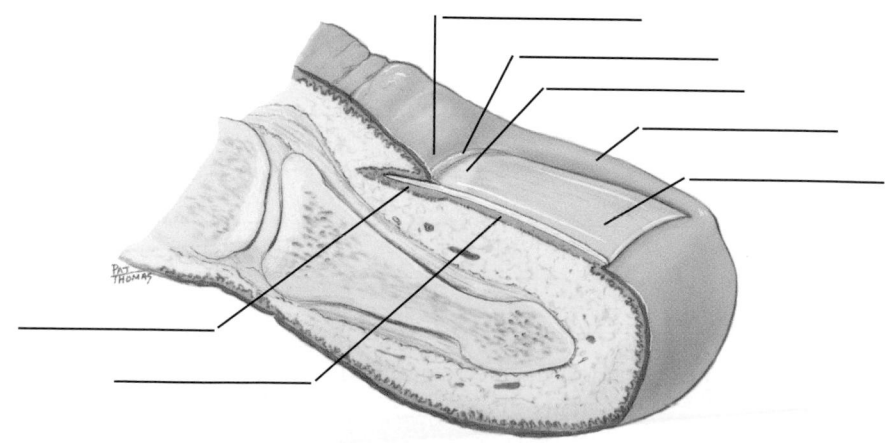

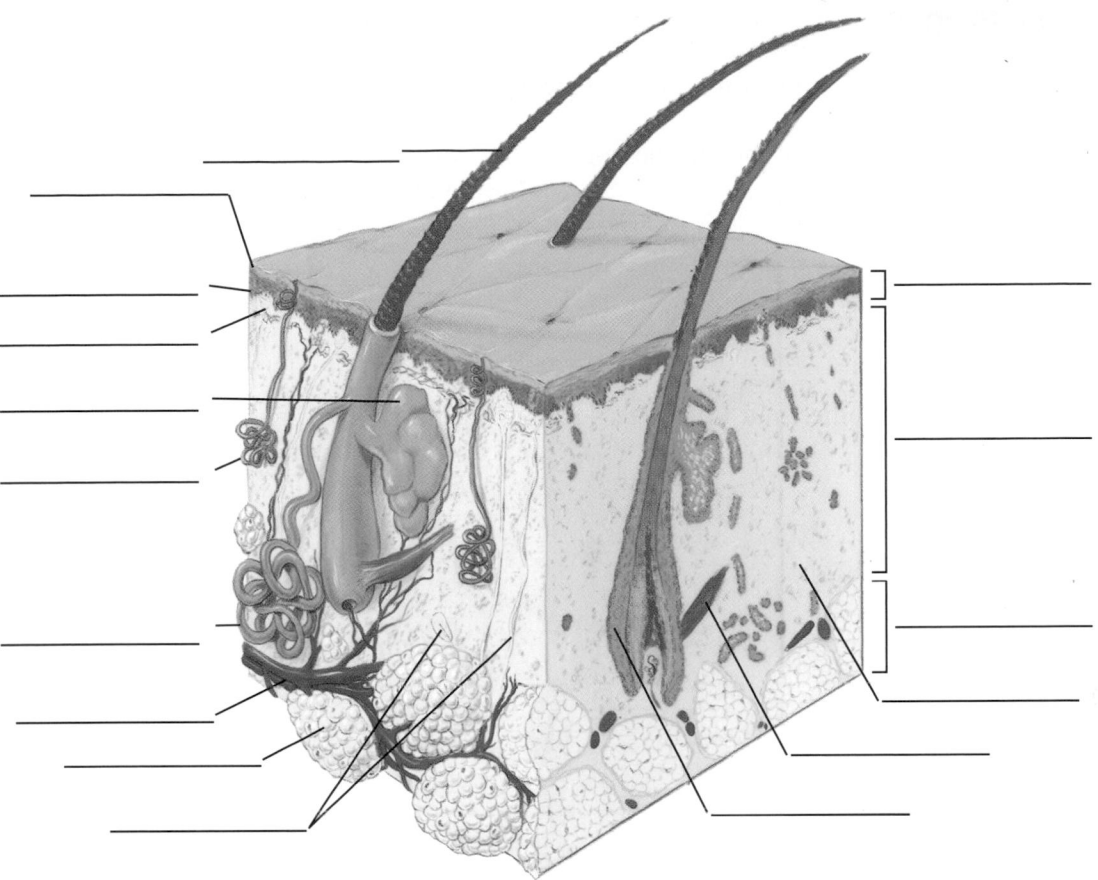

# REVIEW QUESTIONS

This test is for you to check your own mastery of the content. Answers are provided in Appendix A.

1. Select the best description of the secretion of the eccrine glands.

   a. Thick, milky
   b. Dilute saline solution
   c. Protective lipid substance
   d. Keratin

2. To assess for early jaundice, you will assess:

   a. Sclera and hard palate.
   b. Nail beds.
   c. Lips.
   d. All visible skin surfaces.

3. Checking for skin temperature is best accomplished by using:

   a. The palmar surface of the hands.
   b. The ventral surface of the hands.
   c. The fingertips.
   d. The dorsal surface of the hands.

4. Assessing a patient's skin turgor is done to assess which clinical finding?

   a. Edema
   b. Dehydration
   c. Vitiligo
   d. Scleroderma

5. You note a lesion during a skin assessment. Which is the best way to document this finding?

   a. Raised, irregular lesion the size of a quarter, located on dorsum of left hand
   b. Open lesion with no drainage or odor, approximately ¼ inch in diameter
   c. Pedunculated lesion below left scapula with consistent red color and no drainage or odor
   d. Dark brown raised lesion, with irregular border, on dorsum of right foot, 3 cm in size, with no drainage

6. You examine the nail beds of a patient. Which finding indicates a normal angle?

   a. 60 degrees
   b. 100 degrees
   c. 160 degrees
   d. 180 degrees

7. You are assessing capillary refill. The room is warm. Which finding would be considered normal?

   a. ≤1 second
   b. >2 seconds
   c. 2 to 3 seconds
   d. Time is not significant as long as color returns.

8. During a routine visit, M.B., age 78, asks about small, round, flat, brown macules on the hands. What is your best response after assessing the areas?

   a. "These are the result of sun exposure and do not require treatment."
   b. "These are related to exposure to the sun. They may become cancerous."
   c. "These are the skin tags that occur with aging. No treatment is required."
   d. "I'm glad you brought this to my attention. I will arrange for a biopsy."

9. An area of thin shiny skin with decreased visibility of normal skin markings is most likely:

   a. Lichenification.
   b. Plaque.
   c. Atrophy.
   d. Keloid.

10. Flattening of the angle between the nail and its base is:

    a. Found in subacute bacterial endocarditis.
    b. A description of spoon-shaped nails.
    c. Related to calcium deficiency.
    d. Described as clubbing.

11. A configuration of individual lesions arranged in circles or arcs, as occurs with ringworm, is described as a:

    a. Linear lesion.
    b. Clustered lesion.
    c. Annular lesion.
    d. Gyrate lesion.

12. The "A" in the ABCDEF rule for skin cancer stands for:

    a. Accuracy.
    b. Appearance.
    c. Asymmetry.
    d. Attenuated.

13. A risk factor for melanoma is:

    a. Brown eyes
    b. Darkly pigmented skin
    c. Skin that freckles or burns before tanning
    d. Use of sunscreen products

14. Herpes zoster infection (shingles) is characterized by:

    a. A bacterial cause
    b. Lesion on only one side of body; does not cross midline
    c. Absence of pain or edema
    d. Pustular, umbilicated lesions

Match column A to column B; items in column B may be used more than once.

**Column A: Descriptor**

15. _____ Basal cell layer
16. _____ Aids protection by cushioning
17. _____ Collagen
18. _____ Adipose tissue
19. _____ Uniformly thin
20. _____ Stratum corneum
21. _____ Elastic tissue

**Column B: Skin Layer**

a. Epidermis
b. Dermis
c. Subcutaneous layer

**Column A: Descriptor**

22. _____ Pallor
23. _____ Erythema
24. _____ Cyanosis
25. _____ Jaundice

**Column B: Color Change**

a. Intense redness of the skin due to excess blood in the dilated superficial capillaries
b. Bluish mottled color that signifies decreased perfusion
c. Absence of red-pink tones from the oxygenated hemoglobin in blood
d. Increase in bilirubin in the blood causing a yellow color in the skin

**Column A: Descriptor**

26. _____ Tiny, punctate red macules and papules on the cheeks, trunk, chest, back, and buttocks

27. _____ Lower half of body turns red, upper half blanches

28. _____ Transient mottling on trunk and extremities

29. _____ Bluish color around the lips, hands, fingernails, feet, and toenails

30. _____ Large round or oval patch of light brown usually present at birth

31. _____ Yellowing of skin, sclera, and mucous membranes due to increased numbers of red blood cells hemolyzed after birth

32. _____ Yellow-orange color in light-skinned persons from large amounts of foods containing carotene

**Column B: Skin Color Change**

a. Harlequin
b. Erythema toxicum
c. Acrocyanosis
d. Physiologic jaundice
e. Carotenemia
f. Café au lait spot
g. Cutis marmorata

## SKILLS LABORATORY AND CLINICAL SETTING

Usually the clinical examination of the integumentary system is performed along with the examination of each particular body region. The purpose of practicing the steps of this examination separately is so that you begin to think of the skin and its appendages as a separate organ system and so that you learn the components of skin examination.

### Clinical Objectives

1. Inspect and palpate the skin, noting its color, vascularity, edema, moisture, temperature, texture, thickness, mobility, turgor, and any lesions.

2. Inspect the fingernails, noting color, shape, and any lesions.

3. Inspect the hair, noting texture, distribution, and any lesions.

4. Record the history and physical examination findings accurately, reach an assessment of the health state, and develop a plan of care.

### Instructions

Prepare the examination setting. Wash your hands. Practice the steps of the examination on a peer in the skills laboratory, giving appropriate instructions as you proceed. Choosing a peer from an ethnic background other than your own will further heighten your recognition of the range of normal skin tones. Record your findings using the regional write-up sheet that follows. The front of the page is intended as a worksheet; the back of the page is intended for your narrative summary recording using the SOAP format.

   Note the student performance checklist that follows the regional write-up sheet. It lists the essential behaviors that you should display as an examiner, and it may be used by your clinical instructor to evaluate your clinical teaching of the skin self-examination.

# REGIONAL WRITE-UP—SKIN, HAIR, AND NAILS

Date _____

Examiner _____

Patient _____ Age _____ Gender _____

Reason for visit _____

## I. Health History

| | No | Yes, explain |
|---|---|---|
| 1. Any past skin disease? | _____ | _____ |
| 2. Any change in skin color or pigmentation? | _____ | _____ |
| 3. Any changes in a mole? | _____ | _____ |
| 4. Excessive dryness or moisture? | _____ | _____ |
| 5. Any skin itching? | _____ | _____ |
| 6. Any excess bruising? | _____ | _____ |
| 7. Any skin rash or lesions? | _____ | _____ |
| 8. Taking any medications? | _____ | _____ |
| 9. Any recent hair loss? | _____ | _____ |
| 10. Any change in nails? | _____ | _____ |
| 11. Any environmental hazards for skin? | _____ | _____ |
| 12. How do you take care of skin? Sunscreen? | _____ | _____ |
| 13. What is your amount of sun exposure? Indoor tanning? | _____ | _____ |

## II. Physical Examination

### A. Inspect and palpate skin.

Color_____

Pigmentation_____

Temperature_____

Moisture_____ Texture _____

Thickness_____ Any edema _____

Mobility and turgor _____

Vascularity and bruising _____

Any lesions (describe)_____

### B. Inspect and palpate hair.

Color_____

Texture_____Distribution_____

Any lesions (describe) _____

### C. Inspect and palpate nails.

Shape and contour _____

Consistency_____Distribution_____

Color_____

Capillary refill _____

### D. Teach skin self-examination.

## REGIONAL WRITE-UP—SKIN, HAIR, AND NAILS

Summarize your findings using the SOAP format.

**Subjective** (reason for seeking care, health history)

**Objective** (physical examination findings)

Record distribution of any rash or lesions below.

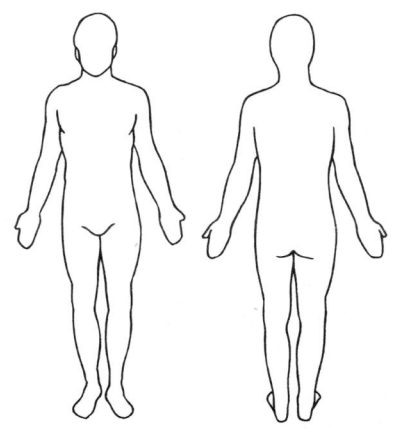

**Assessment** (assessment of problem, diagnosis)

**Plan** (diagnostic evaluation, follow-up care, teaching)

# STUDENT COMPETENCY CHECKLIST

Teaching Skin Self-Examination (SSE)

| | S | U | Comments |
|---|---|---|---|
| I. Cognitive | | | |
|   A. Explain: | | | |
|     1. why skin is examined. | | | |
|     2. who should perform skin self-examination. | | | |
|     3. frequency of skin examination. | | | |
|   B. Define the ABCDEF rule. | | | |
|   C. Describe any equipment the patient may need. | | | |
| II. Performance | | | |
|   A. Explain to patient the need for SSE. | | | |
|   B. Instruct patient on technique of SSE by: | | | |
|     1. demonstrating the order and body positioning for inspecting skin. | | | |
|     2. describing normal skin characteristics. | | | |
|     3. describing abnormal findings to look for. | | | |
|   C. Instruct patient to report unusual findings to provider. | | | |

# NOTES

# Head, Face, Neck, and Regional Lymphatics

## PURPOSE

This chapter helps you learn the location and function of structures in the head and neck, learn to perform inspection and palpation of the head and neck, and record the assessment accurately.

## READING ASSIGNMENT

Jarvis: *Physical Examination and Health Assessment*, 8th ed., Chapter 14, pp. 245-274.

Suggested readings:
Moriarty, M., & Mallick-Searle, T. (2016). Diagnosis and treatment for chronic migraine. *Nurse Pract, 41*(6), 18-32.

## GLOSSARY

Study the following terms after completing the reading assignment. You should be able to cover the definition on the right and define the term out loud.

**Bruit** . . . . . . . . . . . . . . . . . . . . . . blowing, swooshing sound heard through the stethoscope over an area of abnormal blood flow

**Dysphagia** . . . . . . . . . . . . . . . . . . difficulty in swallowing

**Goiter** . . . . . . . . . . . . . . . . . . . . . increase in size of thyroid gland that occurs with hyperthyroidism

**Lymphadenopathy** . . . . . . . . . . enlargement of the lymph nodes due to infection, allergy, or neoplasm

**Macrocephalic** . . . . . . . . . . . . . refers to abnormally large head

**Microcephalic** . . . . . . . . . . . . . . refers to abnormally small head

**Normocephalic** . . . . . . . . . . . . . refers to round symmetric skull that is appropriately related to body size

**Torticollis** . . . . . . . . . . . . . . . . . head tilt due to shortening or spasm of one sternomastoid muscle

**Vertigo** . . . . . . . . . . . . . . . . . . . . illusory sensation of either the room or one's own body spinning; not the same as dizziness

## STUDY GUIDE

After completing the reading assignment and the media assignment, write or draw the answers in the spaces provided.

1. The major neck muscles are the _____.

2. Name the borders of two regions in the neck—the anterior triangle and the posterior triangle.

3. List the facial structures that should appear symmetric when inspecting the head.

4. Describe the characteristics of lymph nodes often associated with:

   Acute infection _____

   Chronic inflammation _____

   Cancer _____

5. Differentiate *caput succedaneum* from *cephalhematoma* in the newborn infant.

6. Describe the tonic neck reflex in the infant.

7. Describe the characteristics of normal cervical lymph nodes during childhood.

8. List the condition(s) associated with parotid gland enlargement.

9. Describe the facial characteristics that occur with Down syndrome.

10. Contrast the facial characteristics of hyperthyroidism versus hypothyroidism.

Fill in the labels indicated on the following illustrations.

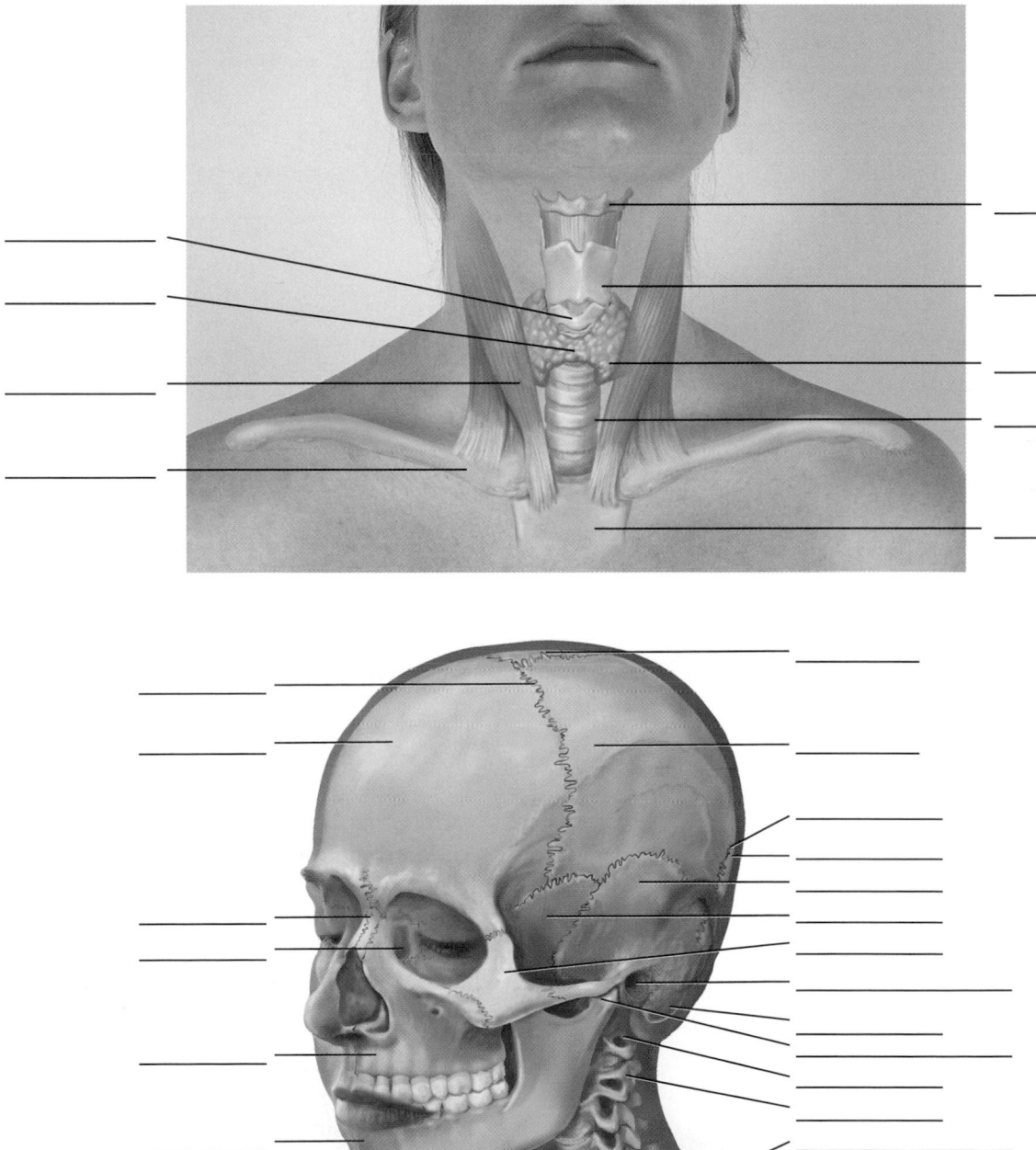

© Pat Thomas, 2018

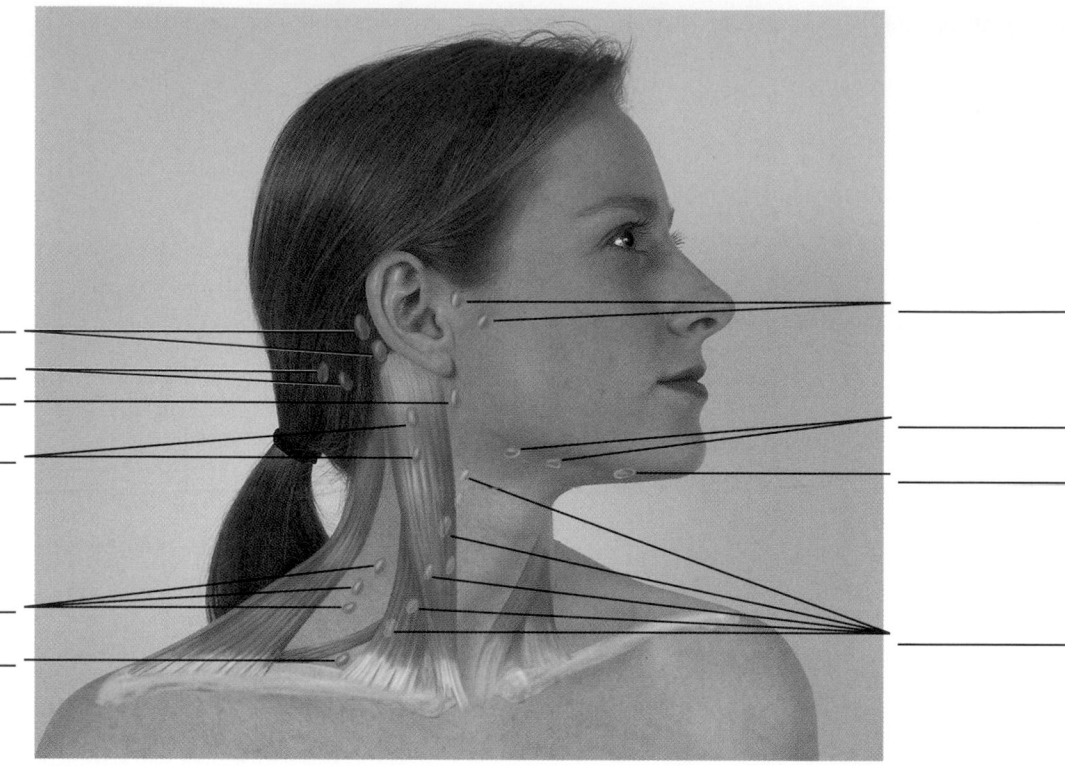

## REVIEW QUESTIONS

This test is for you to check your own mastery of the content. Answers are provided in Appendix A.

1. Which facial bones articulate at a joint instead of a suture?

   a. Zygomatic
   b. Maxilla
   c. Nasal
   d. Mandible

2. Identify the blood vessel that runs diagonally across the sternomastoid muscle.

   a. Temporal artery
   b. Carotid artery
   c. External jugular vein
   d. Internal jugular vein

3. The isthmus of the thyroid gland lies just below the:

   a. Mandible.
   b. Cricoid cartilage.
   c. Hyoid cartilage.
   d. Thyroid cartilage.

4. Which is true regarding cluster headaches?

   a. They may be precipitated by alcohol and daytime napping.
   b. Their usual occurrence is two per month, each lasting 1 to 3 days.
   c. They are characterized as throbbing.
   d. They tend to be supraorbital, retro-orbital, or frontotemporal.

5. Which is least likely to indicate a possible malignancy?

   a. History of radiation therapy to the head, neck, or upper chest
   b. History of using chewing tobacco
   c. History of large alcohol consumption
   d. Marked tenderness

6. Providing resistance while the patient shrugs his or her shoulders is a test of which cranial nerve?

   a. II
   b. V
   c. IX
   d. XI

7. On examination, the newborn's fontanels should feel:

   a. Tense or bulging.
   b. Depressed or sunken.
   c. Firm, slightly concave, and well defined.
   d. Pulsating.

8. If the thyroid gland were enlarged bilaterally, which maneuver would be appropriate for you to assess?

   a. Check for deviation of the trachea.
   b. Listen for a bruit over the carotid arteries.
   c. Listen for a murmur over the aortic area.
   d. Listen for a bruit over the thyroid lobes.

9. It is normal to palpate a few lymph nodes in the neck of a healthy person. What are the characteristics of these nodes?

   a. Mobile, soft, nontender
   b. Large, clumped, tender
   c. Matted, fixed, tender, hard
   d. Matted, fixed, nontender

10. Cephalhematoma is associated with:

    a. Subperiosteal hemorrhage.
    b. Increased intracranial pressure.
    c. Down syndrome.
    d. Cerebral palsy.

11. Normal cervical notes are:

    a. Smaller than 1 cm.
    b. Warm to palpation.
    c. Fixed.
    d. Firm.

12. A throbbing, unilateral pain associated with nausea, vomiting, and photophobia is characteristic of:

    a. Cluster headache.
    b. Subarachnoid hemorrhage.
    c. Migraine headache.
    d. Tension headache.

13. Bell palsy is characterized by:

    a. Unilateral paralysis of complete half of the face.
    b. Bulging eyeballs.
    c. A face that appears masklike.
    d. A puffy, edematous face.

14. You suspect an infant's head is of abnormal size and can use which procedure to verify these findings?

    a. Palpation
    b. Measuring tape
    c. Observing for symmetry of facial features
    d. Noting absence of the tonic neck reflex

Match column A to column B.

**Column A: Lymph Nodes**

15. _____ Preauricular
16. _____ Posterior auricular
17. _____ Occipital
18. _____ Submental
19. _____ Submandibular
20. _____ Jugulodigastric
21. _____ Superficial cervical
22. _____ Deep cervical
23. _____ Posterior cervical
24. _____ Supraclavicular

**Column B: Location**

a. Above and behind the clavicle
b. Deep under the sternomastoid muscle
c. In front of the ear
d. In the posterior triangle along the edge of the trapezius muscle
e. Superficial to the mastoid process
f. At the base of the skull
g. Halfway between the angle and the tip of the mandible
h. Behind the tip of the mandible
i. Under the angle of the mandible
j. Overlying the sternomastoid muscle

## SKILLS LABORATORY AND CLINICAL SETTINGS

The purpose of the clinical component is to practice the steps of the head, face, and neck examination on a peer in the skills laboratory and to achieve the following objectives.

### Clinical Objectives

1. Collect a health history related to pertinent signs and symptoms of the head and neck.
2. Inspect and palpate the skull, noting size, contour, lumps, or tenderness.
3. Inspect the face, noting facial expression, symmetry, skin characteristics, or lesions.
4. Inspect and palpate the neck for symmetry, range of motion, and integrity of lymph nodes, trachea, and thyroid gland.
5. Record the findings systematically, reach an assessment of the health state, and develop a plan of care.

### Instructions

Prepare the examination setting. Wash your hands. Practice the steps of the examination on a peer in the skills laboratory, giving appropriate instructions as you proceed. Record your findings using the regional write-up sheet that follows. The front of the page is intended as a worksheet; the back of the page is intended for your narrative summary recording using the SOAP format.

# REGIONAL WRITE-UP—HEAD, FACE, AND NECK

Date _____

Examiner _____

Patient _____     Age _____ Gender _____

Reason for visit _____

## I. Health History

| | No | Yes, explain |
|---|---|---|
| 1. Any unusually frequent or severe **headaches**? | _____ | |
| 2. Any **head injury**? | _____ | |
| 3. Experienced any **dizziness**? | _____ | |
| 4. Any neck **pain**? | _____ | |
| 5. Any **lumps** or **swelling** in head or neck? | _____ | |
| 6. Any surgery on head or neck? | _____ | |

## II. Physical Examination

### A. Inspect and palpate the skull.

General size and contour _____

Deformities, lumps, tenderness _____

Temporal artery _____

Temporomandibular joint _____

### B. Inspect the face.

Facial expression _____

Symmetry of structures _____

Involuntary movements _____

Edema _____

Masses or lesions _____

Color and texture of skin _____

### C. Inspect the neck.

Symmetry _____

Range of motion, active _____

Test strength of cervical muscles. _____

Abnormal pulsations _____

Enlargement of thyroid _____

Enlargement of lymph and salivary glands _____

### D. Palpate the lymph nodes.

Exact location _____

Size and shape _____

Presence or absence of tenderness _____

Freely movable, adherent to deeper structures, or matted together _____

Presence of surrounding inflammation _____

Texture (hard, soft, firm) _____

### E. Palpate the trachea. _____

### F. Palpate the thyroid gland. _____

### G. Auscultate the thyroid gland (if enlarged). _____

## REGIONAL WRITE-UP—HEAD, FACE, AND NECK

Summarize your findings using the SOAP format.

**Subjective** (reason for seeking care, health history)

**Objective** (physical examination findings)

**Assessment** (assessment of health state or problem, diagnosis)

**Plan** (diagnostic evaluation, follow-up care, patient teaching)

## PURPOSE

This chapter helps you learn the structure and function of the external and internal components of the eyes, learn the methods of examination of vision, external eye, and ocular fundus, and record the assessment accurately.

## READING ASSIGNMENT

Jarvis: *Physical Examination and Health Assessment,* 8th ed., Chapter 15, pp. 275-316.

Suggested readings:
Ossorio, A. (2015). Red eye emergencies in primary care. *Nurse Pract, 40*(12), 47-53.

## GLOSSARY

Study the following terms after completing the reading assignment. You should be able to cover the definition on the right and define the term out loud.

**Accommodation** . . . . . . . . . . . . adaptation of the eye for near vision by increasing the curvature of the lens

**Anisocoria** . . . . . . . . . . . . . . . . . unequal pupil size

**Arcus senilis** . . . . . . . . . . . . . . . gray-white arc or circle around the limbus of the iris that is common with aging

**Argyll Robertson pupil** . . . . . . . pupil does not react to light; does constrict with accommodation

**Astigmatism** . . . . . . . . . . . . . . . . refractive error of vision due to differences in curvature in refractive surfaces of the eye (cornea and lens)

**A-V crossing** . . . . . . . . . . . . . . . . crossing paths of an artery and vein in the ocular fundus

**Bitemporal hemianopsia** . . . . . loss of both temporal visual fields

**Blepharitis** . . . . . . . . . . . . . . . . . inflammation of the glands and eyelash follicles along the margin of the eyelids

**Cataract** . . . . . . . . . . . . . . . . . . . opacity of the lens of the eye that develops slowly with aging and gradually obstructs vision

**Chalazion** . . . . . . . . . . . . . . . . . infection or retention cyst of a meibomian gland, showing as a beady nodule on the eyelid

**Conjunctivitis**. . . . . . . . . . . . . . infection of the conjunctiva, "pinkeye"

**Cotton wool area** . . . . . . . . . . . abnormal soft exudates visible as gray-white areas on the ocular fundus

**Cup-to-disc ratio** . . . . . . . . . . . ratio of the width of the physiologic cup to the width of the optic disc, normally half or less

**Diopter** . . . . . . . . . . . . . . . . . . . unit of strength of the lens settings on the ophthalmoscope that changes focus on the eye structures

**Diplopia**. . . . . . . . . . . . . . . . . . double vision

**Drusen** . . . . . . . . . . . . . . . . . . . benign deposits on the ocular fundus that show as round yellow dots and occur commonly with aging

**Ectropion**. . . . . . . . . . . . . . . . . lower eyelid loose and rolling outward

**Entropion** . . . . . . . . . . . . . . . . lower eyelid rolling inward

**Exophthalmos** . . . . . . . . . . . . . protruding eyeballs

**Fovea** . . . . . . . . . . . . . . . . . . . . area of keenest vision at the center of the macula on the ocular fundus

**Glaucoma** . . . . . . . . . . . . . . . . . a group of eye diseases characterized by increased intraocular pressure

**Hordeolum** . . . . . . . . . . . . . . . . (stye) red, painful pustule that is a localized infection of hair follicle at eyelid margin

**Lid lag** . . . . . . . . . . . . . . . . . . . abnormal white rim of sclera visible between the upper eyelid and the iris when a person moves the eyes downward

**Macula** . . . . . . . . . . . . . . . . . . . round darker area of the ocular fundus that mediates vision only from the central visual field

**Microaneurysm** . . . . . . . . . . . . abnormal finding of round red dots on the ocular fundus that are localized dilations of small vessels

**Miosis**. . . . . . . . . . . . . . . . . . . . constricted pupils

**Mydriasis**. . . . . . . . . . . . . . . . . dilated pupils

**Myopia**. . . . . . . . . . . . . . . . . . . nearsighted; refractive error in which near vision is better than far vision

**Nystagmus**. . . . . . . . . . . . . . . . involuntary, rapid, rhythmic movement of the eyeball

**Optic atrophy** . . . . . . . . . . . . . pallor of the optic disc due to partial or complete death of optic nerve

**Optic disc** . . . . . . . . . . . . . . . . area of ocular fundus in which blood vessels exit and enter

**Papilledema** . . . . . . . . . . . . . . . stasis of blood flow out of the ocular fundus; sign of increased intracranial pressure

**Presbyopia**. . . . . . . . . . . . . . . . decrease in power of accommodation that occurs with aging

**Pterygium** . . . . . . . . . . . . . . . . triangular opaque tissue on the nasal side of the conjunctiva that grows toward the center of the cornea

**Ptosis** . . . . . . . . . . . . . . . . . . . drooping of upper eyelid over the iris and possibly covering the pupil

**Red reflex** . . . . . . . . . . . . . . . . red glow that appears to fill the person's pupil when first visualized through the ophthalmoscope

**Strabismus** . . . . . . . . . . . . . . . (squint, crossed eye) disparity of the eye axes

**Xanthelasma**. . . . . . . . . . . . . . soft, raised yellow plaques occurring on the skin at the inner corners of the eyes

# STUDY GUIDE

After completing the reading assignment and the media assignment, write or draw the answers in the spaces provided.

1. Name the 6 sets of extraocular muscles and the cranial nerve that innervates each one.

2. Name and describe the 3 concentric coats of the eyeball.

3. Name the functions of the ciliary body, the pupil, and the iris.

4. Describe the anterior chamber, the posterior chamber, and the vitreous body.

5. Describe how an image formed on the retina compares with its actual appearance in the outside world.

6. Describe the lacrimal system.

7. Define pupillary light reflex, fixation, and accommodation.

8. Concerning the pupillary light reflex, describe and contrast a direct light reflex with a consensual light reflex.

9. Identify common age-related changes in the eye.

10. Discuss the most common causes of decreased visual function in the older adult.

11. Explain the statement that normal visual acuity is 20/20.

12. Describe the method of testing for presbyopia.

13. To test for accommodation, the person focuses on a distant object and then shifts the gaze to a near object about 6 inches away. At near distance, you would expect the pupils to _____ (dilate/constrict) and the axes of the eyes to _____.

14. Concerning malalignment of the eye axes, contrast *phoria* with *tropia*.

15. Describe abnormal findings of tissue color that are possible on the conjunctiva and sclera, and describe their significance.

16. Describe the method of everting the upper eyelid for examination.

17. Contrast *pinguecula* with *pterygium*.

18. Contrast the use of the negative diopter or red lens settings with the positive diopter or black lens settings on the ophthalmoscope.

19. Explain the rationale for testing for strabismus during early childhood.

20. Describe these findings, and explain their significance: epicanthal fold; pseudostrabismus; ophthalmia neonatorum; Brushfield spots.

21. Describe the following 4 types of red eye, and explain their significance:

    a. Conjunctivitis:

    b. Subconjunctival hemorrhage:

    c. Iritis:

    d. Acute glaucoma:

Fill in the labels indicated on the following illustrations.

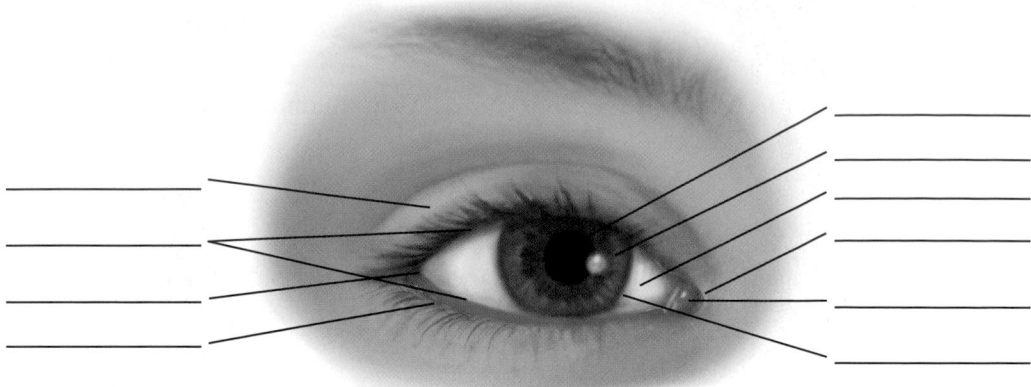

© Pat Thomas, 2006

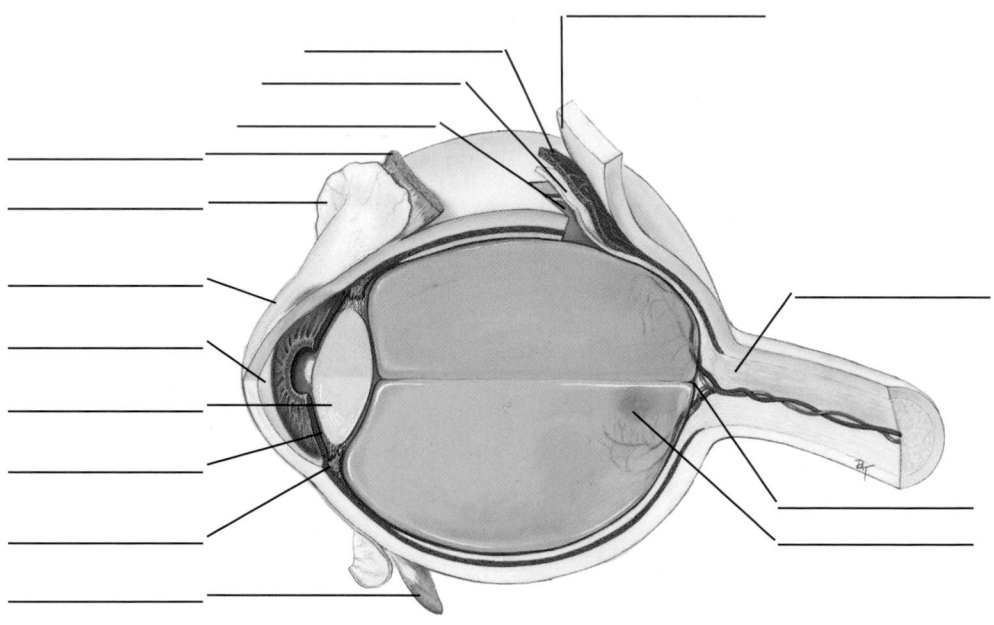

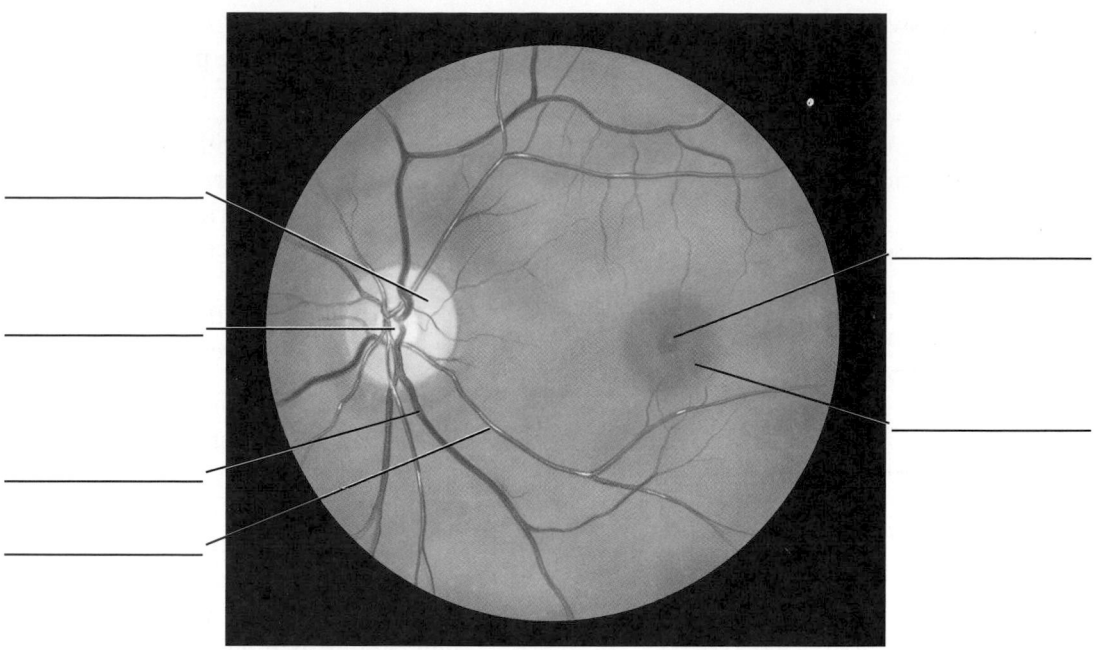

## REVIEW QUESTIONS

This test is for you to check your own mastery of the content. Answers are provided in Appendix A.

1. The palpebral fissure is the:

   a. Border between the cornea and sclera.
   b. Open space between the eyelids.
   c. Angle where the eyelids meet.
   d. Visible on the upper and lower lids at the inner canthus.

2. Which retinal structures can be viewed through the ophthalmoscope?

   a. The optic disc, the retinal vessels, the general background, and the macula
   b. The cornea, the lens, the choroid, and the ciliary body
   c. The optic papilla, the sclera, the retina, and the iris
   d. The pupil, the sclera, the ciliary body, and the macula

3. The examiner records "positive consensual light reflex." This indicates:

   a. Convergence of the axes of the eyeballs.
   b. Simultaneous constriction of the other pupil when one eye is exposed to bright light.
   c. Reflex direction of the eye toward an object attracting a person's attention.
   d. Adaptation of the eye for near vision.

4. The thickening and yellowing of the lens due to aging is described as:

   a. Presbyopia.
   b. Floaters.
   c. Macular degeneration.
   d. Cataract.

5. You must be alert for which eye emergency symptoms?

   a. Floaters
   b. Epiphora
   c. Sudden onset of vision change
   d. Photophobia

6. Visual acuity is assessed with:

   a. The Snellen eye chart.
   b. An ophthalmoscope.
   c. The Hirschberg test.
   d. The Confrontation test.

7. The cover test is used to assess for:

   a. Nystagmus.
   b. Peripheral vision.
   c. Muscle weakness.
   d. Visual acuity.

8. When using the ophthalmoscope, you would:

   a. Remove your own glasses and approach the patient's left eye with your left eye.
   b. Leave the light on in the examining room and remove glasses from the patient.
   c. Remove glasses and set the diopter setting at 0.
   d. Use the smaller white light and instruct the patient to focus on the ophthalmoscope.

9. The 6 eye muscles that control eye movement are innervated by cranial nerves:

   a. II, III, V.
   b. IV, VI, VII.
   c. III, IV, VI.
   d. II, III, VI.

10. Conjunctivitis is associated with:

    a. Absent red reflex.
    b. Reddened conjunctiva.
    c. Impairment of vision.
    d. Fever.

11. A patient has blurred peripheral vision. You suspect glaucoma and assess the visual fields. A patient with normal vision would see your moving finger temporally at:

    a. 50 degrees.
    b. 60 degrees.
    c. 90 degrees.
    d. 180 degrees.

12. A patient is known to be blind in the left eye. What happens to the pupils when the right eye is illuminated by a penlight beam?

    a. No response in both pupils
    b. Both pupils constrict
    c. Right pupil constricts, left has no response
    d. Left pupil constricts, right has no response

13. When using the ophthalmoscope, the interruption of the red reflex occurs when:

    a. There is opacity in the cornea or lens.
    b. The patient has a pathologic process of the optic tract.
    c. The blood vessels are tortuous.
    d. The pupils are constricted.

14. One of the causes of visual impairment in aging adults includes:

    a. Strabismus.
    b. Glaucoma.
    c. Amblyopia.
    d. Retinoblastoma.

15. Documentation of an eye examination can include the term *PERRLA*. What does this mean?

    a. P _____
    b. E _____
    c. R _____
    d. R _____
    e. L _____
    f. A _____

16. What is the cause of the red reflex?

    a. Petechial hemorrhages in the sclera
    b. Diabetic retinopathy
    c. Light reflecting from the retina
    d. Blood in the vitreous

## CRITICAL THINKING EXERCISE

Work with a partner in the lab, but try to pair with someone you do not know well. One person is blind-folded. Each person should guide the other on a campus walk with the following requirements:
1. Go through two different sets of doors.
2. Go up *and* down a set of stairs.
3. Drink at a water fountain.

Walk into buildings with which you are less familiar; this highlights a vision deficit with an unfamiliar environment. Be the blindfolded partner for 7 to 10 minutes and then switch roles. Back in the lab, discuss the following:
1. Frustration levels.
2. How did it feel to be led?
3. How did it feel to lead?
4. What worked? What failed to work?
5. What actions developed your trust in the partner who was leading?
6. How did you handle the doorways? The stairs? The drinking fountain?
7. Did you talk to anyone else on campus? Did you feel self-conscious, as if others were looking at you?
8. What is your takeaway for applying this exercise to your low-vision patients?

## SKILLS LABORATORY AND CLINICAL SETTING

The purpose of the clinical component is to practice the steps of the examination on a peer in the skills laboratory. Note that the first practice session usually takes a long time because there are so many separate steps. Be aware that success with the use of the ophthalmoscope is hard to achieve during the first practice session. Make sure you are holding the instrument correctly, and practice focusing on various objects around the room before you try to look at a person's fundus. When you do examine a peer's eye, make sure to offer occasional rest times. It is very tiring for the "patient" to have the ophthalmoscope light shining in the eye. During the first practice session, aim for finding the red reflex and a retinal vessel or two; if you can locate the optic disc, so much the better.

### Clinical Objectives

1. Collect a health history related to pertinent signs and symptoms of the eye system.

2. Demonstrate and explain the assessment of visual acuity, visual fields, external eye structures, and ocular fundus.

3. Record the history and physical examination findings accurately, reach an assessment of the health state, and develop a plan of care.

### Instructions

Prepare the examination setting. Wash your hands. Practice the steps of the examination on a peer in the skills laboratory, giving appropriate instructions as you proceed. Record your findings using the regional write-up sheet that follows. The front of the page is intended as a worksheet; the back of the page is intended for your narrative summary recording using the SOAP format.

**NOTES**

# REGIONAL WRITE-UP—EYES

Date _____

Examiner _____

Patient _____ Age _____ Gender _____

Reason for visit _____

## I. Health History

| | No | Yes, explain |
|---|---|---|
| 1. Any **difficulty seeing** or blurring? | _____ | _____ |
| 2. Any eye **pain**? | _____ | _____ |
| 3. Any history of **crossed eyes**? | _____ | _____ |
| 4. Any **redness** or **swelling** in eyes? | _____ | _____ |
| 5. Any **watering** or **tearing**? | _____ | _____ |
| 6. Any **injury** or **surgery** to eye? | _____ | _____ |
| 7. Ever tested for **glaucoma**? | _____ | _____ |
| 8. Wear **glasses** or **contact lenses**? | _____ | _____ |
| 9. Ever had vision tested? | _____ | _____ |
| 10. Taking any medications? | _____ | _____ |

## II. Physical Examination

**A. Test visual acuity.**

Snellen eye chart _____

Pocket vision screener for near vision _____

**B. Test visual fields.**

Confrontation test _____

**C. Inspect extraocular muscle function.**

Corneal light reflex _____

Diagnostic positions test _____

**D. Inspect external eye structures.**

General _____

Eyebrows _____

Eyelids and lashes _____

Eyeballs _____

Conjunctiva and sclera _____

Lacrimal gland, puncta _____

**E. Inspect anterior eyeball structures.**

Cornea _____

Iris _____

Pupil size _____

Pupil direct and consensual light reflex _____

Accommodation _____

**F. Inspect ocular fundus.**

Optic disc _____

Vessels _____

General background of fundus _____

Macula _____

## REGIONAL WRITE-UP—EYES

Summarize your findings using the SOAP format.

**Subjective** (reason for seeking care, health history)

**Objective** (physical examination findings)

Record findings on diagram below.

R          L

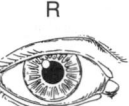 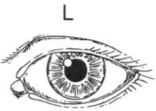

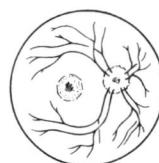 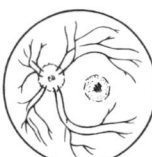

**Assessment** (assessment of problem, diagnosis)

**Plan** (diagnostic evaluation, follow-up care, teaching)

# CHAPTER 16
# Ears

## PURPOSE

This chapter helps you learn the structure and function of the ears, learn the methods of examination of hearing, external ear structures, and tympanic membrane using the otoscope, and record the assessment accurately.

## READING ASSIGNMENT

Jarvis: *Physical Examination and Health Assessment*, 8th ed., Chapter 16, pp. 317-344.

Suggested reading:
Cunningham, L. L., & Tucci, D. L. (2017). Hearing loss in adults. *N Engl J Med, 377*(25), 2465-2473.

## GLOSSARY

Study the following terms after completing the reading assignment. You should be able to cover the definition on the right and define the term out loud.

**Annulus** . . . . . . . . . . . . . . . . . . . outer fibrous rim encircling the eardrum

**Atresia** . . . . . . . . . . . . . . . . . . . congenital absence or closure of ear canal

**Cerumen** . . . . . . . . . . . . . . . . . . yellow waxy material that lubricates and protects the ear canal

**Cochlea** . . . . . . . . . . . . . . . . . . . inner ear structure containing the central hearing apparatus

**Eustachian tube** . . . . . . . . . . . . connects the middle ear with the nasopharynx and allows passage of air

**Helix** . . . . . . . . . . . . . . . . . . . . . superior posterior free rim of the pinna

**Incus** . . . . . . . . . . . . . . . . . . . . . "anvil"; middle of the 3 ossicles of the middle ear

**Malleus** . . . . . . . . . . . . . . . . . . . "hammer"; outermost of the 3 ossicles of the middle ear

**Mastoid** . . . . . . . . . . . . . . . . . . . bony prominence of the skull located just behind the ear

**Organ of Corti** . . . . . . . . . . . . . sensory organ of hearing

**Otalgia** . . . . . . . . . . . . . . . . . . . pain in the ear

**Otitis externa** . . . . . . . . . . . . . . inflammation of the outer ear and ear canal

**Otitis media** . . . . . . . . . . . . . . . inflammation of the middle ear and tympanic membrane

**Otorrhea** . . . . . . . . . . . . . . . . . . discharge from the ear

**Pars flaccida** . . . . . . . . . . . . . . . small, slack, superior section of tympanic membrane

**Pars tensa** . . . . . . . . . . . . . . . . . thick, taut, central-inferior section of tympanic membrane

**Pinna** . . . . . . . . . . . . . . . . . . . . . auricle, or outer ear

**Stapes** . . . . . . . . . . . . . . . . . . . . "stirrup"; innermost of the 3 ossicles of the middle ear

**Tinnitus** . . . . . . . . . . . . . . . . . . . ringing in the ears

**Tympanic membrane** . . . . . . . . "eardrum"; thin, translucent, oval membrane that stretches across the ear canal and separates the middle ear from the outer ear

**Umbo** . . . . . . . . . . . . . . . . . . . . . knob of the malleus that shows through the tympanic membrane

**Vertigo** . . . . . . . . . . . . . . . . . . . . a spinning, twirling sensation

## STUDY GUIDE

After completing the reading assignment and the media assignment, write or draw the answers in the spaces provided.

1. List the 3 functions of the middle ear.

2. Contrast 2 pathways of hearing.

3. Differentiate among the types of hearing loss and give examples.

4. Relate the anatomic differences that place the infant at greater risk for middle ear infections.

5. Describe the whispered voice test of hearing acuity.

6. Explain the positioning of normal ear alignment in the child.

7. Define *otosclerosis* and *presbycusis*.

8. Contrast the motions used to straighten the ear canal when using the otoscope with an infant versus an adult.

9. Describe the appearance of these nodules that could be present on the external ear: Darwin's tubercle, sebaceous cyst, tophi, chondrodermatitis, keloid, carcinoma.

10. Describe the appearance of these conditions that could appear in the ear canal: osteoma, exostosis, furuncle, polyp, foreign body.

11. List the disease state suggested by the following descriptions of the appearance of the eardrum: yellow-amber color, pearly gray color, air-fluid level, distorted light reflex, red color, dense white areas, oval dark areas, black or white dots on drum, blue drum.

Fill in the labels indicated on the following illustrations.

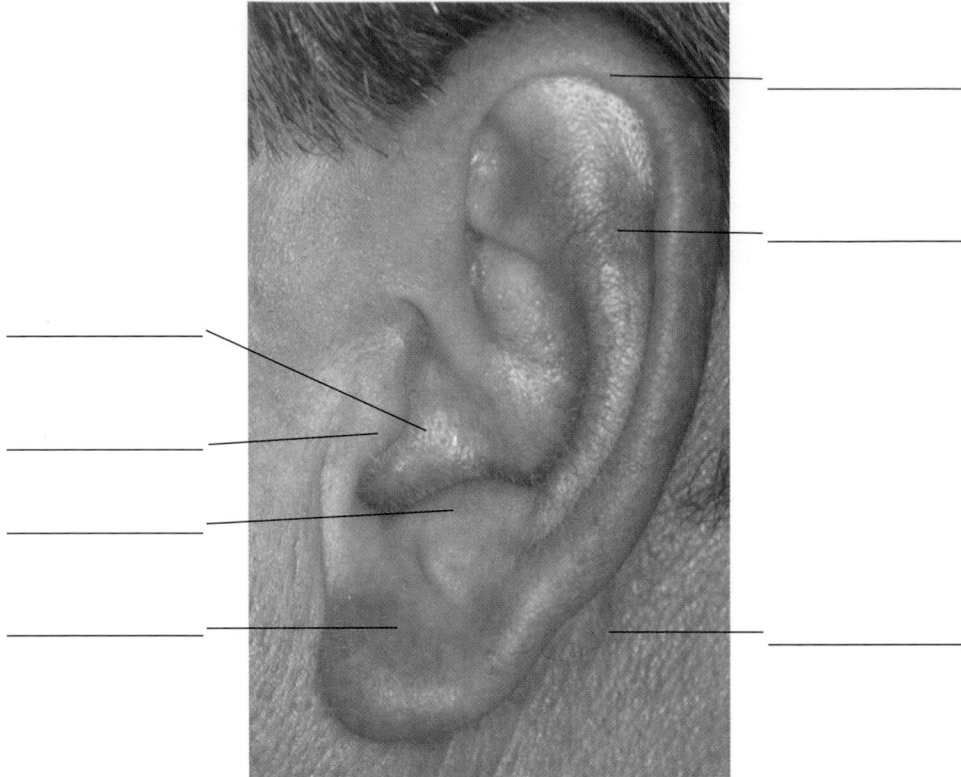

Courtesy Lemmi and Lemmi, 2011.

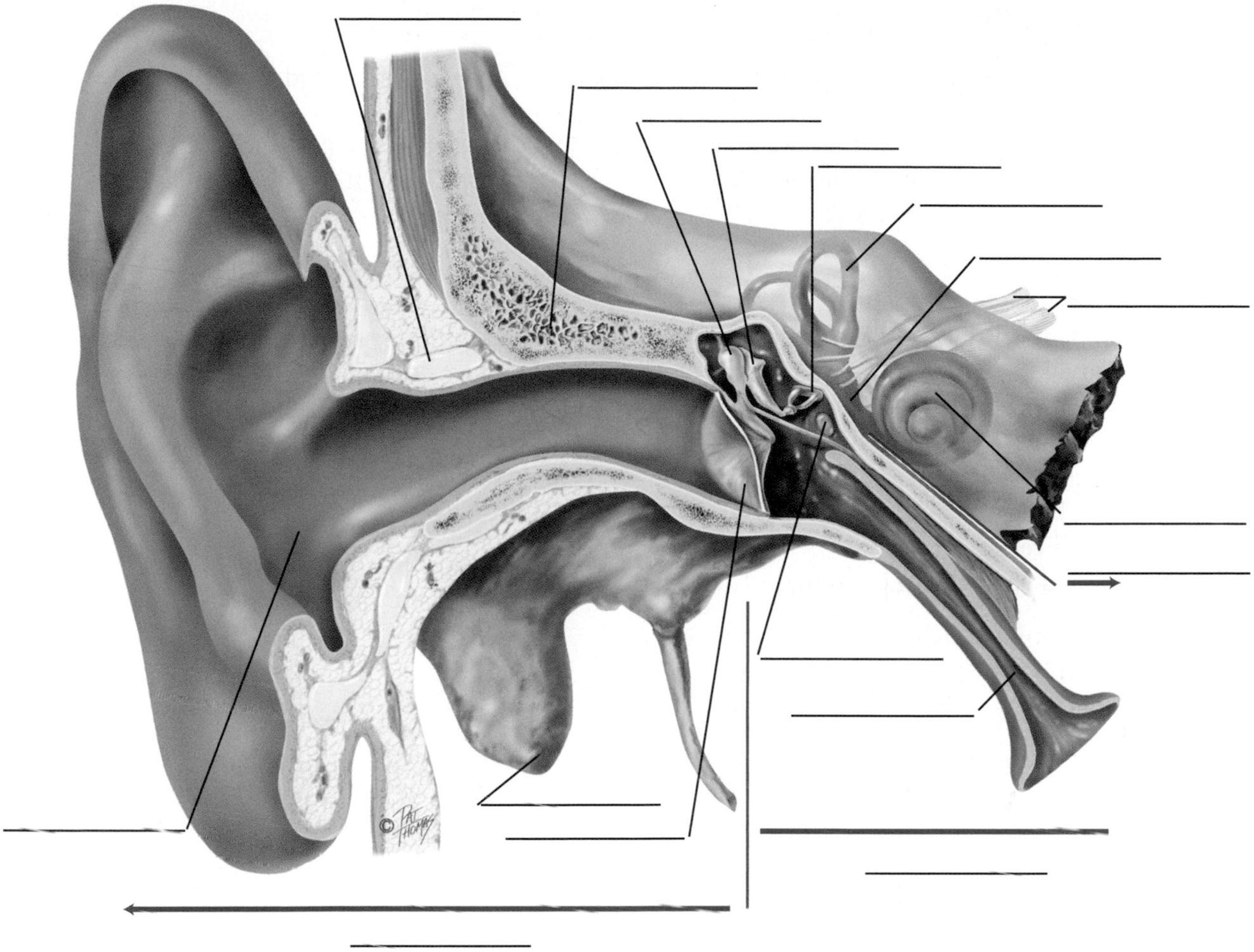

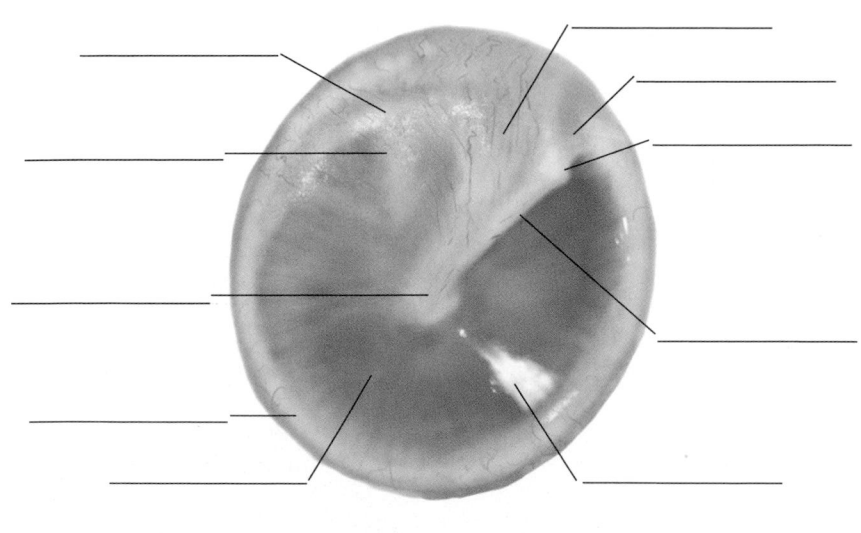

## REVIEW QUESTIONS

This test is for you to check your own mastery of the content. Answers are provided in Appendix A.

1. Using the otoscope, the tympanic membrane is visualized. The color of the membrane is:

   a. Deep pink.
   b. Creamy white.
   c. Pearly gray.
   d. Dependent on the ethnicity of the individual.

2. Sensorineural hearing loss may be related to:

   a. Gradual nerve degeneration.
   b. Foreign bodies.
   c. Impacted cerumen.
   d. Perforated tympanic membrane.

3. Before examining a patient's ear with the otoscope, you would palpate which for tenderness?

   a. Helix, external auditory meatus, and lobule
   b. Mastoid process, tympanic membrane, and malleus
   c. Pinna, pars flaccida, and antitragus
   d. Pinna, tragus, and mastoid process

4. During the otoscopic examination of a child younger than 3 years, the examiner:

   a. Pulls the pinna up and back.
   b. Pulls the pinna down.
   c. Holds the pinna gently but firmly in its normal position.
   d. Tilts the head slightly toward the examiner.

5. In examining the ear of an adult, the canal is straightened by pulling the auricle:

   a. Down and forward.
   b. Down and back.
   c. Up and back.
   d. Up and forward.

6. Darwin tubercle indicates:

   a. An overgrowth of scar tissue.
   b. A blocked sebaceous gland.
   c. A sign of gout called *tophi*.
   d. A congenital, painless nodule at the helix.

7. When assessing a patient's ear with an otoscope, the patient's head should be positioned:

   a. Tilted toward the examiner.
   b. Tilted away from the examiner.
   c. As vertical as possible.
   d. Tilted down.

8. The hearing receptors are located in which region?

   a. Vestibule
   b. Semicircular canals
   c. Middle ear
   d. Cochlea

9. The sensation of vertigo may indicate:

   a. Otitis media.
   b. Pathology in the semicircular canals.
   c. Pathology in the cochlea.
   d. 4th cranial nerve damage.

10. A common cause of a conductive hearing loss is:

    a. Impacted cerumen.
    b. Acute rheumatic fever.
    c. A CVA.
    d. Otitis externa.

11. You are assessing a patient's tympanic membrane and suspect an infection of acute purulent otitis media. Which of the following findings supports this?

    a. Absent light reflex, bluish drum, oval dark areas
    b. Absent light reflex, reddened drum, bulging drum
    c. Oval dark areas on drum
    d. Absent light reflex, air-fluid level, or bubbles behind drum

12. You are teaching a parent of an infant the health promotion activities to reduce the risk for acute otitis media. Which would you include in the teaching plan?

    a. Using pacifiers
    b. Increasing group daycare
    c. Avoiding breastfeeding
    d. Eliminating smoking in the house and car

13. When assessing hearing acuity in a 6-month-old child, the examiner would:

    a. Use an audiometer.
    b. Observe for shyness and withdrawal.
    c. Watch for head turning when saying the child's name.
    d. Test the startle (Moro) reflex.

14. A patient with a head injury has clear, watery drainage from the ear. How should you proceed?

    a. Place a cotton ball loosely at the entrance to the ear canal.
    b. Consider possibility of basal skull fracture and refer immediately.
    c. Perform pneumatic otoscopy to assess for drum hypomobility.
    d. Assess for the presence of a tympanostomy tube in the ear.

## SKILLS LABORATORY AND CLINICAL SETTING

The purpose of the clinical component is to practice the steps of the ear examination on a peer in the skills laboratory or on a patient in the clinical setting. The use of the otoscope is somewhat easier than the use of the ophthalmoscope; however, you still must be sure that you are holding the instrument correctly. Holding the otoscope in an upside-down position seems awkward at first, but it is important to make sure the otoscope tip does not cause pain to the delicate parts of the ear canal. Have someone correct your positioning before you insert the instrument.

### Clinical Objectives

1. Collect a health history related to pertinent signs and symptoms of the ear system.

2. Describe the appearance of the normal outer ear and external ear canal.

3. Describe and demonstrate the correct technique of an otoscopic examination.

4. Describe and perform tests for hearing acuity.

5. Systematically describe the normal tympanic membrane, including position, color, and landmarks.

6. Record the history and physical examination findings accurately, reach an assessment about the health state, and develop a plan of care.

## Instructions

Prepare the examination setting and gather your equipment. Make certain the otoscope light is bright and batteries are freshly charged. Wash your hands. Practice the steps of the examination on a peer in the skills laboratory, giving appropriate instructions as you proceed. Record your findings using the regional write-up sheet that follows. The front of the page is intended as a worksheet; the back of the page is intended for your narrative summary recording using the SOAP format.

## NOTES

# REGIONAL WRITE-UP—EARS

Date _____

Examiner _____

Patient _____ Age _____ Gender _____

Reason for visit _____

I. **Health History (subjective)**

|  | No | Yes, explain |
|---|---|---|
| 1. Any **earache** or ear pain? | _____ | _____ |
| Trauma to head? | _____ | _____ |
| 2. Any ear **infections**? | _____ | _____ |
| Now or in past? | _____ | _____ |
| 3. Any **discharge** from ears? | _____ | _____ |
| 4. Any **hearing loss** now? | _____ | _____ |
| 5. Any **loud noises** at home or job? | _____ | _____ |
| 6. Any **ringing** or **buzzing** in ears? | _____ | _____ |
| Taking any medications? | _____ | _____ |
| 7. Ever felt **vertigo** (spinning)? | _____ | _____ |
| 8. How do you clean your ears? | _____ | _____ |
| 9. Use ear protection from loud noise or while swimming? | _____ | _____ |

II. **Physical Examination (objective)**

A. **Inspect and palpate external ear.**

Size and shape _____

Skin condition _____

Tenderness _____

External auditory meatus _____

B. **Inspect using the otoscope.**

External canal _____

Tympanic membrane _____

Color and characteristics _____

Position _____

Integrity of membrane _____

C. **Test hearing acuity.**

Whispered voice test _____

## REGIONAL WRITE-UP—EARS

Summarize your findings using the SOAP format.

**Subjective** (reason for seeking care, health history)

**Objective** (physical examination findings)          Record findings on diagram below.

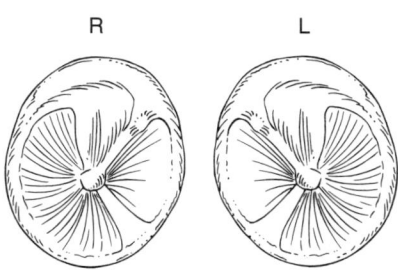

**Assessment** (assessment of health state or problem, diagnosis)

**Plan** (diagnostic evaluation, follow-up care, patient teaching)

# CHAPTER 17

# Nose, Mouth, and Throat

## PURPOSE

This chapter helps you learn the structure and function of the nose, mouth, and throat; learn the methods of inspection and palpation of these structures; and record the assessment accurately.

## READING ASSIGNMENT

Jarvis: *Physical Examination and Health Assessment,* 8th ed., Chapter 17, pp. 345-376.

Suggested readings:
Van Schayck, O. C. P., Williams, S., Barchilon, V., et al. (2017). Treating tobacco dependence: guidance for primary care on life-saving interventions. *NPJ Prim Care Respir Med, 27*(1), 38, doi:10.1038/s41533-017-0039-5.

## GLOSSARY

Study the following terms after completing the reading assignment. You should be able to cover the definition on the right and define the term out loud.

**Aphthous ulcers** . . . . . . . . . . . . "canker sores"; small, painful, round ulcers in the oral mucosa of unknown cause

**Buccal** . . . . . . . . . . . . . . . . . . . . pertaining to the cheek

**Candidiasis** . . . . . . . . . . . . . . . (moniliasis) white, cheesy, curdlike patch on buccal mucosa due to superficial fungal infection

**Caries** . . . . . . . . . . . . . . . . . . . . decay in the teeth

**Cheilitis** . . . . . . . . . . . . . . . . . . red, scaling, shallow, painful fissures at corners of mouth

**Choanal atresia** . . . . . . . . . . . . closure of nasal cavity due to congenital septum between nasal cavity and pharynx

**Crypts** . . . . . . . . . . . . . . . . . . . indentations on surface of tonsils

**Epistaxis** . . . . . . . . . . . . . . . . . nosebleed, usually from anterior septum

**Epulis** . . . . . . . . . . . . . . . . . . . nontender, fibrous nodule of the gum

**Fordyce granules** . . . . . . . . . . . small, isolated, white or yellow papules on oral mucosa

**Gingivitis**. . . . . . . . . . . . . . . . . red, swollen gum margins that bleed easily

**Herpes simplex**. . . . . . . . . . . . . "cold sores"; clear vesicles with red base that evolve into pustules, usually at lip-skin junction

**Koplik spots** . . . . . . . . . . . . . . . small, blue-white spots with red halo over oral mucosa; early sign of measles

**Leukoplakia** . . . . . . . . . . . . . . . chalky white, thick, raised patch on sides of tongue; precancerous

**Malocclusion** . . . . . . . . . . . . . . upper or lower dental arches out of alignment

**Papillae** . . . . . . . . . . . . . . . . . . rough, bumpy elevations on dorsal surface of tongue

**Parotid glands** . . . . . . . . . . . . . pair of salivary glands in the cheeks in front of the ears

**Pharyngitis** . . . . . . . . . . . . . . . . inflammation of the throat

**Plaque** . . . . . . . . . . . . . . . . . . . soft, whitish debris on teeth

**Polyp** . . . . . . . . . . . . . . . . . . . . smooth, pale gray nodules in the nasal cavity due to chronic allergic rhinitis

**Rhinitis** . . . . . . . . . . . . . . . . . . red, swollen inflammation of nasal mucosa

**Thrush**. . . . . . . . . . . . . . . . . . . oral candidiasis in the newborn

**Turbinate**. . . . . . . . . . . . . . . . . one of 3 bony projections into nasal cavity

**Uvula** . . . . . . . . . . . . . . . . . . . . free projection hanging down from the middle of the soft palate

## STUDY GUIDE

After completing the reading assignment and the media assignment, write or draw the answers in the spaces provided.

1.  Name the functions of the nose.



2.  Describe the size and components of the nasal cavity.



3.  List the 4 sets of paranasal sinuses, and describe their function.



4.  List the 3 pairs of salivary glands, including their location and the locations of their duct openings.

5. After tooth loss in the middle or older adult, describe the consequences of chewing with the remaining maloccluded teeth.

6. Describe the appearance of a deviated nasal septum and a perforated septum.

7. Describe the appearance of a torus palatinus, and explain its significance.

8. Contrast the physical appearance and clinical significance of the following: leukoedema; candidiasis, leukoplakia, Fordyce granules.

9. List the 4-point grading scale for the size of tonsils.

10. Describe the appearance and clinical significance of these findings in the infant: sucking tubercle, Epstein pearls, Bednar aphthae.

11. Contrast the appearance of nasal turbinates versus nasal polyps.

12. Describe the appearance and clinical significance of these findings on the tongue: ankyloglossia, fissured tongue, geographic tongue, black hairy tongue, macroglossia.

13. In the space below, sketch a cleft palate and a bifid uvula.

Fill in the labels indicated on the following illustrations.

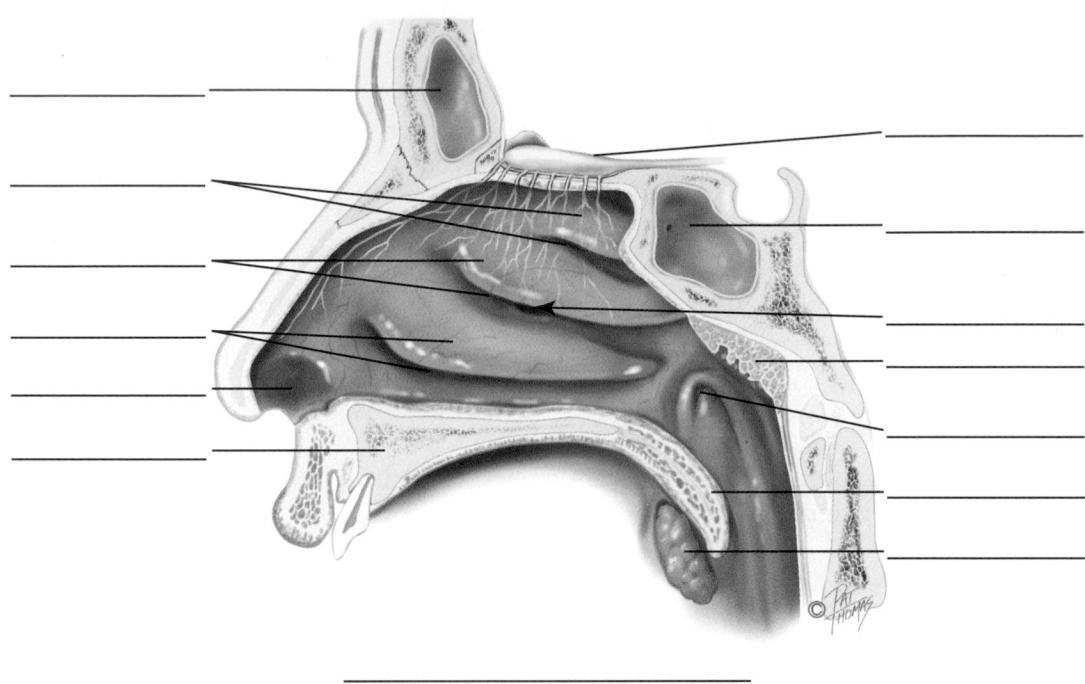

© Pat Thomas, 2006

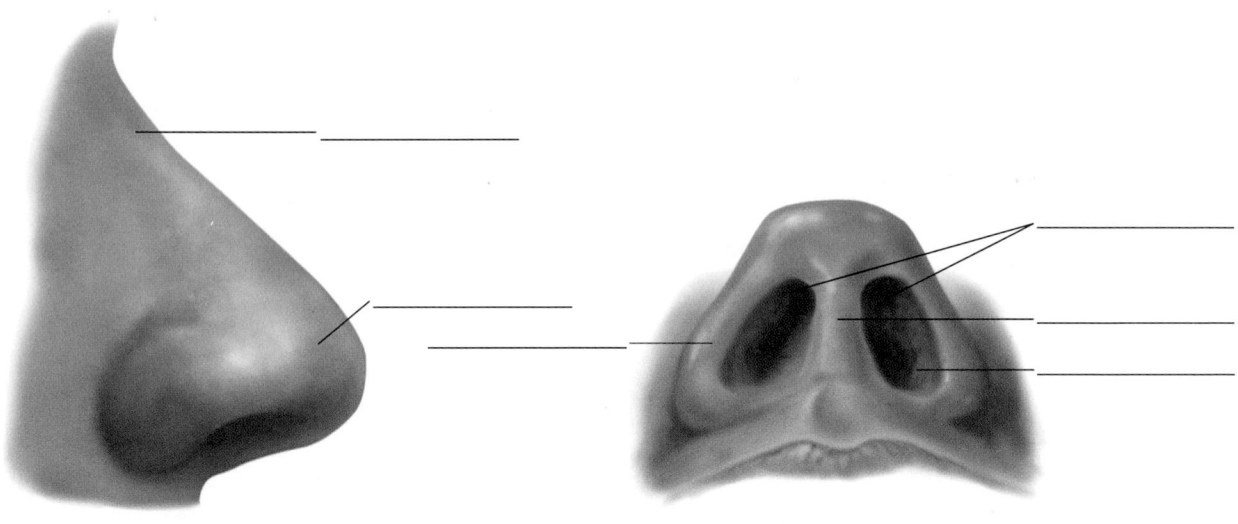

© Pat Thomas, 2006

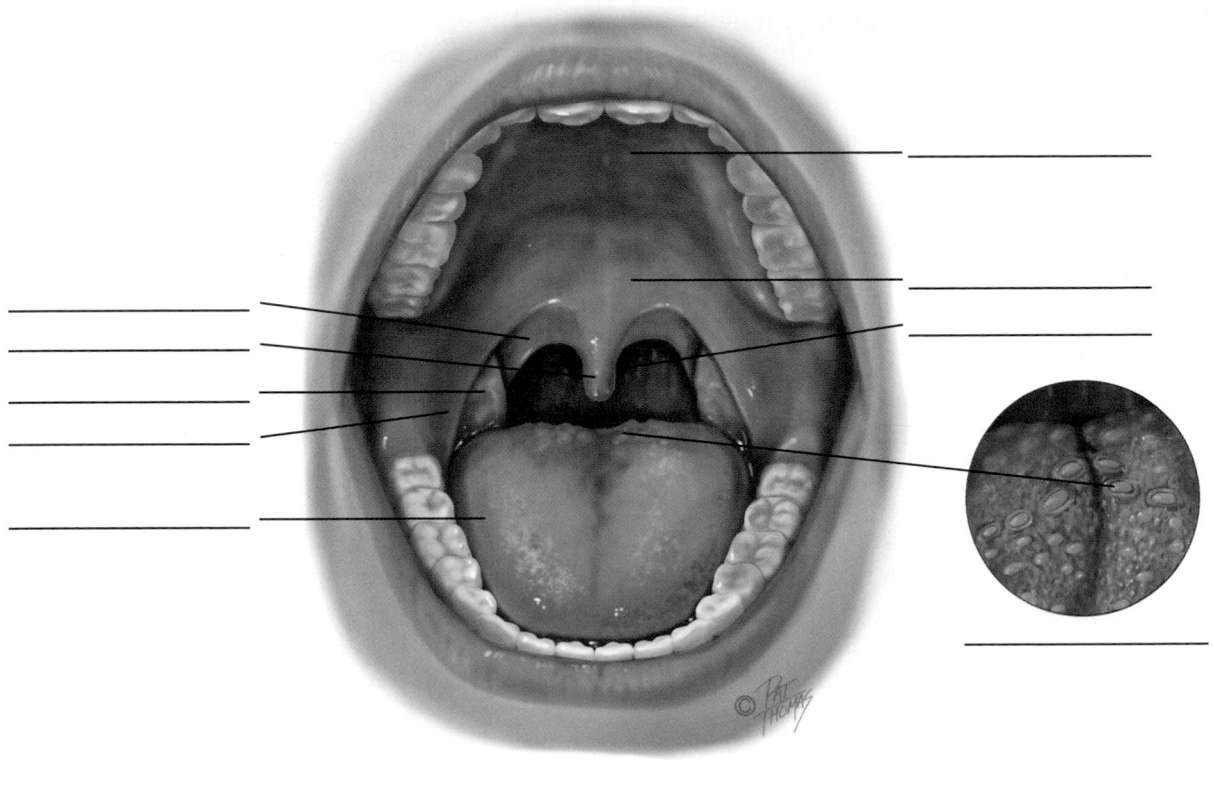

© Pat Thomas, 2006

## REVIEW QUESTIONS

This test is for you to check your own mastery of the content. Answers are provided in Appendix A.

1. What is the most common site of nose bleeds?

   a. The turbinates
   b. The columellae
   c. Kisselbach plexus
   d. The meatus

2. Which sinuses can you assess through examination?

   a. Ethmoid and sphenoid
   b. Frontal and ethmoid
   c. Maxillary and sphenoid
   d. Frontal and maxillary

3. The frenulum is the:

   a. Midline fold of tissue that connects the tongue to the floor of the mouth.
   b. Anterior border of the oral cavity.
   c. Arching roof of the mouth.
   d. Free projection hanging down from the middle of the soft palate.

4. The largest salivary gland is located:

   a. Within the cheeks in front of the ear.
   b. Beneath the mandible at the angle of the jaw.
   c. Within the floor of the mouth under the tongue.
   d. At the base of the tongue.

5. A 70-year-old woman reports dry mouth. The most frequent cause of this is:

   a. The aging process.
   b. Related to medications she may be taking.
   c. The use of dentures.
   d. Related to a diminished sense of smell.

6. During an inspection of a patient's nares, a deviated septum is noted. What should you do next?

   a. Request a consultation with an ear, nose, and throat specialist.
   b. Document the deviation in the medical record in case the person needs to be suctioned.
   c. Teach the person what to do if a nosebleed should occur.
   d. Explore further because polyps frequently accompany a deviated septum.

7. Oral malignancies are most likely to develop:

   a. On the soft palate.
   b. On the tongue.
   c. In the buccal cheek mucosa.
   d. In the mucosal "gutter" under the tongue.

8. The tonsils are graded as 3+. The tonsils would be:

   a. Visible.
   b. Halfway between the tonsillar pillars and uvula.
   c. Touching the uvula.
   d. Touching each other.

9. The function of the nasal turbinates is to:

   a. Warm the inhaled air.
   b. Detect odors.
   c. Stimulate tear formation.
   d. Lighten the weight of the skull bones.

10. The opening of an adult's parotid gland (Stensen's duct) is opposite to:

    a. Lower 2nd molar.
    b. Lower incisors.
    c. Upper incisors.
    d. Upper 2nd molar.

11. A nasal polyp is distinguished from the nasal turbinates by 3 of the following. Which reason is FALSE?

    a. The polyp is highly vascular.
    b. The polyp is movable.
    c. The polyp is pale gray in color.
    d. The polyp is nontender.

12. The examiner notes small, round, white, shiny papules on the hard palate and gums of a 2-month-old infant. What is the significance of this finding?

    a. These are aphthous areas or ulcers that are the result of sucking.
    b. Teeth buds are beginning to appear.
    c. This is a normal finding called *Epstein pearls*.
    d. It indicates the presence of a monilial infection.

13. When assessing the tongue, you should:

    a. Palpate the U-shaped area under the tongue.
    b. Check tongue color for cyanosis.
    c. Use a tongue blade to elevate the tongue while placing a finger under the jaw.
    d. Ask the person to say "ahhh" and note a rise in the midline.

14. You are assessing a 75-year-old patient's oral cavity. Which of the following would most likely be present?

    a. Hypertrophy of the gums
    b. An increased production of saliva
    c. Decreased ability to identify odors
    d. Finer and less prominent nasal hair

15. You are assessing an African-American patient and note a flat, 3-cm, nontender, grayish-white lesion on the left buccal mucosa. Which of the following is most likely?

    a. This lesion is leukoedema and is common in darkly pigmented persons.
    b. This is the result of hyperpigmentation and is normal.
    c. This is torus palatinus and would normally only be found in smokers.
    d. This type of lesion is indicative of cancer and should be tested immediately.

## CRITICAL THINKING EXERCISE

Review the teaching strategies for smoking cessation in the Van Schayck article and in Jarvis: *Physical Examination and Health Assessment*, 8th ed., p. 364 and Fig. 17.25. Plan teaching in your own words, and role-play with a peer in the laboratory setting. Take turns being the "smoker" and the counselor.

## SKILLS LABORATORY AND CLINICAL SETTING

The purpose of the clinical component is to practice the steps of the examination on a peer in the skills laboratory or on a patient in the clinical setting and to achieve the following.

### Clinical Objectives

1. Inspect the external nose.

2. Demonstrate use of the otoscope and nasal attachment to inspect the structures of the nasal cavity.

3. Demonstrate knowledge of infection control practices during inspection and palpation of structures of the mouth and pharynx.

4. Record the history and physical examination findings accurately, reach an assessment of the health state, and develop a plan of care.

### Instructions

Prepare the examination setting, and gather your equipment: gloves, penlight, otoscope with broad nasal speculum, tongue blade, cotton gauze pad.

Wash your hands. Practice the steps of the examination on a peer in the skills laboratory, giving appropriate instructions as you proceed. Record your findings using the regional write-up sheet that follows. The front of the page is intended as a worksheet; the back of the page is intended for your narrative summary recording using the SOAP format.

# NOTES

# REGIONAL WRITE-UP—NOSE, MOUTH, AND THROAT

Date _____

Examiner _____

Patient _____ Age _____ Gender _____

Reason for visit _____

I. **Health History**

| | No | Yes, explain |
|---|---|---|
| A. Nose | | |
| 1. Any nasal **discharge**? | | |
| 2. Unusually frequent or severe colds? | | |
| 3. Any **sinus pain** or sinusitis? | | |
| 4. Any **trauma** or injury to nose? | | |
| 5. Any **nosebleeds**? How often? | | |
| 6. Any **allergies** or hay fever? | | |
| 7. Any change in sense of smell? | | |
| B. Mouth and throat | | |
| 1. Any **sores** in mouth, tongue? | | |
| 2. Any **sore throat**? How often? | | |
| 3. Any **bleeding gums**? Any **toothache?** | | |
| 4. Any **hoarseness**, voice change? | | |
| 5. Any difficulty **swallowing**? | | |
| 6. Any change in sense of taste? | | |
| 7. Do you smoke? How much per day? | | |
| 8. Drink alcohol? How many times per week? Drinks per occasion? | | |
| 9. Use of nasal sprays? Use of nose for illicit drugs? | | |
| 10. Tell me about usual dental care. | | |

II. **Physical Examination**

A. **Inspect and palpate the nose.**

Symmetry _____

Deformity, asymmetry, inflammation _____

Test patency of each nostril _____

Using a nasal speculum, note:

　　Color of nasal mucosa _____

　　Discharge, foreign body _____

　　Septum: deviation, perforation, bleeding _____

　　Turbinates: color, swelling, exudate, polyps _____

B. **Palpate the sinus area.**

Frontal _____

Maxillary _____

C. **Inspect the mouth.**

Lips _____

Teeth and gums _____

Buccal mucosa _____

Palate and uvula _____

Tonsils (grade) _____

Tongue _____

D. **Inspect the throat.**

Tonsils: condition and grade _____

Pharyngeal wall _____

Any breath odor _____

## REGIONAL WRITE-UP—NOSE, MOUTH, AND THROAT

Summarize your findings using the SOAP format.

**Subjective** (reason for seeking care, health history)

**Objective** (physical examination findings)                    Record findings on diagram below.

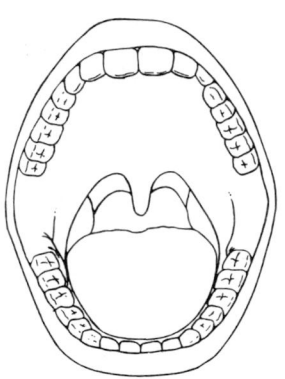

**Assessment** (assessment of health state or problem, diagnosis)

**Plan** (diagnostic evaluation, follow-up care, patient teaching)

# Breasts, Axillae, and Regional Lymphatics

## PURPOSE

This chapter helps you learn the structure and function of the breast, understand the rationale and methods of examination of the breast, accurately record the assessment, and teach breast self-examination.

## READING ASSIGNMENT

Jarvis: *Physical Examination and Health Assessment*, 8th ed., Chapter 18, pp. 377-404.

Suggested readings:
Smania, M. (2017). Evaluation of common breast complaints in primary care. *Nurse Pract, 42*(10), 9-16.

## GLOSSARY

Study the following terms after completing the reading assignment. You should be able to cover the definition on the right and define the term out loud.

**Alveoli** . . . . . . . . . . . . . . . . . . . . smallest structures in the mammary gland

**Areola** . . . . . . . . . . . . . . . . . . . . . darkened area surrounding nipple

**Colostrum** . . . . . . . . . . . . . . . . . thin, yellow fluid, precursor of milk, secreted for a few days after birth

**Cooper ligaments** . . . . . . . . . . suspensory ligaments; fibrous bands extending from the inner breast surface to the chest wall muscles

**Fibroadenoma** . . . . . . . . . . . . . . benign breast mass

**Galactorrhea** . . . . . . . . . . . . . . . persistent white discharge of milk between nursing sessions or after weaning

**Gynecomastia** . . . . . . . . . . . . . . excessive breast development in the male

**Intraductal papilloma** . . . . . . . serosanguineous nipple discharge

**Inverted** . . . . . . . . . . . . . . . . . . . nipples that are depressed or invaginated

**Lactiferous** . . . . . . . . . . . . . . . . conveying milk

**Mastalgia** . . . . . . . . . . . . . . . . . . pain in breast

**Mastitis** . . . . . . . . . . . . . . . . . . . inflammation of the breast

**Montgomery glands** . . . . . . . . sebaceous glands in the areola that secrete protective lipid during lacta-
tion; also called *tubercles of Montgomery*

**Paget disease** . . . . . . . . . . . . . . . intraductal carcinoma in the breast

**Peau d'orange** . . . . . . . . . . . . . . orange peel appearance of breast due to edema

**Retraction** . . . . . . . . . . . . . . . . . dimple or pucker on the skin

**Striae** . . . . . . . . . . . . . . . . . . . . . atrophic pink, purple, or white linear streaks on the breasts, associated with pregnancy, excessive weight gain, or rapid growth during ado-
lescence

**Supernumerary nipple** . . . . . . . minute extra nipple along the embryonic milk line

**Tail of Spence** . . . . . . . . . . . . . . extension of breast tissue into the axilla

**Thelarche** . . . . . . . . . . . . . . . . . beginning of prepubertal breast development

## STUDY GUIDE

After completing the reading assignment and the media assignment, write or draw the answers in the spaces
provided.

1. Identify appropriate history questions to ask regarding the breast examination.

2. Describe the anatomy of the breast.

3. Correlate changes in the female breast with normal developmental stages.

4. Describe the components of the breast examination.

5. List points to include in teaching the breast self-examination.

6. Explain the significance of a supernumerary nipple or breast.

7. Differentiate between the female and male examination procedures and findings.

8. Discuss pathologic changes that may occur in the breast:

    Benign breast disease _____

    Abscess _____

    Acute mastitis _____

    Fibroadenoma _____

    Cancer _____

    Paget disease _____

9. List and describe the characteristics to consider when a mass is noted in the breast.

10. Define gynecomastia.

11. Describe screening mammography and clinical breast examination (CBE) for the diagnosis of breast lesions.

12. List the high-risk and moderate-risk factors that increase the usual risk for breast cancer.

Fill in the labels on the following diagrams.

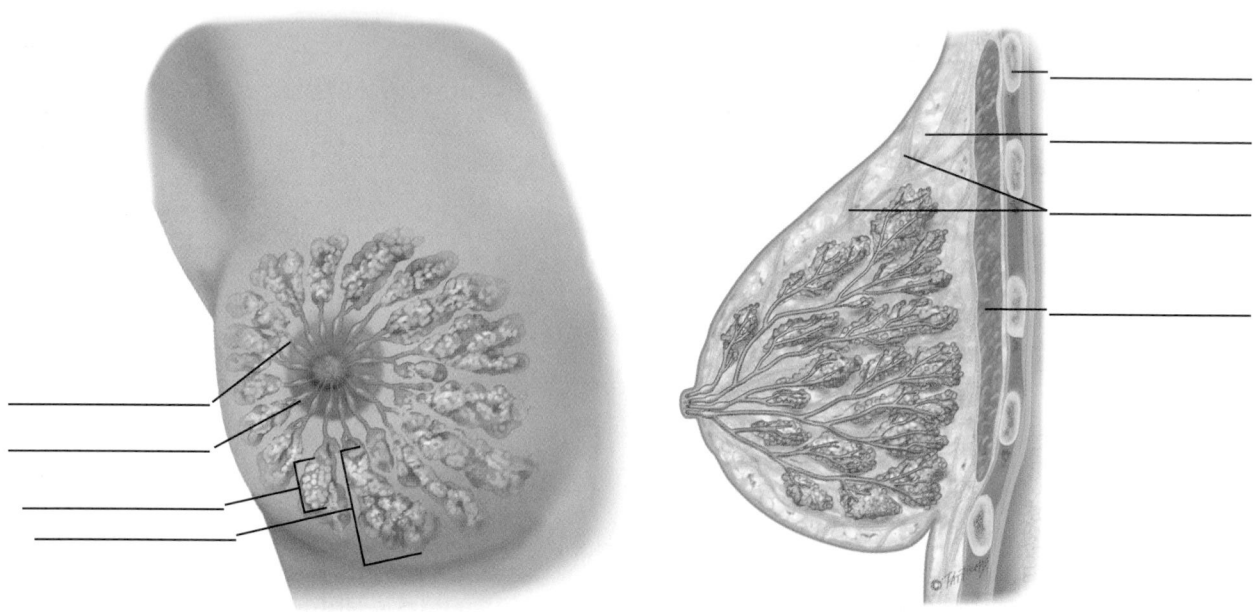

© Pat Thomas, 2006

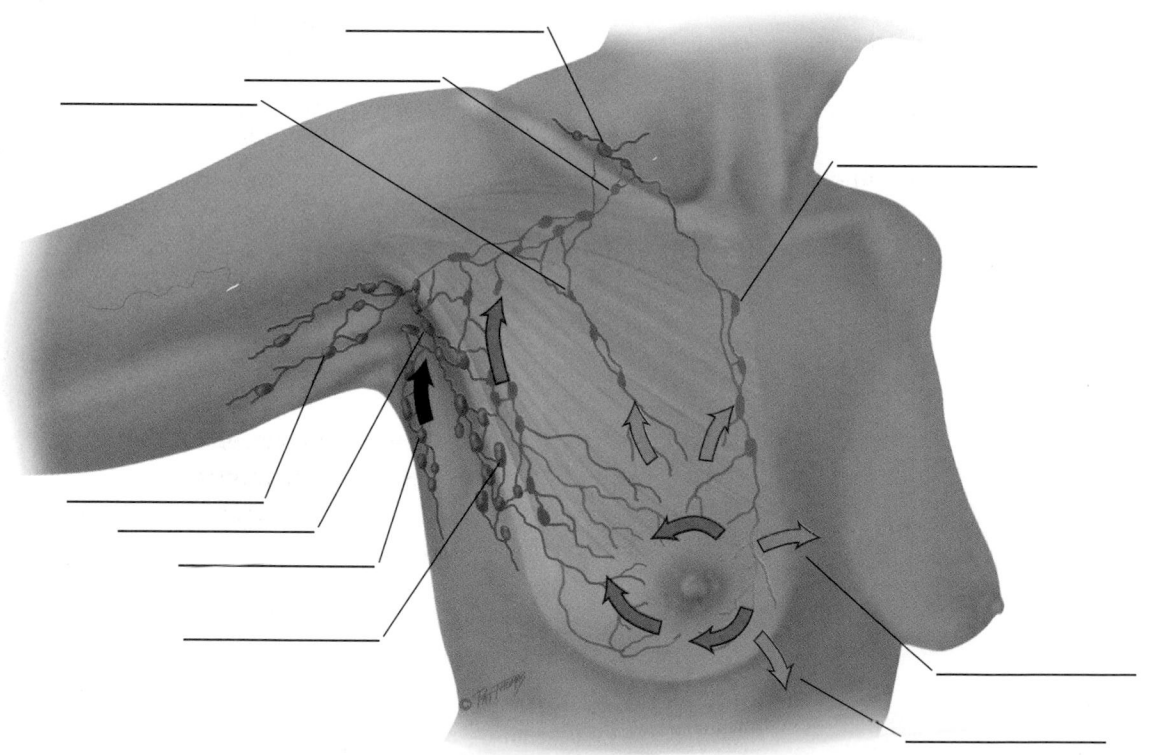

© Pat Thomas, 2006

# REVIEW QUESTIONS

This test is for you to check your own mastery of the content. Answers are provided in Appendix A.

1. The reservoirs for storing milk in the breast are:

   a. Lobules.
   b. Alveoli.
   c. Montgomery glands.
   d. Lactiferous sinuses.

2. What is the most common site of breast tumors?

   a. Upper inner quadrant
   b. Upper outer quadrant
   c. Lower inner quadrant
   d. Lower outer quadrant

3. During a visit for a school physical, the 13-year-old girl being examined questions the asymmetry of her breasts. What is the nurse's best response?

   a. "One breast normally may grow faster than the other during development."
   b. "I will give you a referral for a mammogram."
   c. "You will probably have fibrocystic disease when you are older."
   d. "This may be an indication of hormonal imalance. We will check again in 6 months."

4. When teaching the breast self-examination, you would inform the woman that the best time to conduct breast self-examination is:

   a. At the onset of the menstrual period.
   b. On the 14th day of the menstrual cycle.
   c. On the 4th to 7th day of the cycle.
   d. Just before the menstrual period.

5. You are providing health promotion teaching for a 40-year-old woman. What is the current recommendation for women 40 to 44 years of age and older for breast cancer screening with mammography?

   a. May begin every year
   b. Every 2 years
   c. Twice a year
   d. Only baseline examination needed unless the woman has symptoms

6. You are going to inspect a female patient's breasts for retraction. The best position for this part of the examination is:

   a. Lying supine with arms at the sides.
   b. Leaning forward with hands outstretched.
   c. Sitting with hand pushing onto hips.
   d. One arm at the side, the other arm elevated.

7. A bimanual technique may be the preferred approach for a woman:

   a. Who is pregnant.
   b. Who is having the first breast examination by a health care provider.
   c. With pendulous breasts.
   d. Who has felt a change in the breast during self-examination.

8. During the examination of a 70-year-old man, you note gynecomastia. You would:

   a. Refer for a biopsy.
   b. Refer for a mammogram.
   c. Review the medications for drugs that have gynecomastia as a side effect.
   d. Proceed with the examination. This is a normal part of the aging process.

9. During a breast examination you detect a mass. Which of the following is most consistent with cancer rather than benign breast disease?

    a. Round, firm, well demarcated
    b. Irregular, poorly defined, fixed
    c. Rubbery, mobile, tender
    d. Lobular, clear margins, negative skin retraction

10. During the examination of the breasts of a pregnant woman, you would expect to find:

    a. Peau d'orange.
    b. Nipple retraction.
    c. Unilateral, obvious venous pattern.
    d. Blue vascular pattern over both breasts.

11. Which woman should *not* be referred to a provider for further evaluation?

    a. A 26-year-old with multiple nodules palpated in each breast
    b. A 48-year-old who has a 6-month history of reddened and sore left nipple and areolar area
    c. A 25-year-old with asymmetric breasts and inversion of nipples since adolescence
    d. A 64-year-old with ulcerated area at tip of right nipple; no masses, tenderness, or lymph nodes palpated

12. Any lump found in the breast should be referred for further evaluation. A benign lesion will usually have 3 of the following characteristics. Which one is characteristic of a malignant lesion?

    a. Soft
    b. Well-defined margins
    c. Freely movable
    d. Irregular shape

13. Gynecomastia is:

    a. Enlargement of the male breast.
    b. Presence of mast cells in the male breast.
    c. Cancer of the male breast.
    d. Presence of supernumerary breast on the male chest.

14. Which is the first physical change associated with puberty in girls?

    a. Areolar elevation
    b. Breast bud development
    c. Height spurt
    d. Pubic hair development

15. During the examination of a 30-year-old woman, she asks about "the 2 large moles" that are below her left breast. After examining the area, how do you respond?

    a. "I think you should be examined by a dermatologist."
    b. "This is a normal finding of supernumerary nipples that are not developed."
    c. "These are Montgomery glands, which are common."
    d. "Is there a possibility you are pregnant?"

## SKILLS LABORATORY AND CLINICAL SETTING

The purpose of the clinical component is to practice the steps of the assessment on a peer in the skills laboratory and to achieve the following.

### Clinical Objectives

1. Demonstrate knowledge of the symptoms related to the breasts and axillae by obtaining a health history.

2. Perform inspection and palpation of the breasts, with the woman in sitting and supine positions, using proper technique and providing appropriate draping.

3. Teach breast self-examination to a woman, or list the points to include in teaching breast self-examination.

4. Record the history and physical examination findings accurately, reach an assessment of the health state, and develop a plan of care.

### Instructions

Gather the health history on a peer or a woman in the clinical area. Gather any equipment (small pillow, centimeter ruler, handout on breast self-examination). Then practice the steps of the breast examination. Record your findings on the regional write-up sheet that follows. The front of the page is intended as a worksheet; the back of the page is intended for your narrative summary recording using the SOAP format.

Note the student performance checklist that follows the regional write-up sheet. It lists the essential behaviors you should display as an examiner, and it may be used by your clinical instructor to evaluate your clinical teaching of breast self-examination.

Using a computer or electronic device, enter: www.cancer.gov/bcrisktool/default/aspx. This Breast Cancer Risk Assessment is an interactive tool to help estimate a woman's risk for developing breast cancer. It has been updated for African-American women and for Asian and Pacific Islander women. The model does not apply to women with a history of breast cancer or chest irradiation or women younger than 35 years. Practice using the tool in your laboratory setting. The screen should look like this:

**Before using the tool, please note the following:**

> The Breast Cancer Risk Assessment Tool was designed for use by health professionals. If you are not a health professional, you are encouraged to discuss the results and your personal risk of breast cancer with your doctor.

> Although the tool may accurately estimate a woman's risk of developing breast cancer, these risk estimates do not allow one to say precisely which woman will develop breast cancer. In fact, the distribution of risk estimates for women who develop breast cancer overlaps the estimates of risk for women who do not.

> The tool should not be used to calculate breast cancer risk for women who have already had a diagnosis of breast cancer, lobular carcinoma in situ (LCIS), or ductal carcinoma in situ (DCIS).

> The BCRA risk calculator may be updated periodically as new data or research becomes available.

> Although the tool has been used with success in clinics for women with strong family histories of breast cancer, more specific methods of estimating risk are appropriate for women known to have breast cancer–producing mutations in the BRCA1 or BRCA2 genes.

> Other factors may also affect risk and are not accounted for by the tool. These factors include previous radiation therapy to the chest for the treatment of Hodgkin lymphoma or women who have recently immigrated to the United States from certain regions of Asia where breast cancer risk is low. Further, the tool may not be appropriate for women living outside the United States. The tool's risk calculations assume that a woman is screened for breast cancer as in the general U.S. population. A woman who does not have mammograms will have a somewhat lower chance of a diagnosis of breast cancer.

www.cancer.gov/bcrisktool/default.aspx

**Risk Tool**

(Click a question number for a brief explanation, or read all explanations.)

1.  Does the woman have a medical history of any breast cancer or of ductal carcinoma in situ (DCIS) or lobular carcinoma in situ (LCIS) or has she received previous radiation therapy to the chest for treatment of Hodgkin lymphoma?     Select

2.  Does the woman have a mutation in either the BRCA1 or BRCA2 gene, or a diagnosis of a genetic syndrome that may be associated with elevated risk of breast cancer?     Select

3.  What is the woman's age?
    *This tool only calculates risk for women 35 years of age or older.*     Select

4.  What was the woman's age at the time of her first menstrual period?     Select

5.  What was the woman's age at the time of her first live birth of a child?     Select

6.  How many of the woman's first-degree relatives - mother, sisters, daughters - have had breast cancer?     Select

7.  Has the woman ever had a breast biopsy?     Select

    7a. How many breast biopsies (positive or negative) has the woman had?     Select

    7b. Has the woman had at least one breast biopsy with atypical hyperplasia?     Select

8.  What is the woman's race/ethnicity?     Select

    8a. What is the sub race/ethnicity?     Select

**Calculate Risk >**

# REGIONAL WRITE-UP—BREASTS AND AXILLAE

Date _____

Last Menstrual Period _____

Patient _____ Age _____ Gender _____

Reason for visit _____

## I. Health History

|  | No | Yes, explain |
|---|---|---|
| 1. Any **pain** or tenderness in breasts? | | |
| 2. Any **lump** or thickening in breasts? | | |
| 3. Any **discharge** from nipples? | | |
| 4. Any **rash** on breasts? | | |
| 5. Any **swelling** in the breasts? | | |
| 6. Any **trauma**, injury, or radiation to breasts? | | |
| 7. Any **history** of breast disease? | | |
| 8. Ever had **surgery** on breasts? | | |
| 9. List medications: | | |
| 10. Ever been taught breast self-examination? | | |
| 11. Ever had mammography? When? | | |

12. Past health:
   a. Age at menses _____    b. Age at first birth _____
   c. Age at menopause _____    d. Take hormone therapy? _____
   e. Usual number of alcoholic drinks/week _____

## II. Physical Examination
### A. Inspection
   1. Breast symmetry _____
      Skin color and condition _____
      Lesions _____
      Rash or edema _____
   2. Areolae and nipples
      Direction _____
      Discharge _____
   3. Response to arm movement _____
   4. Axillae _____
### B. Palpation
   1. Breast texture _____
      Masses _____
      Tenderness _____
   2. Areolae and nipples
      Masses _____
      Discharge _____
   3. Axillae and lymph nodes
      Size _____    Shape _____
      Consistency _____    Mobility _____
      Discrete or matted _____    Tenderness _____
### C. Teach breast self-examination

## REGIONAL WRITE-UP—BREASTS AND AXILLAE

Summarize your findings using the SOAP format.

**Subjective** (reason for seeking care, health history)

**Objective** (physical examination findings)                    Record findings on diagram below.

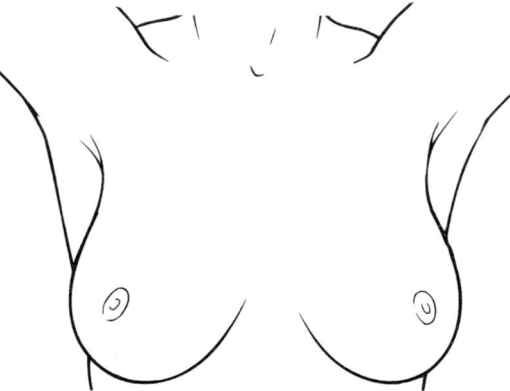

**Assessment** (assessment of health state or problem, diagnosis)

**Plan** (diagnostic evaluation, follow-up care, teaching)

# STUDENT COMPETENCY CHECKLIST

## Teaching Breast Self-Examination (BSE)

| | S | U | Comments |
|---|---|---|---|
| A. Cognitive | | | |
| 1. Explain the following: | | | |
| a. Why breasts are examined | | | |
| (1) in the shower. | | | |
| (2) before a mirror. | | | |
| (3) supine with pillow under side of breast being examined. | | | |
| b. Who should do breast examination | | | |
| c. Frequency options of breast examination | | | |
| d. Best time of the month to do breast examination and rationale | | | |
| 2. State the area of breast where most lumps are found. | | | |
| 3. Give two reasons a person may not report significant findings to the health care provider. | | | |
| B. Performance | | | |
| 1. Explains to woman need for BSE | | | |
| 2. Instructs woman on technique of BSE by: | | | |
| a. inspecting and bilaterally comparing breasts in front of mirror. | | | |
| b. noting new or unusual rash or redness on skin and areola. | | | |
| c. palpating breast in a systemic manner, using pads of three fingers and with woman's arm raised overhead. | | | |
| d. palpating tail of Spence and axilla. | | | |
| e. gently compressing nipples. | | | |
| 3. Instructs woman to report unusual findings to the health professional at once | | | |
| 4. Asks woman to do return demonstration | | | |

# NOTES

# CHAPTER
# 19

# Thorax and Lungs

## PURPOSE

This chapter helps you learn the structure and function of the thorax and lungs, understand the methods of examination of the respiratory system, identify lung sounds that are normal, describe the characteristics of adventitious lung sounds, and accurately record the assessment. At the end of this unit you will be able to perform a complete physical examination of the respiratory system.

## READING ASSIGNMENT

Jarvis: *Physical Examination and Health Assessment*, 8th ed., Chapter 19, pp. 405-450.

Suggested readings:
Durham, C. O., Fowler, T., Smith, W., et al. (2017). Adult asthma: diagnosis and treatment. *Nurse Pract,* *42*(11), 16-25.
Jain, S., Self, W. H., Wunderink, R. G., et al. (2015). Community-acquired pneumonia requiring hospitalization among U.S. adults. *N Engl J Med, 373*(5), 415-426.

## GLOSSARY

Study the following terms after completing the reading assignment. You should be able to cover the definition on the right and define the term out loud.

**Alveoli** . . . . . . . . . . . . . . . . . . . . functional units of the lung; the thin-walled chambers surrounded by networks of capillaries that are the site of respiratory exchange of carbon dioxide and oxygen

**Angle of Louis** . . . . . . . . . . . . . manubriosternal angle, the articulation of the manubrium and body of the sternum, continuous with the second rib

**Apnea** . . . . . . . . . . . . . . . . . . . . . . cessation of breathing

**Asthma** . . . . . . . . . . . . . . . . . . . . an abnormal respiratory condition associated with allergic hypersensitivity to certain inhaled allergens, characterized by inflammation, bronchospasm, wheezing, and dyspnea

**Atelectasis** . . . . . . . . . . . . . . . . . an abnormal respiratory condition characterized by collapsed, shrunken, deflated sections of alveoli

**Bradypnea** . . . . . . . . . . . . . . . . . slow breathing, fewer than 10 breaths per minute, regular rate

**Bronchiole** . . . . . . . . . . . . . . . one of the smaller respiratory passageways into which the segmental bronchi divide

**Bronchitis** . . . . . . . . . . . . . . . . inflammation of the bronchi with partial obstruction of bronchi due to excessive mucus secretion

**Bronchophony** . . . . . . . . . . . . . the spoken voice sound heard through the stethoscope, which sounds soft, muffled, and indistinct over normal lung tissue

**Bronchovesicular** . . . . . . . . . . . the normal breath sound heard over major bronchi, characterized by moderate pitch and an equal duration of inspiration and expiration

**Chronic obstructive
pulmonary disease (COPD)** . . . a functional category of abnormal respiratory conditions characterized by airflow obstruction (e.g., emphysema, chronic bronchitis)

**Cilia** . . . . . . . . . . . . . . . . . . . . . millions of hairlike cells lining the tracheobronchial tree

**Consolidation** . . . . . . . . . . . . . . the solidification of portions of lung tissue as it fills up with infectious exudate, as in pneumonia

**Crackles** . . . . . . . . . . . . . . . . . . (rales) abnormal, discontinuous, adventitious lung sounds heard on inspiration

**Crepitus** . . . . . . . . . . . . . . . . . . coarse, crackling sensation palpable over the skin when air abnormally escapes from the lung and enters the subcutaneous tissue

**Dead space** . . . . . . . . . . . . . . . . passageways that transport air but are not available for gaseous exchange (e.g., trachea, bronchi)

**Dyspnea** . . . . . . . . . . . . . . . . . . difficult, labored breathing

**Emphysema** . . . . . . . . . . . . . . . . chronic obstructive pulmonary disease characterized by enlargement of alveoli distal to terminal bronchioles

**Fissure** . . . . . . . . . . . . . . . . . . . . the narrow crack dividing the lobes of the lungs

**Fremitus** . . . . . . . . . . . . . . . . . . a palpable vibration from the spoken voice felt over the chest wall

**Friction rub** . . . . . . . . . . . . . . . a coarse, grating, adventitious lung sound heard when the pleurae are inflamed

**Hypercapnia** . . . . . . . . . . . . . . . (hypercarbia) increased levels of carbon dioxide in the blood

**Hyperventilation** . . . . . . . . . . . increased rate and depth of breathing

**Hypoxemia** . . . . . . . . . . . . . . . . decreased level of oxygen in the blood

**Intercostal space** . . . . . . . . . . . space between the ribs

**Kussmaul respiration** . . . . . . . type of hyperventilation that occurs with diabetic ketoacidosis

**Orthopnea** . . . . . . . . . . . . . . . . ability to breathe easily only in an upright position

**Paroxysmal nocturnal
dyspnea** . . . . . . . . . . . . . . . . . . sudden awakening from sleeping, with shortness of breath

**Percussion** . . . . . . . . . . . . . . . . striking over the chest wall with short, sharp blows of the fingers to determine the size and density of the underlying organ

**Pleural effusion** . . . . . . . . . . . abnormal fluid between the layers of the pleura

**Rhonchi**. . . . . . . . . . . . . . . . . . . low-pitched, musical, snoring, adventitious lung sounds caused by airflow obstruction from secretions

**Tachypnea**. . . . . . . . . . . . . . . . . rapid, shallow breathing; more than 24 breaths per minute

**Vesicular** . . . . . . . . . . . . . . . . . . refers to soft, low-pitched, normal breath sounds heard over peripheral lung fields

**Wheeze**. . . . . . . . . . . . . . . . . . . high-pitched, musical, squeaking adventitious lung sound

**Xiphoid process**. . . . . . . . . . . . sword-shaped lower tip of the sternum

## STUDY GUIDE

After completing the reading assignment and the media assignment, write or draw your answers in the spaces provided.

1. Describe the most important points about the health history for the respiratory system.

2. Describe the pleura and its function.

3. List the structures that compose the respiratory dead space.

4. Summarize the mechanics of respiration.

5. List the elements included in the inspection of the respiratory system.

6. Discuss the significance of a barrel chest.

7. List and describe common thoracic deformities.

8. List and describe 3 types of normal breath sounds.

9. Define 2 types of adventitious breath sounds.

10. The manubriosternal angle is also called _____.

    Why is it a useful landmark?

11. How many degrees is the normal costal angle? _____

12. When comparing the anteroposterior diameter of the chest with the transverse diameter, what is the expected ratio? What is the significance of this?

13. What is the tripod position?

14. List 3 factors that affect the normal intensity of tactile fremitus.

    1. _____

    2. _____

    3. _____

15. During percussion, which sound would you expect to predominate over normal lung tissue?

16. List 5 factors that can cause extraneous noise during auscultation.

    1. _____
    2. _____
    3. _____
    4. _____
    5. _____

17. Describe the 3 types of normal breath sounds.

| Name | Location | Description |
|------|----------|-------------|
| | | |
| | | |
| | | |

Fill in the labels indicated on the following illustration.

© Pat Thomas, 2010

Jarvis, Carolyn: PHYSICAL EXAMINATION AND HEALTH ASSESSMENT: Study Guide and Laboratory Manual, Eighth Edition.

Study the lobes of the lungs and label their landmarks on the following two illustrations.

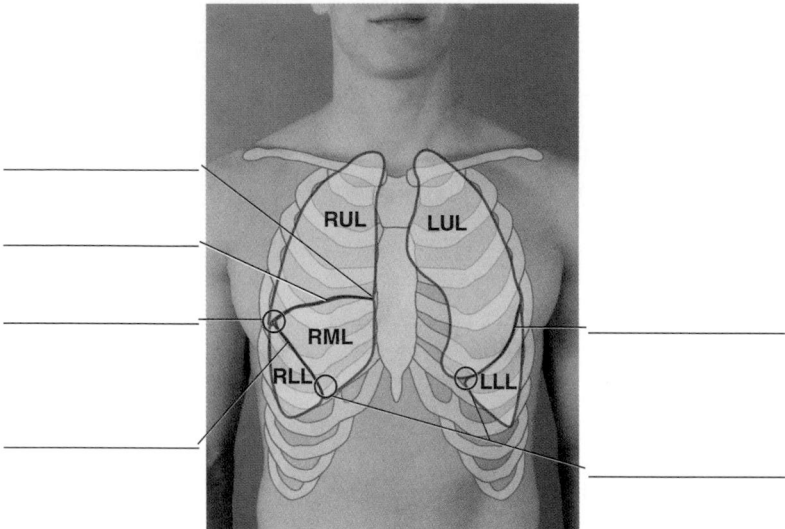

© Pat Thomas, 2010

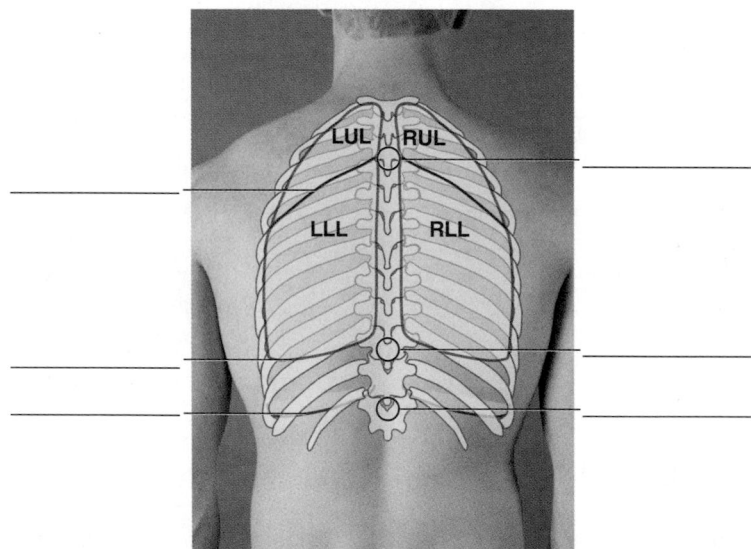

© Pat Thomas, 2010

Label the normal location of the three types of breath sounds on the posterior and anterior chest walls.

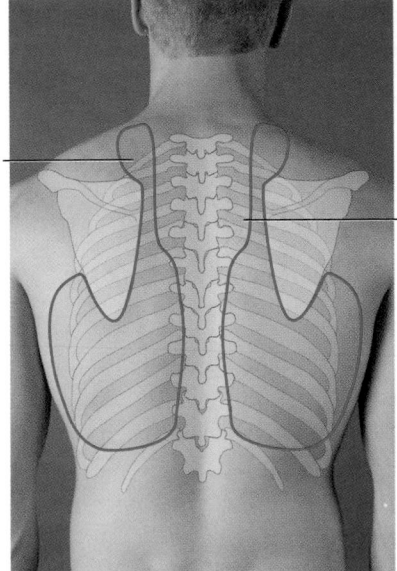

© Pat Thomas, 2010

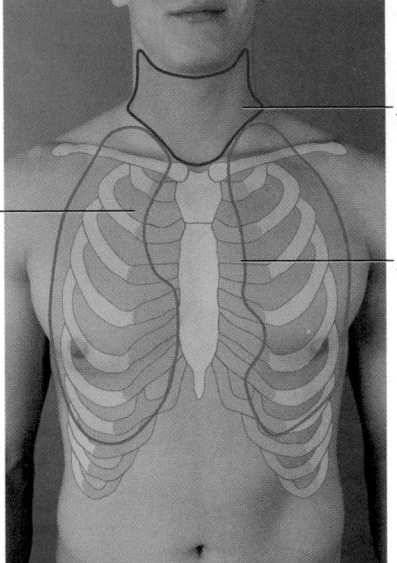

© Pat Thomas, 2010

## REVIEW QUESTIONS

This test is for you to check your own mastery of the content. Answers are provided in Appendix A.

1. The manubriosternal angle is:

   a. The articulation of the manubrium and the body of the sternum.
   b. A hollow, U-shaped depression just above the sternum.
   c. Also known as the *breastbone*.
   d. A term synonymous with costochondral junction.

2. Select the correct description of the left lung.

   a. Narrower than the right lung with three lobes
   b. Narrower than the right lung with two lobes
   c. Wider than the right lung with two lobes
   d. Shorter than the right lung with three lobes

3. You assess a patient who reports a cough. The characteristic timing of the cough of chronic bronchitis is described as:

   a. Continuous throughout the day.
   b. Productive cough for at least 3 months of the year for 2 consecutive years.
   c. Occurring in the afternoon or evening because of exposure to irritants at work.
   d. Occurring in the early morning.

4. Which of the following assessments best confirms symmetric chest expansion?

   a. Placing hands on the posterolateral chest wall with thumbs at the level of T9 or T10 and then sliding the hands up to pinch a small fold of skin between the thumbs
   b. Inspection of the shape and configuration of the chest wall
   c. Placing the palmar surface of the fingers of one hand against the chest and having the person repeat the words "ninety-nine"
   d. Percussion of the posterior chest

5. You are auscultating breath sounds on a patient. Which of the following best describes how to proceed?

   a. Hold the bell of the stethoscope against the chest wall; listen to the entire right field and then the entire left field.
   b. Hold the diaphragm of the stethoscope against the chest wall; listen to one full respiration in each location, being sure to do side-to-side comparisons.
   c. Listen from the apices to the bases of each lung field using the bell of the stethoscope.
   d. Select the bell or diaphragm depending on the quality of sounds heard; listen for one respiration in each location, moving from side to side.

6. Select the best description of bronchovesicular breath sounds.

   a. High-pitched, of longer duration on inspiration than expiration
   b. Moderate-pitched, inspiration equal to expiration
   c. Low-pitched, inspiration greater than expiration
   d. Rustling sound, like the wind in the trees

7. After examining a patient, you note: fever, increased respiratory rate, chest expansion decreased on left side, dull to percussion over left lower lobe, breath sounds louder with fine crackles over left lower lobe. These findings are consistent with:

   a. Bronchitis.
   b. Asthma.
   c. Pleural effusion.
   d. Lobar pneumonia.

8. On examining a patient's nails, you note that the angle of the nail base is >160 degrees and that the nail base feels spongy to palpation. These findings are consistent with:

   a. Acute respiratory distress syndrome.
   b. Normal findings for the nails.
   c. Congenital heart disease and COPD.
   d. Atelectasis.

9. On auscultating a patient, you note a coarse, low-pitched sound during both inspiration and expiration. This patient reports pain with breathing. These findings are consistent with:

   a. Fine crackles.
   b. Wheezes.
   c. Atelectatic crackles.
   d. Pleural friction rub.

10. To use the technique of egophony, ask the patient to:

    a. Take several deep breaths and then hold for 5 seconds.
    b. Say "eeeeee" each time the stethoscope is moved.
    c. Repeat the phrase "ninety-nine" each time the stethoscope is moved.
    d. Whisper a phrase as auscultation is performed.

11. When examining for tactile fremitus, it is important to:

    a. Ask the patient to breathe quickly.
    b. Ask the patient to cough.
    c. Palpate the chest symmetrically.
    d. Use the bell of the stethoscope.

12. Pulse oximetry measures:

    a. Arterial oxygen saturation of hemoglobin.
    b. Venous oxygen saturation of hemoglobin.
    c. Combined saturation of arterial and venous blood.
    d. Carboxyhemoglobin levels.

13. A pleural friction rub is best detected by:

    a. Observation.
    b. Palpation.
    c. Auscultation.
    d. Percussion.

14. A patient has a barrel-shaped chest, characterized by:

    a. Equal anteroposterior transverse diameter and ribs being horizontal.
    b. Anteroposterior transverse diameter of 1:2 and an elliptic shape.
    c. Anteroposterior transverse diameter of 2:1 and ribs being elevated.
    d. Anteroposterior transverse diameter of 3:7 and ribs sloping back.

Match column A to column B.

**Column A: Lung Borders**

15. _____ Apex
16. _____ Base
17. _____ Lateral left
18. _____ Lateral right
19. _____ Posterior apex

**Column B: Location**

a. Rests on the diaphragm
b. C7
c. Sixth rib, midclavicular line
d. Fifth intercostal
e. 3 to 4 cm above the inner third of the clavicles

Match column A to column B.

**Column A: Configurations of the Thorax**

20. _____ Normal chest
21. _____ Barrel chest
22. _____ Pectus excavatum
23. _____ Pectus carinatum
24. _____ Scoliosis
25. _____ Kyphosis

**Column B: Description**

a. Anteroposterior = transverse diameter
b. Exaggerated posterior curvature of thoracic spine
c. Lateral S-shaped curvature of the thoracic and lumbar spines
d. Sunken sternum and adjacent cartilages
e. Elliptic shape with an anteroposterior to transverse diameter in the ratio of 1:2
f. Forward protrusion of the sternum with ribs sloping back at either side

## CRITICAL THINKING EXERCISE

Spend 10 to 15 minutes with the lung sounds simulator in your Skills Laboratory. Or use various websites on the Internet to access audio recordings of healthy lung sounds, as well as adventitious sounds, at various locations over the lungs. One Internet source is *https://www.easyauscultation.com/lung-sounds*.

## SKILLS LABORATORY AND CLINICAL SETTING

The purpose of the clinical component is to practice the regional examination on a peer in the skills laboratory or on a patient in the clinical setting and to achieve the following.

### Clinical Objectives

1. Demonstrate knowledge of the symptoms related to the respiratory system by obtaining a regional health history from a peer or patient.

2. Correctly locate anatomic landmarks on the thorax of a peer.

3. Using a grease pencil, and with peer's permission, draw lobes or landmarks of the lungs on a peer's thorax.

4. Demonstrate correct techniques for inspection, palpation, percussion, and auscultation of the respiratory system.

5. Demonstrate the technique for estimation of diaphragmatic excursion.

6. Record the history and physical examination findings accurately, reach an assessment of the health state, and develop a plan of care.

### Instructions

Gather your equipment. Wash your hands. Clean the stethoscope endpiece with an alcohol wipe. Practice the steps of the examination of the thorax and lungs on a peer or on a patient in the clinical area. Record your findings using the regional write-up sheet. The front of the sheet is intended as a worksheet; the back of the sheet is intended for a narrative summary using the SOAP format.

# REGIONAL WRITE-UP—THORAX AND LUNGS

Date _____

Examiner _____

**Patient** _____ Age _____ Gender _____

**Reason for visit** _____

## I. Health History

| | No | Yes, explain |
|---|---|---|
| 1. Do you have a **cough?** | _____ | _____ |
| 2. Any shortness of **breath?** | _____ | _____ |
| 3. Any **chest pain** with breathing? | _____ | _____ |
| 4. Any **past history** of lung diseases? | _____ | _____ |
| 5. Ever **smoke** cigarettes? What age did you start? How many per day? For how long? Ever tried to quit? | _____ | _____ |
| 6. Any living or work conditions that affect your breathing? | _____ | _____ |
| 7. Last TB skin test, chest radiography, flu vaccine? | _____ | _____ |

## II. Physical Examination

### A. Inspection

1. Thoracic cage _____ Any deformity? _____
2. Respiratory rate and pattern _____ Use accessory muscles? _____
3. Skin and nails _____
4. Person's position _____
5. Person's facial expression _____
6. Level of consciousness _____

### B. Palpation

1. Confirm symmetric chest expansion _____
2. Tactile fremitus _____
3. Skin temperature and moisture _____
4. Detect any lumps, masses, tenderness _____
5. Trachea _____

### C. Percussion

1. Determine percussion note that predominates over lung fields _____

### D. Auscultation

1. Listen: posterior, lateral, anterior _____
2. Any abnormal breath sounds? _____
   If so, perform bronchophony _____
   Whispered pectoriloquy _____,
   Egophony _____
3. Any adventitious sounds? _____

## REGIONAL WRITE-UP—THORAX AND LUNGS

Summarize your findings using the SOAP format.

**Subjective** (reason for seeking care, health history)

**Objective** (physical examination findings)     Use the drawing to record your findings.

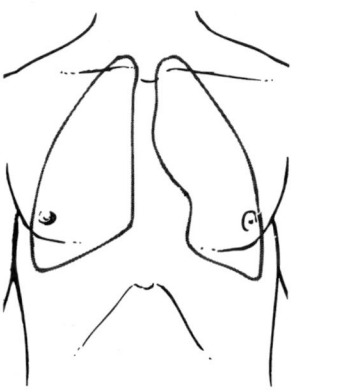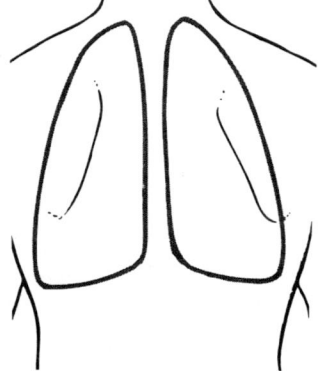

**Assessment** (assessment of health state or problem, diagnosis)

**Plan** (diagnostic evaluation, follow-up care, teaching)

# CHAPTER 20

# Heart and Neck Vessels

## PURPOSE

This chapter helps you learn the structure and function of the heart, valves, and great vessels, understand the cardiac cycle, describe the heart sounds, understand the rationale and methods of examination of the heart, and accurately record the assessment. At the end of this chapter you should be able to perform a complete assessment of the heart and neck vessels.

## READING ASSIGNMENT

Jarvis: *Physical Examination and Health Assessment,* 8th ed., Chapter 20, pp. 451-500.

Suggested readings:
Campo, D. L. (2016). Recognizing myocardial infarction in women. *Am J Nurs, 116*(9), 46-49.
Melnyk, B. M., Orosilini, L., Gawlik, K., et al. (2016). The Million Hearts initiative: guidelines and best practices. *Nurse Pract, 41*(2), 46-53.

## GLOSSARY

Study the following terms after completing the reading assignment. You should be able to cover the definition on the right and define the term out loud.

**Angina pectoris** . . . . . . . . . . . . . acute chest pain that occurs when myocardial demand exceeds its oxygen supply

**Aortic regurgitation** . . . . . . . . (aortic insufficiency) incompetent aortic valve that allows backward flow of blood into left ventricle during diastole

**Aortic stenosis** . . . . . . . . . . . . . . calcification of aortic valve cusps that restricts forward flow of blood during systole

**Aortic valve** . . . . . . . . . . . . . . . . . the left semilunar valve separating the left ventricle and the aorta

**Apex of the heart** . . . . . . . . . . . tip of the heart pointing down toward the 5th left intercostal space

**Apical impulse** . . . . . . . . . . . . . . point of maximal impulse (PMI); pulsation created as the left ventricle rotates against the chest wall during systole, normally at the 5th left intercostal space in the midclavicular line

**Base of the heart** . . . . . . . . . . . broader area of heart's outline located at the 3rd right and left intercostal spaces

**Bell (of the stethoscope)**...... cup-shaped endpiece used for soft, low-pitched heart sounds

**Bradycardia**............... slow heart rate, less than 50 beats per minute in the adult

**Clubbing** ................... bulbous enlargement of distal phalanges of fingers and toes that occurs with chronic cyanotic heart and lung conditions

**Coarctation of aorta** ........ severe narrowing of the descending aorta, a congenital heart defect

**Cor pulmonale**............. right ventricular hypertrophy and heart failure due to pulmonary hypertension

**Cyanosis**................... dusky blue mottling of the skin and mucous membranes due to excessive amount of reduced hemoglobin in the blood

**Diaphragm (of the stethoscope)**......... flat endpiece of the stethoscope used for hearing relatively high-pitched heart sounds

**Diastole** ................... the heart's filling phase

**Dyspnea**................... difficult, labored breathing

**Edema** ................... swelling of legs or dependent body part due to increased interstitial fluid

**Erb's point**................ traditional auscultatory area in the 3rd left intercostal space

**First heart sound (S$_1$)** ........ occurs with closure of the atrioventricular valves signaling the beginning of systole

**Fourth heart sound (S$_4$)** ...... S$_4$ gallop, atrial gallop; very soft, low-pitched ventricular filling sound that occurs in late diastole

**Gallop rhythm** ............. the addition of a 3rd or a 4th heart sound; makes the rhythm sound like the cadence of a galloping horse

**Inching** ................... technique of moving the stethoscope incrementally across the precordium through the auscultatory areas while listening to the heart sounds

**Left ventricular hypertrophy (LVH)** ......... increase in thickness of myocardial wall that occurs when the heart pumps against chronic outflow obstruction (e.g., aortic stenosis)

**Midclavicular line (MCL)**..... imaginary vertical line bisecting the middle of the clavicle in each hemithorax

**Mitral regurgitation** ........ mitral insufficiency; incompetent mitral valve allows regurgitation of blood back into left atrium during systole

**Mitral stenosis** ............. calcified mitral valve impedes forward flow of blood into left ventricle during diastole

**Mitral valve**................ left atrioventricular valve separating the left atrium and ventricle

**Palpitation** ................ uncomfortable awareness of rapid or irregular heart rate

**Paradoxical splitting**........ opposite of a normal split S$_2$ so that the split is heard in expiration, and in inspiration the sounds fuse to one sound

**Pericardial friction rub** ...... high-pitched, scratchy extracardiac sound heard when the precordium is inflamed

Jarvis, Carolyn: PHYSICAL EXAMINATION AND HEALTH ASSESSMENT: Study Guide and Laboratory Manual, Eighth Edition.
Copyright © 2020, 2016, 2012, 2008, 2004, 2000, 1996 by Elsevier Inc. All rights reserved.

**Physiologic splitting**........normal variation in $S_2$ heard as two separate components during inspiration

**Precordium**.................area of the chest wall overlying the heart and great vessels

**Pulmonic regurgitation**......pulmonic insufficiency; backflow of blood through incompetent pulmonic valve into the right ventricle

**Pulmonic stenosis**...........calcification of pulmonic valve that restricts forward flow of blood during systole

**Pulmonic valve**..............right semilunar valve separating the right ventricle and pulmonary artery

**Second heart sound ($S_2$)**......occurs with closure of the semilunar valves, aortic and pulmonic; signals the end of systole

**Summation gallop**...........abnormal mid-diastolic heart sound heard when both the pathologic $S_3$ and $S_4$ are present

**Syncope**....................temporary loss of consciousness due to decreased cerebral blood flow (fainting); caused by ventricular asystole, pronounced bradycardia, or ventricular fibrillation

**Systole** .....................the heart's pumping phase

**Tachycardia**.................rapid heart rate, greater than 95 beats per minute in the adult

**Third heart sound ($S_3$)** .......soft, low-pitched ventricular filling sound that occurs in early diastole ($S_3$ gallop) and may be an early sign of heart failure

**Thrill** ......................palpable vibration on the chest wall accompanying severe heart murmur

**Tricuspid valve**..............right atrioventricular valve separating the right atrium and ventricle

## STUDY GUIDE

After completing the reading assignment and the media assignment, write or draw the answers in the spaces provided.

1. Define the apical impulse and describe its normal location, size, and duration.

Which *abnormal* conditions may affect the location of the apical impulse?

2. Explain the mechanism producing normal first and second heart sounds.

3. Describe the effect of respiration on the heart sounds.

4. Describe the characteristics of the **first heart sound** and its intensity at the apex of the heart and at the base.

5. Describe the characteristics of the **second heart sound** and its intensity at the apex of the heart and at the base.

6. Explain the physiologic mechanism for normal splitting of $S_2$ in the pulmonic valve area.

7. Define the **third heart sound.** When in the cardiac cycle does it occur? Describe its intensity, quality, location in which it is heard, and method of auscultation.

8. Differentiate a physiologic $S_3$ from a pathologic $S_3$.

9. Define the **fourth heart sound.** When in the cardiac cycle does it occur? Describe its intensity, quality, location in which it is heard, and method of auscultation.

10. Explain the position of the valves during the cardiac cycle in diastole, isometric contraction, systole, and isometric relaxation.

11. Define venous pressure and jugular venous pulse.

12. Differentiate between carotid artery pulsation and jugular vein pulsation.

13. List the major risk factors for heart disease and stroke as identified in this text.

14. Define bruit, and discuss what it indicates.

15. State 4 guidelines to distinguish $S_1$ from $S_2$.

    1. _____
    2. _____
    3. _____
    4. _____

16. Define pulse deficit, and discuss what it indicates.

17. Define preload and afterload.

18. List the characteristics to explore when you hear a murmur, including the grading scale of murmurs.

19. Discuss the characteristics of an innocent or functional murmur.

Fill in the labels indicated on the following illustrations.

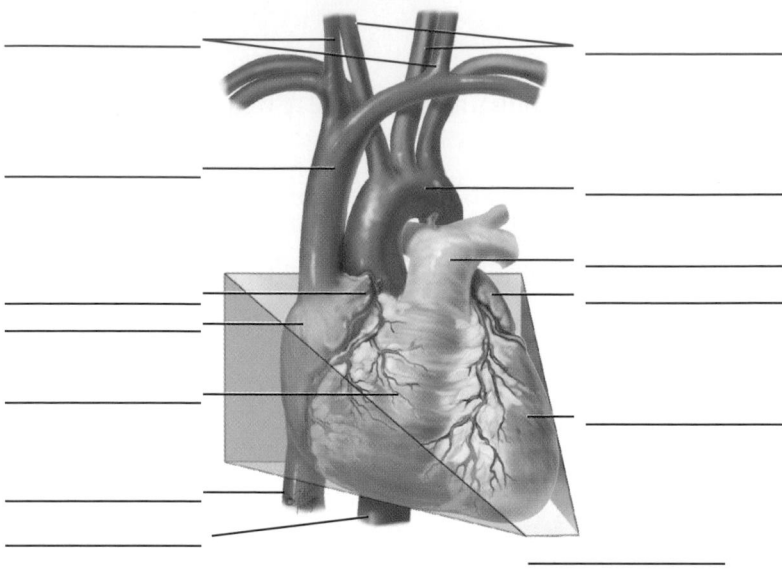

© Pat Thomas, 2006

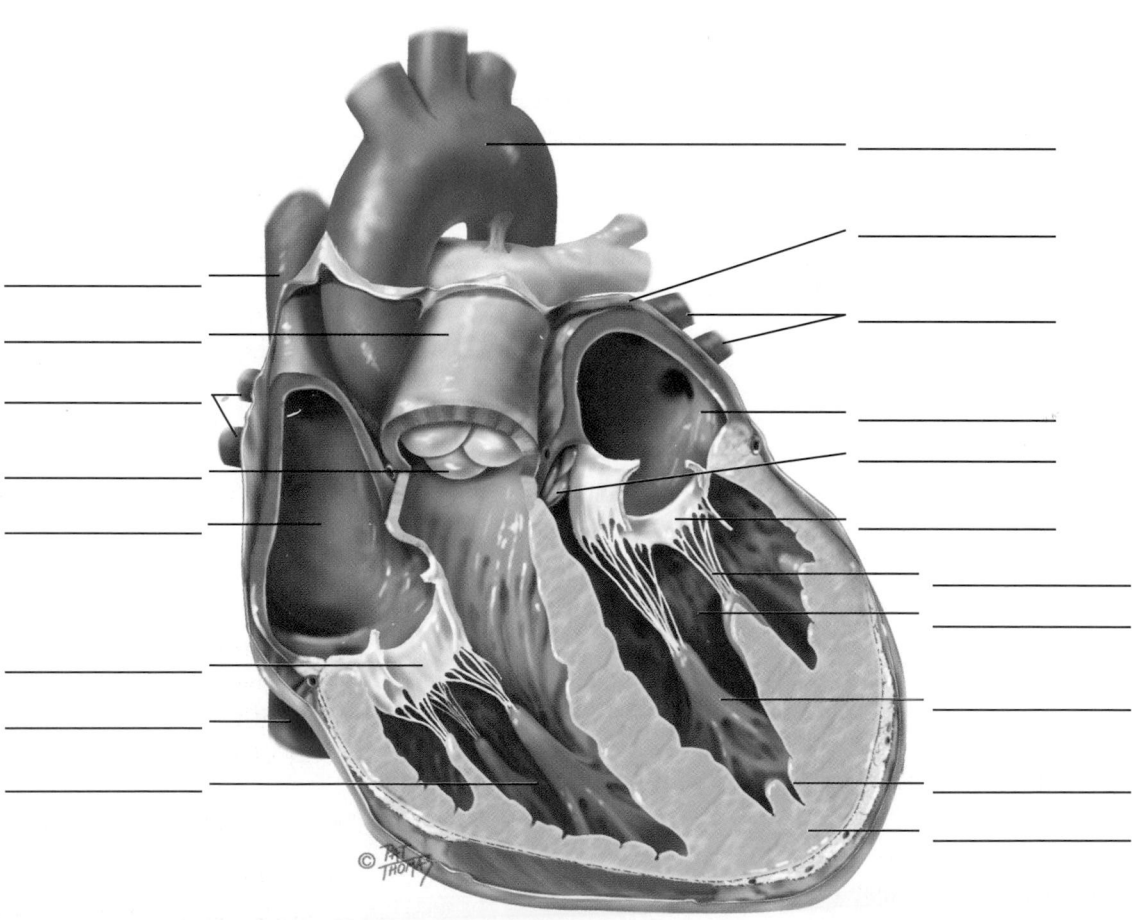

© Pat Thomas, 2010

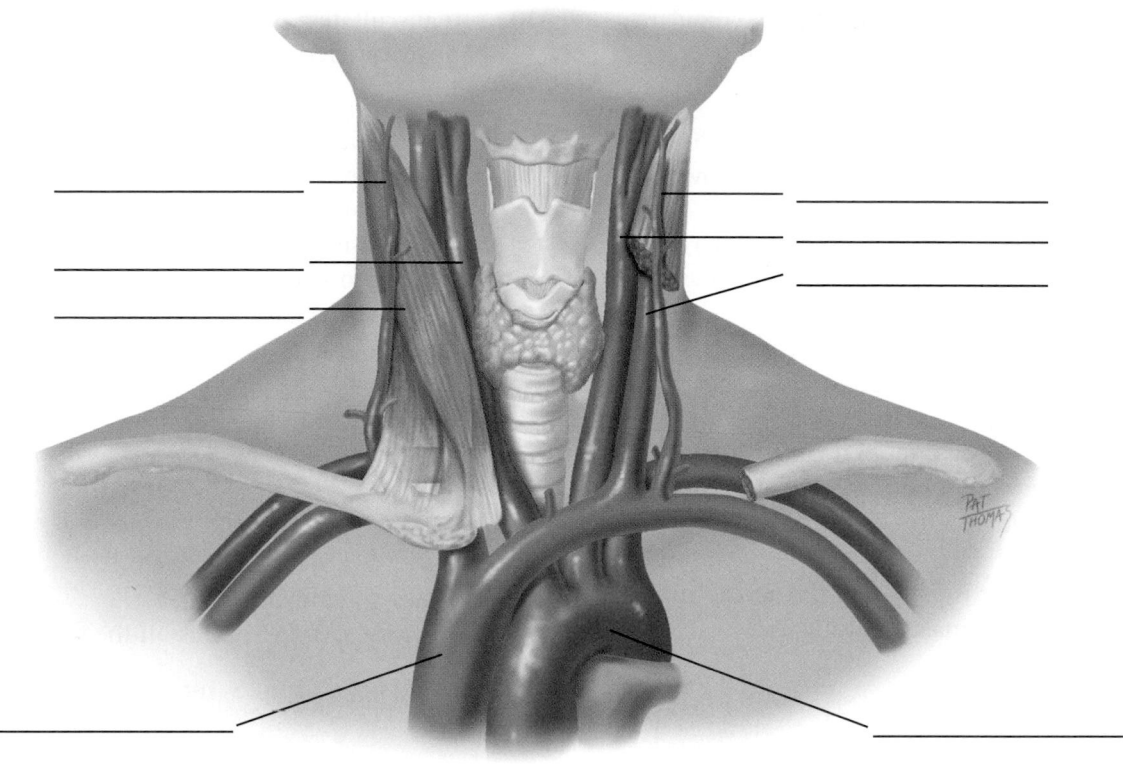

© Pat Thomas, 2010

## REVIEW QUESTIONS

This test is for you to check your own mastery of the content. Answers are provided in Appendix A.

1. The precordium is:

   a. A synonym for the mediastinum.
   b. The area on the chest where the apical impulse is felt.
   c. The area on the anterior chest overlying the heart and great vessels.
   d. A synonym for the area where the superior and inferior venae cavae return unoxygenated venous blood to the right side of the heart.

2. Select the best description of the tricuspid valve.

   a. Left semilunar valve
   b. Right atrioventricular valve
   c. Left atrioventricular valve
   d. Right semilunar valve

3. The function of the pulmonic valve is to:

   a. Divide the left atrium and left ventricle.
   b. Guard the opening between the right atrium and right ventricle.
   c. Protect the orifice between the right ventricle and the pulmonary artery.
   d. Guard the entrance to the aorta from the left ventricle.

4. Atrial systole occurs:

   a. During ventricular systole.
   b. During ventricular diastole.
   c. Concurrently with ventricular systole.
   d. Independently of ventricular function.

5. The second heart sound is the result of:

   a. Opening of the mitral and tricuspid valves.
   b. Closing of the mitral and tricuspid valves.
   c. Opening of the aortic and pulmonic valves.
   d. Closing of the aortic and pulmonic valves.

6. The examiner is has estimated the jugular venous pressure. Identify the finding that is abnormal.

   a. Patient elevated to 30 degrees, internal jugular vein pulsation at 1 cm above sternal angle
   b. Patient elevated to 30 degrees, internal jugular vein pulsation at 2 cm above sternal angle
   c. Patient elevated to 40 degrees, internal jugular vein pulsation at 1 cm above sternal angle
   d. Patient elevated to 45 degrees, internal jugular vein pulsation at 4 cm above sternal angle

7. The examiner is palpating the apical impulse. Which is a normal-sized impulse?

   a. Less than 1 cm
   b. Approximately $1 \times 2$ cm
   c. 3 cm
   d. Varies depending on the size of the person

8. The nurse auscultates the pulmonic valve area in which region?

   a. Second right interspace
   b. Second left interspace
   c. Left lower sternal border
   d. Fifth interspace, left midclavicular line

9. Which description would differentiate a split $S_2$ from $S_3$?

   a. $S_3$ is lower pitched and is heard at the apex.
   b. $S_2$ is heard at the left lower sternal border.
   c. The timing of $S_2$ varies with respirations.
   d. $S_3$ is heard at the base; the timing varies with respirations.

10. You auscultate a patient to rule out a pericardial friction rub. Which assessment technique is most appropriate?

    a. Listen with the diaphragm, patient sitting up and leaning forward, breath held in expiration.
    b. Listen using the bell with the patient leaning forward.
    c. Listen at the base during normal respiration.
    d. Listen with the diaphragm, patient turned to the left side.

11. When auscultating the heart, your first step is to:

    a. Identify $S_1$ and $S_2$.
    b. Listen for $S_3$ and $S_4$.
    c. Listen for murmurs.
    d. Identify all four sounds on the first round.

12. You will hear a split $S_2$ most clearly in which area?

    a. Apical
    b. Pulmonic
    c. Tricuspid
    d. Aortic

13. The stethoscope bell should be pressed lightly against the skin so that:

    a. Chest hair doesn't simulate crackles.
    b. High-pitched sounds can be heard better.
    c. The bell does not act as a diaphragm.
    d. The bell does not interfere with amplification of heart sounds.

14. A murmur is heard after $S_1$ and before $S_2$. This murmur would be classified as:

    a. Diastolic (possibly benign).
    b. Diastolic (always pathologic).
    c. Systolic (possibly benign).
    d. Systolic (always pathologic).

15. When assessing the carotid artery, the nurse should palpate:

   a. Bilaterally at the same time while standing behind the patient.
   b. Medial to the sternomastoid muscle, one side at a time.
   c. For a bruit while asking the patient to hold his or her breath briefly.
   d. For unilateral distention while turning the patient's head to one side.

16. Fill in the blanks.

   $S_1$ is best heard at the _____ of the heart, whereas $S_2$ is loudest at the _____ of the heart. $S_1$ coincides with the pulse in the _____ and coincides with the _____ wave if the patient is on an ECG monitor.

Match column A to column B

**Column A**

17. _____ Tough, fibrous, double-walled sac that surrounds and protects the heart
18. _____ Thin layer of endothelial tissue that lines the inner surface of the heart chambers and valves
19. _____ Reservoir for holding blood
20. _____ Ensures smooth, friction-free movement of the heart muscle
21. _____ Muscular pumping chamber
22. _____ Muscular wall of the heart

**Column B**

a. Pericardial fluid
b. Ventricle
c. Endocardium
d. Myocardium
e. Pericardium
f. Atrium

## CRITICAL THINKING EXERCISE

Calculate 10-year and long-term cardiovascular disease risk.
First try these online calculators yourself, and then interview a man older than 40 years and a woman older than 40 years, perhaps members of your family. Consider the multiple traditional cardiovascular risk factors for asymptomatic adults without a clinical history of cardiovascular disease. Obtain a global risk score using the tools given below, which are based on Framingham data.
- Framingham 10-year and 30-year risk calculator:
   http://www.framinghamheartstudy.org/risk/hrdcoronary.html
      http://www.globalrph.com/10_year_risk.htm
- Stroke risk calculator (Cleveland Clinic):
   http://my.clevelandclinic.org/p2/stroke-risk-calculator.aspx
- Or, use the printed version given on the next page.

## Men

### Estimate of 10-Year Risk for Men
(Framingham Point Scores)

| Age | Points |
|-----|--------|
| 20-34 | -9 |
| 35-39 | -4 |
| 40-44 | 0 |
| 45-49 | 3 |
| 50-54 | 6 |
| 55-59 | 8 |
| 60-64 | 10 |
| 65-69 | 11 |
| 70-74 | 12 |
| 75-79 | 13 |

| Total Cholesterol | Points | | | | |
|------|---------|---------|---------|---------|---------|
|  | Age 20-39 | Age 40-49 | Age 50-59 | Age 60-69 | Age 70-79 |
| <160 | 0 | 0 | 0 | 0 | 0 |
| 160-199 | 4 | 3 | 2 | 1 | 0 |
| 200-239 | 7 | 5 | 3 | 1 | 0 |
| 240-279 | 9 | 6 | 4 | 2 | 1 |
| ≥280 | 11 | 8 | 5 | 3 | 1 |

| | Points | | | | |
|------|---------|---------|---------|---------|---------|
|  | Age 20-39 | Age 40-49 | Age 50-59 | Age 60-69 | Age 70-79 |
| Nonsmoker | 0 | 0 | 0 | 0 | 0 |
| Smoker | 8 | 5 | 3 | 1 | 1 |

| HDL (mg/dL) | Points |
|-----|--------|
| ≥60 | -1 |
| 50-59 | 0 |
| 40-49 | 1 |
| <40 | 2 |

| Systolic BP (mm Hg) | If Untreated | If Treated |
|------|------|------|
| <120 | 0 | 0 |
| 120-129 | 0 | 1 |
| 130-139 | 1 | 2 |
| 140-159 | 1 | 2 |
| ≥160 | 2 | 3 |

| Point Total | 10-Year Risk % |
|------|------|
| <0 | < 1 |
| 0 | 1 |
| 1 | 1 |
| 2 | 1 |
| 3 | 1 |
| 4 | 1 |
| 5 | 2 |
| 6 | 2 |
| 7 | 3 |
| 8 | 4 |
| 9 | 5 |
| 10 | 6 |
| 11 | 8 |
| 12 | 10 |
| 13 | 12 |
| 14 | 16 |
| 15 | 20 |
| 16 | 25 |
| ≥17 | ≥ 30 |

**10-Year risk _____ %**

## Women

### Estimate of 10-Year Risk for Women
(Framingham Point Scores)

| Age | Points |
|-----|--------|
| 20-34 | -7 |
| 35-39 | -3 |
| 40-44 | 0 |
| 45-49 | 3 |
| 50-54 | 6 |
| 55-59 | 8 |
| 60-64 | 10 |
| 65-69 | 12 |
| 70-74 | 14 |
| 75-79 | 16 |

| Total Cholesterol | Points | | | | |
|------|---------|---------|---------|---------|---------|
|  | Age 20-39 | Age 40-49 | Age 50-59 | Age 60-69 | Age 70-79 |
| <160 | 0 | 0 | 0 | 0 | 0 |
| 160-199 | 4 | 3 | 2 | 1 | 1 |
| 200-239 | 8 | 6 | 4 | 2 | 1 |
| 240-279 | 11 | 8 | 5 | 3 | 2 |
| ≥280 | 13 | 10 | 7 | 4 | 2 |

| | Points | | | | |
|------|---------|---------|---------|---------|---------|
|  | Age 20-39 | Age 40-49 | Age 50-59 | Age 60-69 | Age 70-79 |
| Nonsmoker | 0 | 0 | 0 | 0 | 0 |
| Smoker | 9 | 7 | 4 | 2 | 1 |

| HDL (mg/dL) | Points |
|-----|--------|
| ≥60 | -1 |
| 50-59 | 0 |
| 40-49 | 1 |
| <40 | 2 |

| Systolic BP (mm Hg) | If Untreated | If Treated |
|------|------|------|
| <120 | 0 | 0 |
| 120-129 | 1 | 3 |
| 130-139 | 2 | 4 |
| 140-159 | 3 | 5 |
| ≥160 | 4 | 6 |

| Point Total | 10-Year Risk % |
|------|------|
| < 9 | < 1 |
| 9 | 1 |
| 10 | 1 |
| 11 | 1 |
| 12 | 1 |
| 13 | 2 |
| 14 | 2 |
| 15 | 3 |
| 16 | 4 |
| 17 | 5 |
| 18 | 6 |
| 19 | 8 |
| 20 | 11 |
| 21 | 14 |
| 22 | 17 |
| 23 | 22 |
| 24 | 27 |
| ≥25 | ≥ 30 |

**10-Year risk _____ %**

U.S. DEPARTMENT OF HEALTH AND HUMAN SERVICES
Public Health Service
National Institutes of Health
National Heart, Lung, and Blood Institute

NIH Publication No. 01-3305
May 2001

## SKILLS LABORATORY AND CLINICAL SETTING

The purpose of the clinical component is to practice the regional examination on a peer in the skills laboratory or on a patient in the clinical setting to achieve the following.

### Clinical Objectives

1. Demonstrate knowledge of cardiovascular symptoms by obtaining a regional health history from a peer or patient.

2. Correctly locate anatomic landmarks on the chest wall of a peer.

3. Using a grease pencil, and with peer's permission, outline borders of the heart and label auscultatory areas on a peer's chest wall.

4. Demonstrate correct technique for inspection and palpation of the neck vessels.

5. Demonstrate correct techniques for inspection, palpation, and auscultation of the precordium.

6. Record the history and physical examination findings accurately, reach an assessment of the health state, and develop a plan of care.

### Instructions

Gather your equipment. Wash your hands. Clean the stethoscope endpiece with an alcohol wipe. Practice the steps of the examination of the cardiovascular system on a peer or on a patient in the clinical area. Record your findings using the regional write-up sheet that follows. The front of the page is intended as a worksheet; the back of the page is intended for your narrative recording using the SOAP format.

**NOTES**

# REGIONAL WRITE-UP—CARDIOVASCULAR SYSTEM

Date _____

Examiner _____

Patient _____ Age _____ Gender _____

Reason for visit _____

I. **Health History**

| | No | Yes, explain |
|---|---|---|
| 1. Any **chest pain** or tightness? | | |
| 2. Any **shortness of breath**? | | |
| 3. Use more than one pillow to sleep? | | |
| 4. Do you have a **cough**? | | |
| 5. Do you seem to **tire easily**? | | |
| 6. Facial skin ever turn blue or ashen? | | |
| 7. Any **swelling** of feet or legs? | | |
| 8. Awaken at night to urinate? | | |
| 9. Any past history of heart disease? | | |
| 10. Any family history of heart disease? | | |
| 11. Any change in usual daily activities? | | |
| 12. Current medications? | | |
| 13. Smoking? How many per day? Alcohol use? Number of drinks per day? | | |

14. Assess cardiac risk factors: diabetes, hypertension, smoking, high cholesterol, obesity, sedentary lifestyle, age _____

II. **Physical Examination**

A. **Carotid arteries**

Palpate R _____ L _____
(absent, weak, moderate, bounding)

B. **Jugular venous system**

External jugular veins (circle one):
- collapsed supine
- meniscus visible at _____ bed elevated

Internal jugular venous pulsations:
- not visible
- visible at _____ bed elevated

C. **Precordium—inspect and palpate.**

1. Skin color and condition _____
2. Chest wall pulsations _____
3. Heave or lift _____
4. Apical impulse in the _____ at _____
   Size _____

D. **Auscultation**

1. Identify anatomic areas where you will listen.
2. Rate and rhythm _____
3. Identify $S_1$ and $S_2$ in diagram at right and note any variation.
   Fill in any murmur below:

   $S_1$     $S_2$     $S_1$     $S_2$
   $S_1$ _____
   $S_2$ _____

4. Listen in systole and diastole:
Extra heart sounds _____
Systolic murmur _____
Diastolic murmur _____

## REGIONAL WRITE-UP—CARDIOVASCULAR SYSTEM

Summarize your findings using the SOAP format.

**Subjective** (reason for seeking care, health history)

**Objective** (physical examination findings)

Record findings using diagram.

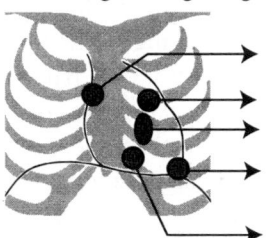

**Assessment** (assessment of health state or problem, diagnosis)

**Plan** (diagnostic evaluation, follow-up care, patient teaching)

# Peripheral Vascular System and Lymphatic System

## PURPOSE

This chapter helps you learn the structure and function of the peripheral vascular system and the lymphatic system; locate the peripheral pulse sites; understand the rationale and methods of examination of the peripheral vascular and lymphatic systems; and accurately record the assessment. At the end of this chapter you should be able to perform a complete assessment of the peripheral vascular and lymphatic systems.

## READING ASSIGNMENT

Jarvis: *Physical Examination and Health Assessment,* 8th ed., Chapter 21, pp. 501-528.

Suggested readings:
Kullo, I. J., & Rooke, T. W. (2016). Peripheral artery disease. *N Engl J Med, 374*(9), 861-870.
Roberts, S. H., & Lawrence, S. M. (2017). Venous thromboembolism. *Am J Nurs, 117*(5), 38-48.

## GLOSSARY

Study the following terms after completing the reading assignment. You should be able to cover the definition on the right and define the term out loud.

**Allen test** . . . . . . . . . . . . . . . . . . test that determines the patency of the radial and ulnar arteries by compressing one artery site and observing return of skin color as evidence of patency of the other artery

**Aneurysm** . . . . . . . . . . . . . . . . . defect or sac formed by dilation in artery wall due to atherosclerosis, trauma, or congenital defect

**Arrhythmia** . . . . . . . . . . . . . . . variation from the heart's regular rhythm

**Arteriosclerosis** . . . . . . . . . . . . thickening and loss of elasticity of the arterial walls

**Atherosclerosis** . . . . . . . . . . . . . plaques of fatty deposits formed in the inner layer (intima) of the arteries

**Bradycardia** . . . . . . . . . . . . . . . . slow heart rate, less than 50 beats per minute in the adult

**Bruit** . . . . . . . . . . . . . . . . . . . . . . blowing, swooshing sound heard through a stethoscope when an artery is partially occluded

**Cyanosis**. . . . . . . . . . . . . . . . . . dusky blue mottling of the skin and mucous membranes due to excessive amount of reduced hemoglobin in the blood

**Diastole** . . . . . . . . . . . . . . . . . . the heart's filling phase

**Ischemia** . . . . . . . . . . . . . . . . . deficiency of arterial blood to a body part due to constriction or obstruction of a blood vessel

**Lymph nodes** . . . . . . . . . . . . . . small oval clumps of lymphatic tissue located at grouped intervals along lymphatic vessels

**Lymphedema** . . . . . . . . . . . . . . swelling of extremity due to obstructed lymph channel, nonpitting

**Pitting edema**. . . . . . . . . . . . . . indentation left after examiner depresses the skin over swollen edematous tissue

**Profile sign** . . . . . . . . . . . . . . . viewing the finger from the side to detect early clubbing

**Pulse**. . . . . . . . . . . . . . . . . . . . . pressure wave created by each heartbeat, palpable at body sites where the artery lies close to the skin and over a bone

**Pulsus alternans**. . . . . . . . . . . . regular rhythm, but force of pulse varies with alternating beats of large and small amplitude

**Pulsus bigeminus**. . . . . . . . . . . irregular rhythm; every other beat is premature; premature beats have weakened amplitude

**Pulsus paradoxus**. . . . . . . . . . . beats have weaker amplitude with respiratory inspiration, stronger with expiration

**Systole** . . . . . . . . . . . . . . . . . . . the heart's pumping phase

**Tachycardia**. . . . . . . . . . . . . . . rapid heart rate, more than 95 beats per minute in the adult

**Thrombophlebitis** . . . . . . . . . . inflammation of the vein associated with thrombus formation

**Ulcer**. . . . . . . . . . . . . . . . . . . . . open skin lesion extending into dermis, with sloughing of necrotic inflammatory tissue

**Varicose veins**. . . . . . . . . . . . . . dilated tortuous veins with incompetent valves

## STUDY GUIDE

After completing the reading assignment and the media assignment, write or draw the answers in the spaces provided.

1. Describe the structure and function of arteries and veins.

2. List the pulse sites accessible to examination.

3. Describe 3 mechanisms that help return venous blood to the heart.

4. Define the term *capacitance vessels,* and explain its significance.

5. List the risk factors for venous stasis.

6. Describe the function of the lymphatic system.

7. Describe the function of the lymph nodes.

8. Name the related organs in the lymphatic system.

9. List the symptom areas to address during history taking of the peripheral vascular system.

10. Fill in the grading scale for assessing the force of an arterial pulse: 0 _____; 1+ _____; 2+ _____; 3+ _____

11. List the skin characteristics expected with arterial insufficiency to the lower legs.

12. Compare the characteristics of leg ulcers associated with arterial insufficiency with ulcers with venous insufficiency.

13. Fill in the description of the grading scale for pitting edema:

    1+ _____

    2+ _____

    3+ _____

    4+ _____

14. Describe the technique for using the Doppler ultrasonic probe to detect peripheral pulses.

15. Raynaud phenomenon has associated progressive tricolor changes of the skin from _____ to _____ and then to _____. State the mechanism for each of these color changes.

Fill in the labels indicated on the following arteries and name the pulse sites.

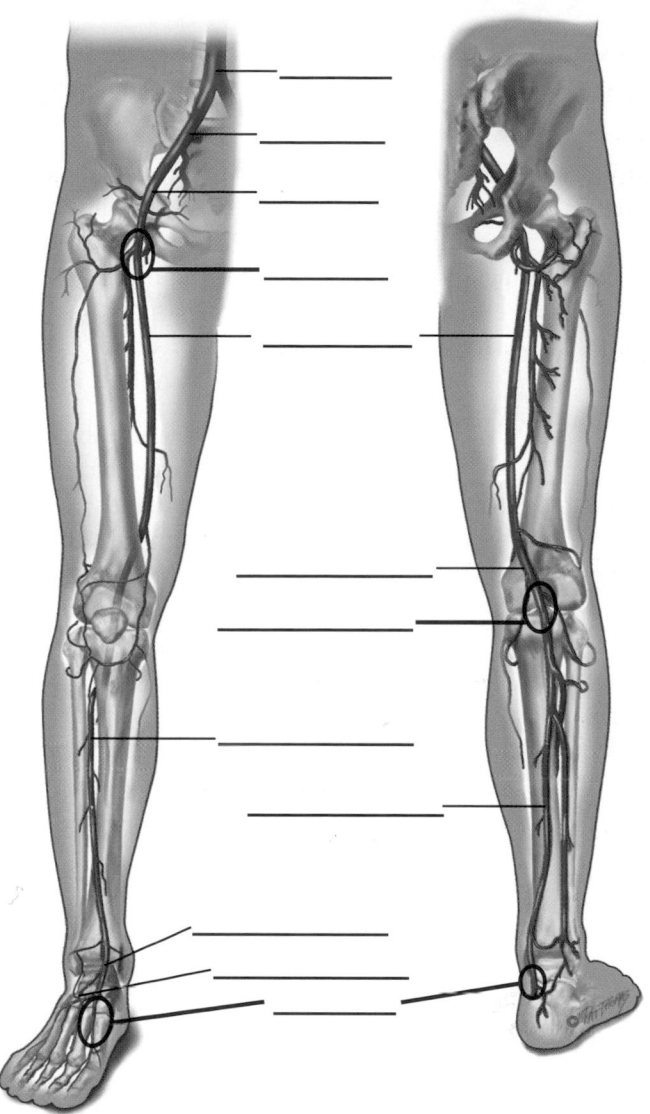

@ Pat Thomas, 2010

## REVIEW QUESTIONS

This test is for you to check your own mastery of the content. Answers are provided in Appendix A.

1. A function of the venous system includes:

   a. Holding more blood when blood volume increases.
   b. Conserving fluid and plasma proteins that leak out of the capillaries.
   c. Forming a major part of the immune system that defends the body against disease.
   d. Absorbing lipids from the intestinal tract.

2. Which of the following organs aid the lymphatic system?

   a. Liver, lymph nodes, and stomach
   b. Pancreas, small intestine, and thymus
   c. Spleen, tonsils, and thymus
   d. Pancreas, spleen, and tonsils

3. Ms. T. has come for a prenatal visit. She reports dependent edema, varicosities in the legs, and hemorrhoids. What is the best response?

   a. "If these symptoms persist, we will perform an amniocentesis."
   b. "If these symptoms persist, we will discuss having you hospitalized."
   c. "The symptoms are caused by the pressure of the growing uterus on the veins. They are usual conditions of pregnancy."
   d. "At this time, the symptoms are a minor inconvenience. You should learn to accept them."

4. A patient's pulse with an amplitude of 3+ indicates:

   a. Irregular, with 3 premature beats.
   b. Increased, full.
   c. Normal.
   d. Weak.

5. Inspection of a person's right hand reveals a red swollen area. To further assess for infection, you would palpate the:

   a. Cervical node.
   b. Axillary node.
   c. Epitrochlear node.
   d. Inguinal node.

6. To screen for deep vein thrombosis, you would:

   a. Measure the circumference of the ankle.
   b. Check the temperature with the palm of the hand.
   c. Compress the dorsalis pedis pulse, looking for blood return.
   d. Measure the widest point with a tape measure.

7. During the examination of the lower extremities, you are unable to palpate the popliteal pulse. You should:

   a. Proceed with the examination. It is often impossible to palpate this pulse.
   b. Refer the patient to a vascular surgeon for further evaluation.
   c. Schedule the patient for a venogram.
   d. Schedule the patient for an arteriogram.

8. You assess a patient who has 4+ edema of the right leg. What is the best way to document this finding?

   a. Mild pitting, no perceptible swelling of the leg
   b. Moderate pitting, indentation subsides rapidly
   c. Deep pitting, leg looks swollen
   d. Very deep pitting, indentation lasts a long time

9. You assess a patient for arterial deficit in the lower extremities. After raising the legs 12 inches off the table and then having the person sit up and dangle the leg, the color should return in:

   a. 5 seconds or less.
   b. 10 seconds or less.
   c. 15 seconds.
   d. 30 seconds.

10. A 54-year-old woman with 5 children has varicose veins of the lower extremities. Her most characteristic sign is:

    a. Reduced arterial circulation.
    b. Blanching, deathlike appearance of the extremities on elevation.
    c. Loss of hair on feet and toes.
    d. Dilated, tortuous superficial bluish vessels.

11. Atrophic skin changes that occur with peripheral arterial insufficiency include:

    a. Thin, shiny skin with loss of hair.
    b. Brown discoloration.
    c. Thick, leathery skin.
    d. Slow-healing blisters on the skin.

12. Intermittent claudication includes:

    a. Muscular pain relieved by exercise.
    b. Neurologic pain relieved by exercise.
    c. Muscular pain brought on by exercise.
    d. Neurologic pain brought on by exercise.

13. A known risk factor for venous ulcer development is:

    a. Obesity.
    b. Male gender.
    c. History of hypertension.
    d. Daily aspirin therapy.

14. Arteriosclerosis is caused by:

    a. Deposition of fatty plaques on the intima of the arteries.
    b. Loss of elasticity of the walls of blood vessels.
    c. Loss of lymphatic tissue that occurs in the aging process.
    d. Progressive enlargement of the intramuscular calf veins.

15. Raynaud phenomenon occurs:

    a. When the patient's extremities are exposed to heat and compression.
    b. In hands and feet as a result of exposure to cold, vibration, and stress.
    c. After removal of lymph nodes or damage to lymph nodes and channels.
    d. As a result of leg cramps due to excessive walking or climbing stairs.

## CRITICAL THINKING EXERCISE

Study the 2 photos below regarding foot and leg ulcers. The pathogenesis of these ulcers could be arterial (ischemic) dysfunction or venous (stasis) dysfunction. Choose which is which. To support your thinking, state the Subjective (history) symptoms and the Objective signs that would accompany these ulcers.

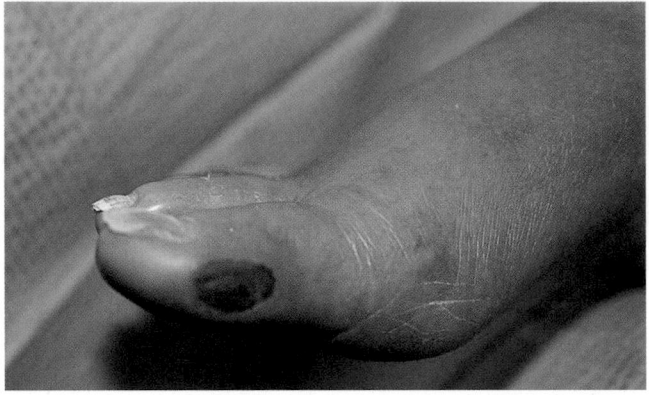

From Dockery, G. L. (1997). *Cutaneous disorders of the lower extremity*. Philadelphia: Saunders.

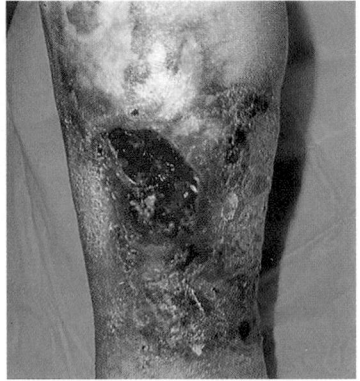

From Lookingbill, D. P., & Marks, J. G. (1993). *Principles of dermatology* (2nd ed.). Philadelphia: Saunders.

# SKILLS LABORATORY AND CLINICAL SETTING

The purpose of the clinical component is to practice the regional examination on a peer in the skills laboratory or on a patient in the clinical setting to achieve the following.

## Clinical Objectives

1. Demonstrate knowledge of the symptoms related to the peripheral vascular system by obtaining a regional health history from a peer or patient.

2. Demonstrate palpation of peripheral arterial pulses (brachial, radial, femoral, popliteal, posterior tibial, dorsalis pedis) by assessing amplitude and symmetry, noting any signs of arterial insufficiency.

3. Demonstrate inspection and palpation of peripheral veins by noting any signs of venous insufficiency.

4. Demonstrate palpation of lymphatic system by identifying enlargement, clumping, or abnormal firmness of regional lymph nodes.

5. Demonstrate correct technique for performing the following additional tests when indicated: Allen test, Doppler ultrasonic stethoscope, computing the ankle-brachial index (ABI).

6. Record the history and physical examination findings accurately, reach an assessment of the health state, and develop a plan of care.

## Instructions

Gather your equipment. Wash your hands. Practice the steps of the examination of the peripheral vascular system on a peer or on a patient in the clinical setting, giving appropriate instructions as you proceed. Record your findings using the regional write-up sheets that follow. The first part is intended as a worksheet; the last page is intended for your narrative summary recording using the SOAP format. Note that the peripheral examination and cardiovascular examination usually are practiced together.

## NOTES

## REGIONAL WRITE-UP—PERIPHERAL VASCULAR SYSTEM

Date _____

Examiner _____

Patient _____ Age _____ Gender _____

Reason for visit _____

### I.  Health History

| | No | Yes, explain |
|---|---|---|
| 1. Any leg **pain** (cramps)? Where? | | |
| 2. Any **skin changes** in arms or legs? | | |
| 3. Any sores or **lesions** in arms or legs? | | |
| 4. Any **swelling** in the legs? | | |
| 5. Any **swollen glands**? Where? | | |
| 6. What medications are you taking? | | |
| 7. Do you smoke cigarettes? How many per day? Ever tried to quit? | | |

### II.  Physical Examination

#### A.  Arms, Inspect:

Color of skin and nail beds _____

Symmetry _____

Lesions _____

Edema _____ Clubbing _____

Palpate

    Temperature _____ Texture _____

    Capillary refill _____

    Locate and grade pulses (record below)

    Check epitrochlear lymph nodes _____

    Modified Allen test (if indicated) _____

#### B.  Legs, Inspect:

Color _____ Hair distribution _____

Venous pattern, varicosities _____

Swelling, edema _____ Atrophy _____

If so, measure calf circumference in centimeters: R _____ L _____

Skin lesions or ulcers _____

Palpate

    Temperature _____

    Calf tenderness _____

    Inguinal lymph nodes _____

    Locate and grade pulses (record below) _____

    Check pretibial edema (grade if present) _____

    Auscultate for bruit (if indicated) _____

## REGIONAL WRITE-UP—PERIPHERAL VASCULAR SYSTEM

| | Brachial | Radial | Femoral | Popliteal | Dorsalis pedis | P. tibial |
|---|---|---|---|---|---|---|
| R | | | | | | |
| L | | | | | | |

0 = absent, 1+ = weak, 2+ = normal, 3+ = full, bounding

## C. Ankle-Brachial Index (ABI)

Use Doppler ultrasonic probe and locate pulse sites: brachial, dorsalis pedis, posterior tibial. Compute ABI.

**Ankle-Brachial Index Interpretation**
Above 0.90: Normal or borderline
0.71 – 0.89: Mild PAD
0.41 – 0.70: Moderate PAD
0.00 – 0.40: Severe PAD

**Right arm:**
Systolic pressure ☐☐☐ mm Hg

**Left arm:**
Systolic pressure ☐☐☐ mm Hg

**Right ankle:**
**Systolic pressure**
Posterior tibial (PT) ☐☐☐ mm Hg
Dorsalis pedis (DP) ☐☐☐ mm Hg

**Left ankle:**
**Systolic pressure**
Posterior tibial (PT) ☐☐☐ mm Hg
Dorsalis pedis (DP) ☐☐☐ mm Hg

*Right ABI equals ratio of:*

$$\frac{\text{Higher of the right ankle pressures (PT or DP)} \;\boxed{\phantom{00}}\; \text{mm Hg}}{\text{Higher arm pressure (right or left arm)} \;\boxed{\phantom{00}}\; \text{mm Hg}} = \boxed{\phantom{0}}.\boxed{\phantom{00}}$$

*Left ABI equals ratio of:*

$$\frac{\text{Higher of the left ankle pressures (PT or DP)} \;\boxed{\phantom{00}}\; \text{mm Hg}}{\text{Higher arm pressure (right or left arm)} \;\boxed{\phantom{00}}\; \text{mm Hg}} = \boxed{\phantom{0}}.\boxed{\phantom{00}}$$

From AACN (2009). AACN Advanced Critical Care Nursing (ed. 1). Philadelphia: Saunders.

## REGIONAL WRITE-UP—PERIPHERAL VASCULAR SYSTEM

Summarize your findings using the SOAP format.

**Subjective** (reason for seeking care, health history)

**Objective** (physical examination findings)                    Record pulses on diagram below.

**Assessment** (assessment of health state or problem, diagnosis)

**Plan** (diagnostic evaluation, follow-up care, teaching)

## NOTES

## PURPOSE

This chapter helps you learn the structure and function of the abdominal organs; know the location of the abdominal organs; discriminate normal bowel sounds; understand the rationale and methods of examination of the abdomen; and accurately record the assessment. At the end of this chapter you should be able to perform a complete assessment of the abdomen.

## READING ASSIGNMENT

Jarvis: *Physical Examination and Health Assessment,* 8th ed., Chapter 22, pp. 529-568.

Suggested reading:
Saccomano, S. J., & Ferrara, L. R. (2013). Evaluation of acute abdominal pain. *Nurse Pract, 38*(11), 46-53.

## GLOSSARY

Study the following terms after completing the reading assignment. You should be able to cover the definition on the right and define the term out loud.

**Aneurysm** . . . . . . . . . . . . . . . . . defect or sac formed by dilation in artery wall due to atherosclerosis, trauma, or congenital defect

**Anorexia** . . . . . . . . . . . . . . . . . . loss of appetite for food

**Ascites** . . . . . . . . . . . . . . . . . . . abnormal accumulation of serous fluid within the peritoneal cavity, associated with heart failure, cirrhosis, cancer, or portal hypertension

**Borborygmi** . . . . . . . . . . . . . . . loud, gurgling bowel sounds signaling increased motility or hyperperistalsis; occurs with early bowel obstruction, gastroenteritis, diarrhea

**Bruit** . . . . . . . . . . . . . . . . . . . . . blowing, swooshing sound heard through a stethoscope when an artery is partially occluded

**Cecum** . . . . . . . . . . . . . . . . . . . first or proximal part of large intestine

**Cholecystitis** . . . . . . . . . . . . . . . inflammation of the gallbladder

**Costal margin** . . . . . . . . . . . . . . lower border of rib margin formed by the medial edges of the 8th, 9th, and 10th ribs

**Costovertebral angle (CVA)** . . . angle formed by the 12th rib and the vertebral column on the posterior thorax, overlying the kidney

**Diastasis recti**. . . . . . . . . . . . . .midline longitudinal ridge in the abdomen, a separation of abdominal rectus muscles

**Dysphagia** . . . . . . . . . . . . . . . . .difficulty swallowing

**Epigastrium** . . . . . . . . . . . . . . .name of abdominal region between the costal margins

**Hepatomegaly** . . . . . . . . . . . . .abnormal enlargement of liver

**Hernia** . . . . . . . . . . . . . . . . . . . .abnormal protrusion of bowel through weakening in abdominal musculature

**Inguinal ligament** . . . . . . . . . .ligament extending from pubic bone to anterior superior iliac spine, forming lower border of abdomen

**Linea alba** . . . . . . . . . . . . . . . . .midline tendinous seam joining the abdominal muscles

**Paralytic ileus**. . . . . . . . . . . . . .complete absence of peristaltic movement that may follow abdominal surgery or complete bowel obstruction

**Peritoneal friction rub** . . . . . . .rough grating sound heard through the stethoscope over the site of peritoneal inflammation

**Peritoneum**. . . . . . . . . . . . . . . . .double envelope of serous membrane that lines the abdominal wall and covers the surface of most abdominal organs

**Peritonitis**. . . . . . . . . . . . . . . . . .inflammation of peritoneum

**Pyloric stenosis** . . . . . . . . . . . .congenital narrowing of pyloric sphincter, forming outflow obstruction of stomach

**Pyrosis**. . . . . . . . . . . . . . . . . . . .heartburn; burning sensation in upper abdomen due to reflux of gastric acid

**Rectus abdominis muscles**. . . .midline abdominal muscles extending from rib cage to pubic bone

**Scaphoid** . . . . . . . . . . . . . . . . . .abnormally sunken abdominal wall, as with malnutrition or underweight

**Splenomegaly**. . . . . . . . . . . . . .abnormal enlargement of spleen

**Striae** . . . . . . . . . . . . . . . . . . . .(lineae albicantes) silvery white or pink scar tissue formed by stretching of abdominal skin as with pregnancy or obesity

**Suprapubic** . . . . . . . . . . . . . . . .name of abdominal region just superior to pubic bone

**Tympany** . . . . . . . . . . . . . . . . . .high-pitched, musical, drumlike percussion note heard when percussing over the stomach and intestine

**Umbilicus** . . . . . . . . . . . . . . . . .depression on the abdomen marking site of entry of umbilical cord

**Viscera**. . . . . . . . . . . . . . . . . . . .internal organs

## STUDY GUIDE

After completing the reading assignment and the media assignment, write or draw the answers in the spaces provided.

1. Describe the proper positioning and preparation of the patient for the abdominal examination.

2. Discuss inspection of the abdomen, including findings that you should note.

3. State the rationale for performing auscultation of the abdomen before palpation or percussion.

4. Describe the procedure for auscultation of bowel sounds.

5. Differentiate the following abdominal sounds: normal, hyperactive, and hypoactive bowel sounds; succession splash; bruit.

6. List 4 conditions that may alter normal percussion notes heard over the abdomen.

7. Name the organs that are normally palpable in the abdomen.

8. Differentiate between light and deep palpation, and explain the purpose of each.

List 2 abnormalities that may be detected by light palpation and 2 that may be detected by deep palpation.

9. Contrast rigidity with voluntary guarding.

10. Contrast visceral pain and somatic (parietal) pain.

11. Describe rebound tenderness.

12. Distinguish abdominal wall masses from intra-abdominal masses.

13. Describe the procedure and rationale for determining costovertebral angle (CVA) tenderness.

Fill in the labels indicated on the following illustrations.

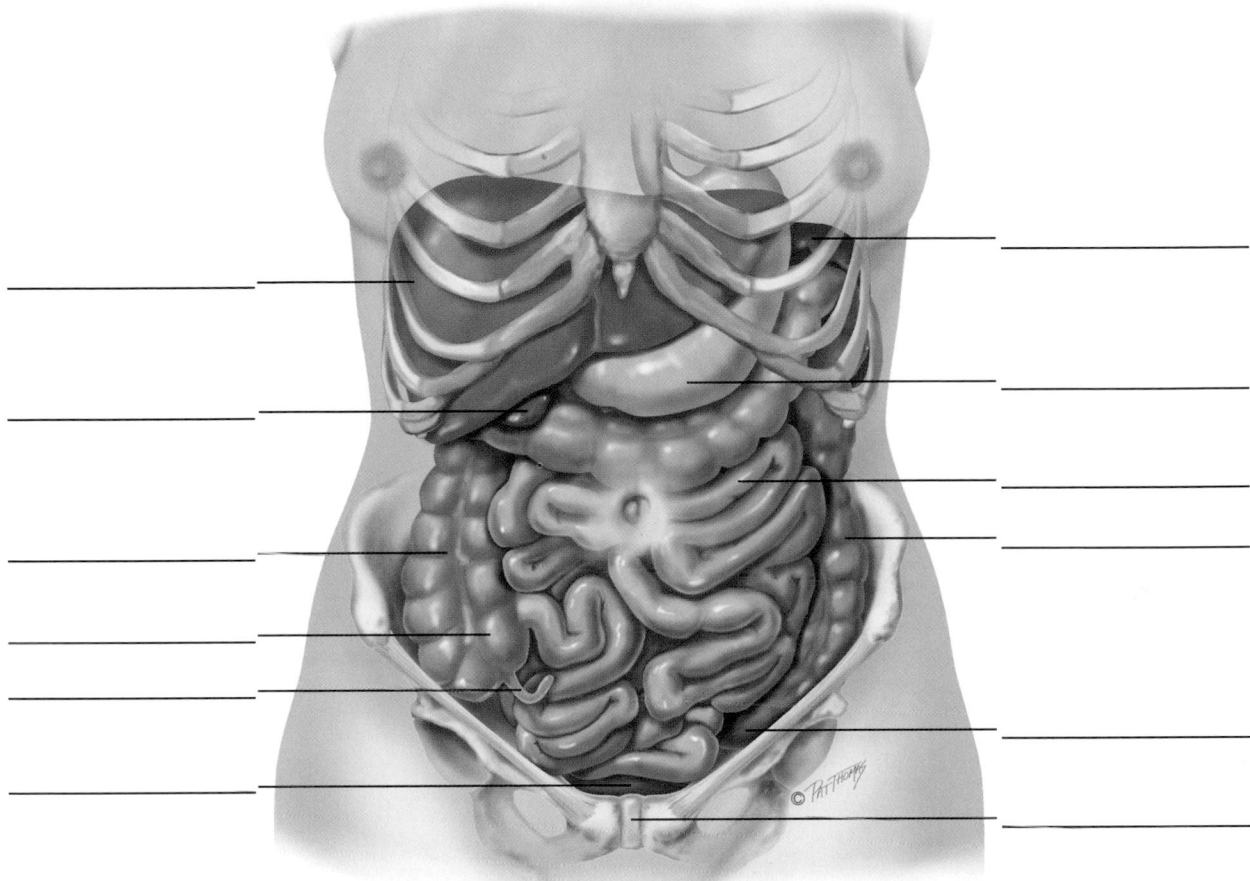

@ Pat Thomas, 2010

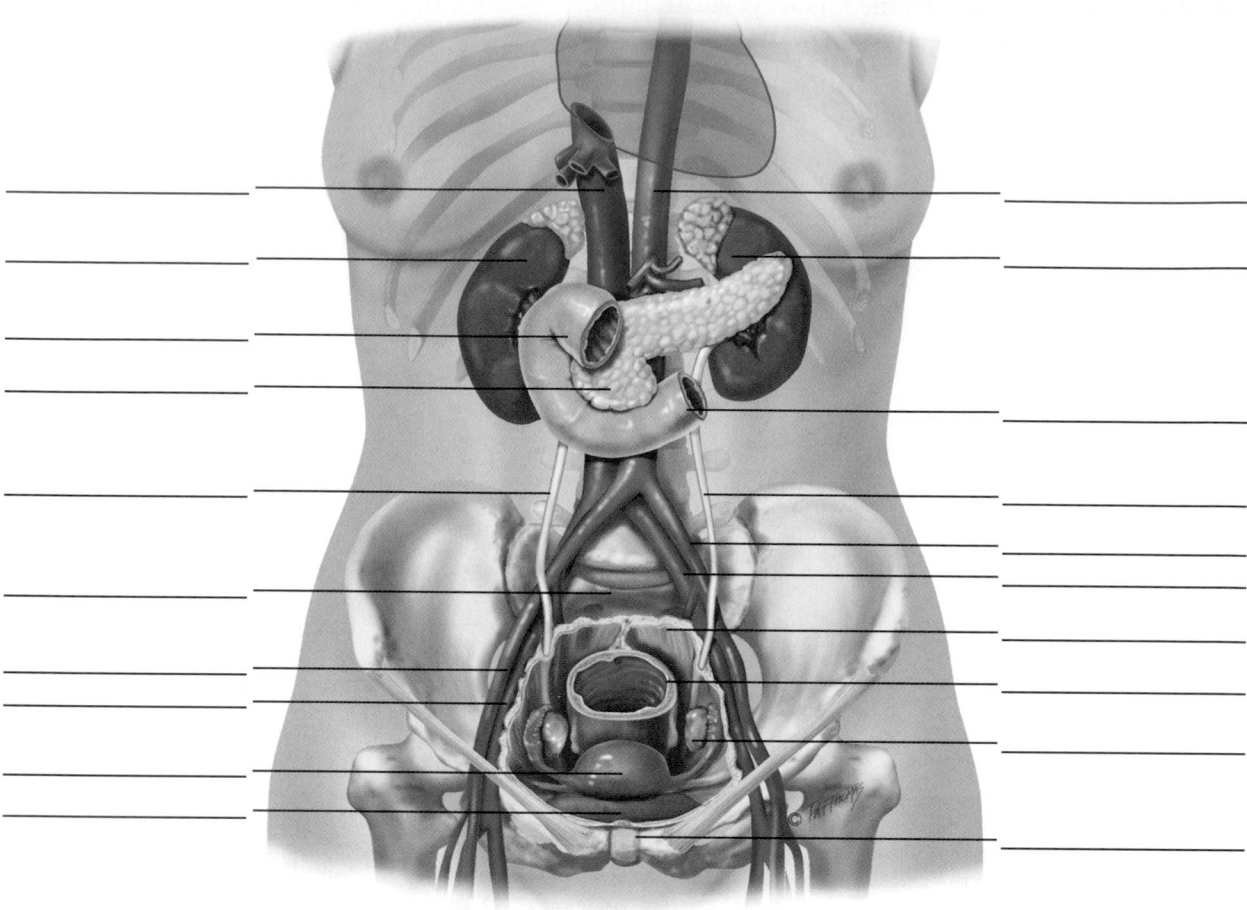

@ Pat Thomas, 2006

## REVIEW QUESTIONS

This test is for you to check your own mastery of the content. Answers are provided in Appendix A.

1. Select the sequence of techniques used during an examination of the abdomen.

   a. Percussion, inspection, palpation, auscultation
   b. Inspection, palpation, percussion, auscultation
   c. Inspection, auscultation, percussion, palpation
   d. Auscultation, inspection, palpation, percussion

2. Which of the following can be noted through inspection of a patient's abdomen?

   a. Fluid waves and abdominal rigidity
   b. Umbilical eversion and Murphy sign
   c. Venous pattern, peristaltic waves, and abdominal contour
   d. Peritoneal irritation, general tympany, and peristaltic waves

3. Right upper quadrant tenderness may indicate pathology in the:

   a. Liver, pancreas, or ascending colon.
   b. Liver and stomach.
   c. Sigmoid colon, spleen, or rectum.
   d. Appendix or ileocecal valve.

4. Hyperactive bowel sounds are:

   a. High-pitched.
   b. Rushing.
   c. Tinkling.
   d. All of the above.

5. The absence of bowel sounds is established after listening for:

   a. 1 full minute.
   b. 3 full minutes.
   c. 5 full minutes.
   d. None of the above.

6. Auscultation of the abdomen may reveal bruits of the _____ arteries.

   a. Aortic, renal, iliac, and femoral
   b. Jugular, aortic, carotid, and femoral
   c. Pulmonic, aortic, and portal
   d. Renal, iliac, internal jugular, and basilic

7. The left upper quadrant (LUQ) contains the:

   a. Liver.
   b. Appendix.
   c. Left ovary.
   d. Spleen.

8. A woman has striae on the abdomen. Which color indicates long-standing striae?

   a. Pink
   b. Blue
   c. Purple-blue
   d. Silvery white

9. Auscultating the abdomen is begun in the right lower quadrant (RLQ) because:

   a. Bowel sounds are always normally present here.
   b. Peristalsis through the descending colon is usually active.
   c. This is the location of the pyloric sphincter.
   d. Vascular sounds are best heard in this area.

10. Shifting dullness is a test for:

    a. Ascites.
    b. Splenic enlargement.
    c. Inflammation of the kidney.
    d. Hepatomegaly.

11. Tenderness during abdominal palpation is expected when palpating the:

    a. Liver edge.
    b. Spleen.
    c. Sigmoid colon.
    d. Kidneys.

12. A positive Murphy sign is best described as:

    a. The pain felt when the examiner's hand is rapidly removed from an inflamed appendix.
    b. Pain felt when taking a deep breath when the examiner's fingers are on the approximate location of the inflamed gallbladder.
    c. A sharp pain felt by the patient when one hand of the examiner is used to thump the other at the costovertebral angle.
    d. This is not a valid examination technique.

13. A positive Blumberg sign indicates:

    a. Possible aortic aneurysm.
    b. Presence of renal artery stenosis.
    c. Enlarged, nodular liver.
    d. Peritoneal inflammation.

## CRITICAL THINKING EXERCISE

Your patient is complaining of abdominal pain. Study Table 22.3, Common Sites of Referred Abdominal Pain, on p. 562 in Jarvis: *Physical Examination and Health Assessment,* 8th ed. Choose two conditions and list important subjective data to help determine what might be wrong with your patient.

## SKILLS LABORATORY AND CLINICAL SETTING

The purpose of the clinical component is to practice the regional examination on a peer in the skills laboratory or on a patient in the clinical setting and to achieve the following.

### Clinical Objectives

1. Demonstrate correct knowledge of the abdominal symptoms by obtaining a regional health history from a peer or patient.

2. Demonstrate correct inspection of the abdomen by inspection, auscultation, percussion, and palpation.

3. Demonstrate correct technique of performing the following additional tests when indicated: fluid wave, rebound tenderness, inspiratory arrest.

4. Record the history and physical examination findings accurately, reach an assessment of the health state, and develop a plan of care.

### Instructions

Gather your equipment. Wash your hands. Assess the patient's comfort before starting. Practice the steps of the examination on a peer or on a patient in the clinical setting, giving appropriate instructions as you proceed. Record your findings using the regional write-up sheets that follow. The front of the page is intended as a worksheet; the back of the page is intended for your narrative summary recording using the SOAP format.

# REGIONAL WRITE-UP—ABDOMEN

Date _____

Examiner _____

Patient _____ Age _____ Gender _____

Reason for visit _____

## I. Health History

| | No | Yes, explain |
|---|---|---|
| 1. Any change in **appetite**? Loss? | | |
| 2. Any difficulty **swallowing**? | | |
| 3. Any foods you **cannot tolerate**? | | |
| 4. Any **abdominal pain**? | | |
| 5. Any **nausea or vomiting**? | | |
| 6. How often are **bowel movements**? | | |
| 7. Any past history of **GI disease**? | | |

8. What **medications** are you taking?

9. Tell me all food you ate in the last **24 hours,** starting with:

breakfast         snack         lunch         snack         dinner         snack

## II. Physical Examination

### A. Inspection

Contour of abdomen _____ General symmetry _____

Skin color and condition _____

Pulsation or movement _____

Umbilicus _____

State of hydration and nutrition _____

Person's facial expression and position in bed _____

### B. Auscultation

Bowel sounds _____

Note any vascular sounds. _____

### C. Percussion

Percuss in all four quadrants. _____

If suspect ascites, test for fluid wave and shifting dullness. _____

### D. Palpation

Light palpation in all four quadrants

Muscle wall _____ Tenderness _____

Enlarged organs _____

Masses _____

Deep palpation in all four quadrants

Masses _____

Contour of liver _____ Spleen _____

Kidneys _____ Aorta _____

Rebound tenderness _____

CVA tenderness _____

# REGIONAL WRITE-UP—ABDOMEN

Summarize your findings using the SOAP format.

**Subjective** (reason for seeking care, health history)

**Objective** (physical examination findings)

Record findings on diagram.

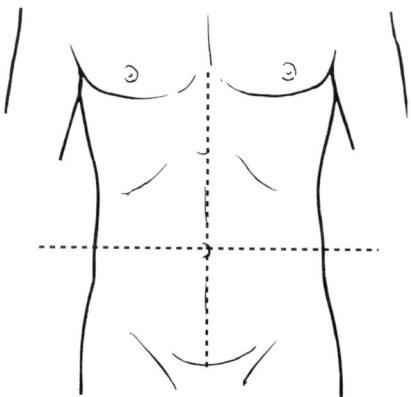

**Assessment** (assessment of health state or problem, diagnosis)

**Plan** (diagnostic evaluation, follow-up care, teaching)

# CHAPTER 23

# Musculoskeletal System

## PURPOSE

This chapter helps you learn the structure and function of the various joints in the body, know their normal ranges of motion, position the patient comfortably during the examination, understand the rationale and methods of examination of the musculoskeletal system, assess functional ability, and accurately record the assessment. At the end of this chapter you should be able to perform a complete assessment of the musculoskeletal system.

## READING ASSIGNMENT

Jarvis: *Physical Examination and Health Assessment,* 8th ed., Chapter 23, pp. 569-624.

Suggested reading:
Black, D. M., & Rosen, C. J. (2016). Postmenopausal osteoporosis. *New Engl J Med, 374*(3), 254-262.

## GLOSSARY

Study the following terms after completing the reading assignment. You should be able to cover the definition on the right and define the term out loud.

**Abduction** . . . . . . . . . . . . . . . . . . moving a body part away from an axis or the median line

**Adduction** . . . . . . . . . . . . . . . . . . moving a body part toward the center or toward the median line

**Ankylosis** . . . . . . . . . . . . . . . . . . immobility, consolidation, and fixation of a joint because of disease, injury, or surgery; most often due to chronic rheumatoid arthritis

**Ataxia** . . . . . . . . . . . . . . . . . . . . . inability to perform coordinated movements

**Bursa** . . . . . . . . . . . . . . . . . . . . . . enclosed sac filled with viscous fluid located in joint areas of potential friction

**Circumduction** . . . . . . . . . . . . . moving the arm in a circle around the shoulder

**Crepitation** . . . . . . . . . . . . . . . . dry crackling sound or sensation due to grating of the ends of damaged bone

**Dorsal** . . . . . . . . . . . . . . . . . . . . . directed toward or located on the surface

**Dupuytren contracture** . . . . . . flexion contracture of the fingers due to chronic hyperplasia of the palmar fascia

**Eversion** . . . . . . . . . . . . . . . . . . . moving the sole of the foot outward at the ankle

**Extension**.................straightening a limb at a joint

**Flexion**...................bending a limb at a joint

**Ganglion** ................round, cystic, nontender nodule overlying a tendon sheath or joint capsule, usually on dorsum of wrist

**Hallux valgus** ..............lateral or outward deviation of the great toe

**Inversion**..................moving the sole of the foot inward at the ankle

**Kyphosis** .................outward or convex curvature of the thoracic spine; hunchback

**Ligament**..................fibrous band running directly from one bone to another bone that strengthens the joint

**Lordosis**..................inward or concave curvature of the lumbar spine

**Nucleus pulposus**...........center of the intervertebral disc

**Olecranon process**..........bony projection of the ulna at the elbow

**Patella** ...................kneecap

**Plantar**...................refers to the surface of the sole of the foot

**Pronation** ................turning the forearm so that the palm is down

**Protraction** ...............moving a body part forward and parallel to the ground

**Range of motion (ROM)**......extent of movement of a joint

**Retraction**.................moving a body part backward and parallel to the ground

**Rheumatoid arthritis** .......chronic systemic inflammatory disease of joints and surrounding connective tissue

**Sciatica**...................nerve pain along the course of the sciatic nerve that travels down from the back or thigh through the leg and into the foot

**Scoliosis**..................**S**-shaped curvature of the thoracic spine

**Supination** ...............turning the forearm so that the palm is up

**Talipes equinovarus** ........(clubfoot) congenital deformity of the foot in which it is plantar flexed and inverted

**Tendon**...................strong fibrous cord that attaches a skeletal muscle to a bone

**Torticollis** ................wryneck; contraction of the cervical neck muscles, producing torsion of the neck

## STUDY GUIDE

After completing the reading assignment and the media assignment, write the answers in the spaces provided.

1. Differentiate synovial from nonsynovial joints.


2. List 4 signs that suggest acute inflammation in a joint.


3. Differentiate the following:

    Dislocation  _____

    Subluxation  _____

    Contracture  _____

    Ankylosis  _____

4. Differentiate testing of active range of motion versus passive range of motion.


5. Explain the method for measuring leg length.


6. Describe the Ortolani maneuver for checking an infant's hips.


7. When performing a functional assessment for an older adult, state the common adaptations that the older adult makes when attempting these maneuvers:

    Walking  _____

    Climbing up stairs  _____

    Walking down stairs  _____

    Picking up object from floor  _____

    Rising up from sitting in chair  _____

    _____

Rising up from lying in bed  _____

_____

8. Draw and describe swan neck deformity and boutonnière deformity in rheumatoid arthritis.

9. Contrast Bouchard nodes with Heberden nodes in osteoarthritis.

Fill in the labels indicated on the following illustrations.

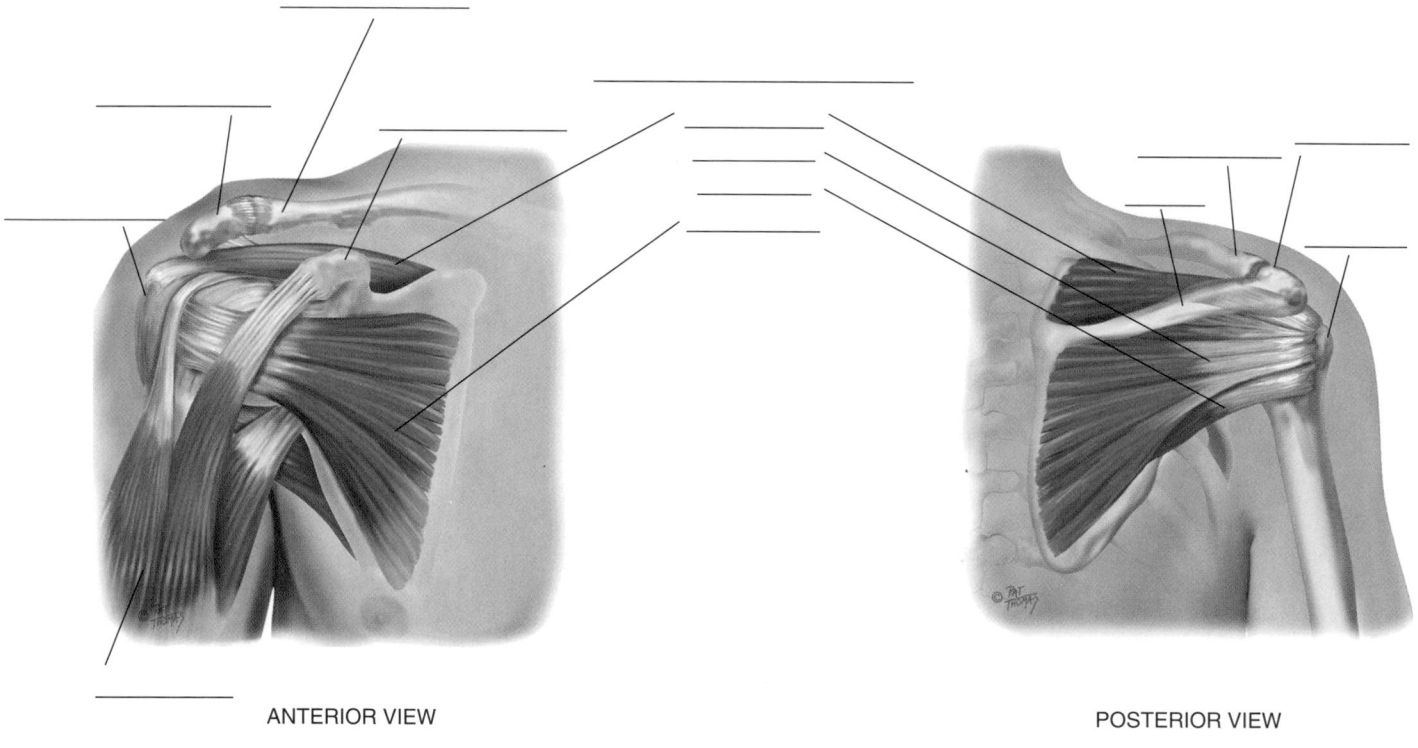

ANTERIOR VIEW                                                    POSTERIOR VIEW

(© Pat Thomas, 2018.)

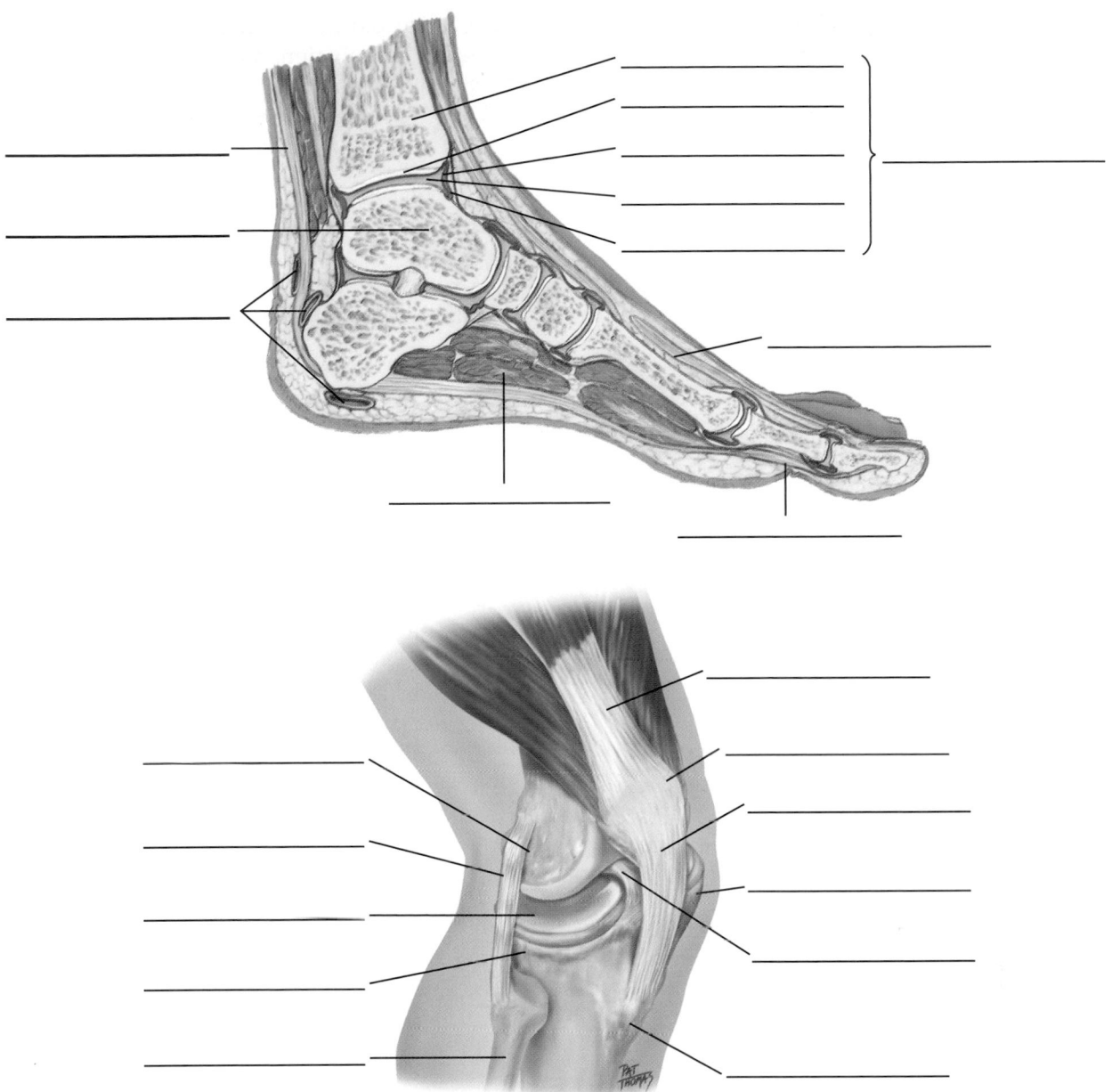

## REVIEW QUESTIONS

This test is for you to check your own mastery of the content. Answers are provided in Appendix A.

1. During the assessment of the spine, the patient would be asked to:

   a. Adduct and extend.
   b. Supinate, evert, and retract.
   c. Extend, adduct, invert, and rotate.
   d. Flex, extend, abduct, and rotate.

2. Pronation and supination of the hand and forearm are the result of the articulation of the:

   a. Scapula and clavicle.
   b. Radius and ulna.
   c. Patella and condyle of fibula.
   d. Femur and acetabulum.

3. Anterior and posterior stability are provided to the knee joint by the:

   a. Medial and lateral menisci.
   b. Patellar tendon and ligament.
   c. Medial collateral ligament and quadriceps muscle.
   d. Anterior and posterior cruciate ligaments.

4. A 70-year-old woman has come for a health examination. Which of the following is a common age-related change in the curvature of the spinal column?

   a. Lordosis
   b. Scoliosis
   c. Kyphosis
   d. Lateral scoliosis

5. Examination of the shoulder includes 4 motions. These are:

   a. Forward flexion, internal rotation, abduction, and external rotation.
   b. Abduction, adduction, pronation, and supination.
   c. Circumduction, inversion, eversion, and rotation.
   d. Elevation, retraction, protraction, and circumduction.

6. The bulge sign is a test for:

   a. Swelling in the suprapatellar pouch.
   b. Carpal tunnel syndrome.
   c. Heberden nodes.
   d. Olecranon bursa inflammation.

7. The examiner measures a patient's legs for length discrepancy. Which is a normal finding?

   a. No difference in measurements
   b. 0.5 cm difference
   c. Within 1 cm of each other
   d. 2 cm difference

8. A 2-year-old child comes to the clinic for a health examination. A common finding for this age group is:

   a. Kyphosis.
   b. Lordosis.
   c. Scoliosis.
   d. No deviation is normal.

9. A positive Phalen test and Tinel sign are found in a patient with:

   a. A torn meniscus.
   b. Hallux valgus.
   c. Carpal tunnel syndrome.
   d. Tennis elbow.

10. When assessing an infant, the examiner completes the Ortolani maneuver by:

    a. Lifting the newborn and noting a C-shaped curvature of the spine.
    b. Gently lifting and abducting the infant's flexed knees while palpating the greater trochanter with the fingers.
    c. Comparing the height of the tops of the knees when the knees are flexed up.
    d. Palpating the length of the clavicles.

11. Hematopoiesis takes place in which of the following?

    a. Liver
    b. Spleen
    c. Kidneys
    d. Bone marrow

12. Fibrous bands running directly from one bone to another that strengthen the joint and help prevent movement in undesirable directions are known as:

    a. Bursa.
    b. Tendons.
    c. Cartilage.
    d. Ligaments.

Match column A to column B.

| Column A: Movement | Column B: Description |
|---|---|

13. _____ Flexion

14. _____ Extension

15. _____ Abduction

16. _____ Adduction

17. _____ Pronation

18. _____ Supination

19. _____ Circumduction

20. _____ Inversion

21. _____ Eversion

22. _____ Rotation

23. _____ Protraction

24. _____ Retraction

25. _____ Elevation

26. _____ Depression

a. Turning the forearm so that the palm is up

b. Bending a limb at a joint

c. Lowering a body part

d. Turning the forearm so that the palm is down

e. Straightening a limb at a joint

f. Raising a body part

g. Moving a limb away from the midline of the body

h. Moving a body part backward and parallel to the ground

i. Moving a limb toward the midline of the body

j. Moving the arm in a circle around the shoulder

k. Moving the sole of the foot outward at the ankle

l. Moving a body part forward and parallel to the ground

m. Moving the sole of the foot inward at the ankle

n. Moving the head around a central axis

## CRITICAL THINKING EXERCISE

The FRAX assessment tool is a computerized fracture risk algorithm developed by the World Health Organization and is available at *www.shef.ac.uk/FRAX*. To increase your experience and comfort with this tool, enter the website on your computer, click the calculation tool tab at the top of the page, and pick the correct regional version (e.g., U.S. Caucasian version).

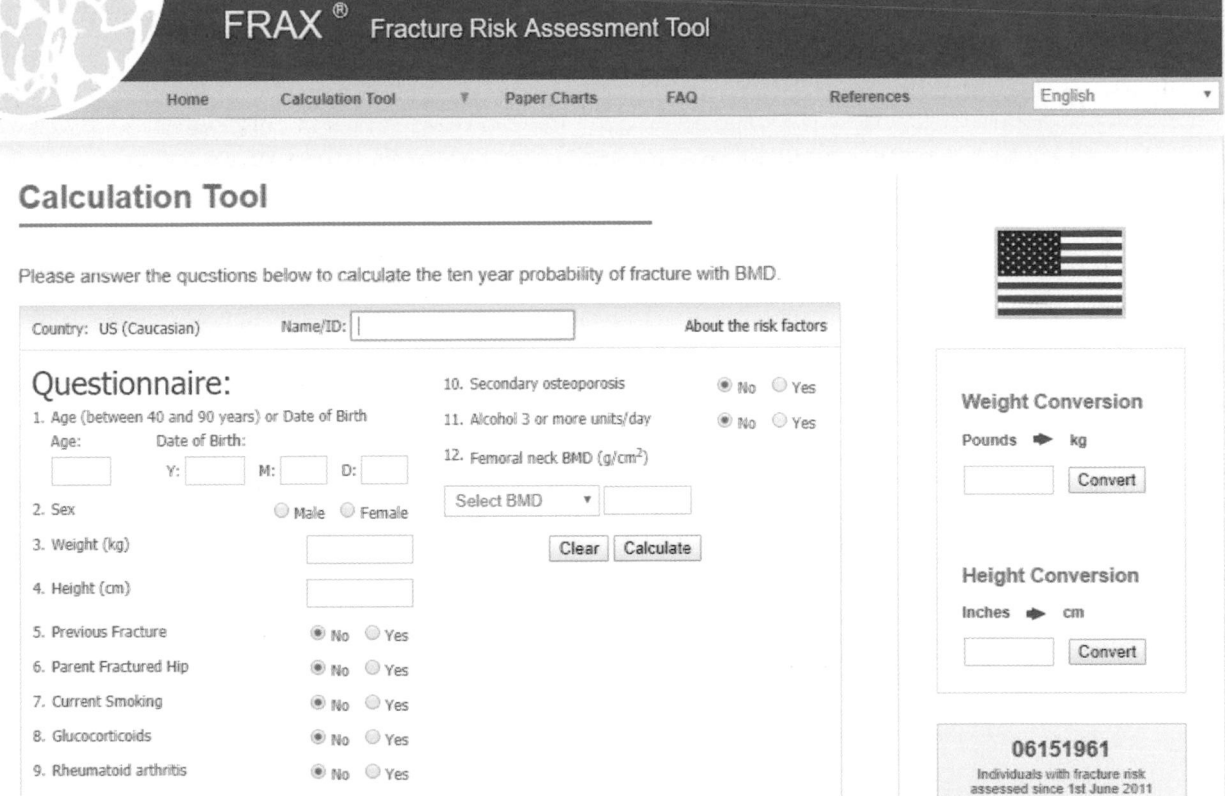

(© Centre for Metabolic Bone Diseases at the University of Sheffield.)

Enter the following data to determine fracture risk: C.M. is an 81-year-old white female, height 5 feet 7 inches, weight 124 lbs. (NOTE: The tool includes a feature that converts height and weight to kg and cm; it will also calculate body mass index, shown in the red results box.) C.M. has no previous fracture, no smoking or glucocorticoid use, and alcohol use of 1 to 2 units per day. She has osteoporosis with a femoral neck T-score of −2.0. (Enter in field for question 12.)

The FRAX outcome gives you a 10-year absolute risk by percentages of hip fracture and major osteoporotic fracture. Write a teaching plan for C.M., including risk management and follow-up care. Present the plan to a peer, using simple, understandable layperson terms.

## SKILLS LABORATORY AND CLINICAL SETTING

The purpose of the clinical component is to practice the regional musculoskeletal examination on a peer in the skills laboratory or on a patient in the clinical setting to achieve the following.

### Clinical Objectives

1. Demonstrate knowledge of the musculoskeletal symptoms by obtaining a regional health history from a peer or patient.

2. Demonstrate inspection and palpation of the musculoskeletal system by assessing the muscles, bones, and joints for size, symmetry, swelling, nodules, deformities, atrophy, and active range of motion.

3. Assess the person's ability to carry out functional activities of daily living.

4. Record the history and physical examination findings accurately, reach an assessment about the health state, and develop a plan of care.

## INSTRUCTIONS

Gather your equipment. Wash your hands. Practice the steps of the examination on a peer or on a patient in the clinical setting, giving appropriate instructions as you proceed and maintaining the safety of the person during movement. Record your findings using the regional write-up sheet that follows. The first section is intended as a worksheet; the last page is intended for your narrative summary recording using the SOAP format.

# REGIONAL WRITE-UP—MUSCULOSKELETAL SYSTEM

Date _____

Examiner _____

Patient _____    Age _____  Gender _____

Reason for visit _____

## I. Health History

| | No | Yes, explain |
|---|---|---|
| 1. Any **pain** in the joints? | | |
| 2. Any **stiffness** in the joints? | | |
| 3. Any **swelling, heat, redness** in joints? | | |
| 4. Any **limitation of movement**? | | |
| 5. Any **muscle pain** or cramping? | | |
| 6. Any **deformity** of bone or joint? | | |
| 7. Any **accidents or trauma** to bones or joints? | | |
| 8. Ever had **back pain**? | | |
| 9. Any problems with **ADL:** | | |
| Bathing, toileting, dressing? | | |
| Grooming, eating, mobility? | | |
| Communicating? | | |

## II. Physical Examination

### A. Cervical spine

1. Inspect size, contour _____ Deformity _____
2. Palpate for temperature _____ Pain _____
   Swelling or mass _____
3. Active range of motion
   Flexion _____ Extension _____
   Lateral bending right _____ Left _____
   Right rotation _____ Left _____

### B. Shoulders

1. Inspect size, contour _____ Color, swelling _____
   Mass or deformity _____
2. Palpate for temperature _____ Pain _____
   Swelling or mass _____
3. Active range of motion
   Flexion _____ Extension _____
   Abduction _____ Adduction _____
   Internal rotation _____ External rotation _____

### C. Elbows

1. Inspect for size, contour _____ Color, swelling _____
   Mass or deformity _____
2. Palpate for temperature _____ Pain _____
   Swelling or mass _____
3. Active range of motion
   Flexion _____ Extension _____
   Pronation _____ Supination _____

**D. Wrists and hands**

   1. Inspect for size, contour _____ Color, swelling _____
      Mass or deformity

   2. Palpate for temperature _____ Pain _____
      Swelling or mass _____

   3. Active range of motion
      Wrist extension _____ Flexion _____
      Finger extension _____ Flexion _____
      Ulnar deviation _____ Radial deviation _____
      Fingers spread _____ Make fist _____
      Touch thumb to each finger _____

**E. Hips**

   1. Inspect for size, contour _____ Color, swelling _____
      Mass or deformity _____

   2. Palpate for temperature _____ Pain _____
      Swelling or mass _____

   3. Active range of motion
      Extension _____ Flexion _____
      External rotation _____ Internal rotation _____
      Abduction _____ Adduction _____

**F. Knees**

   1. Inspect size, contour _____ Color, swelling _____
      Mass or deformity _____

   2. Palpate for temperature _____ Pain _____
      Swelling or mass _____

   3. Active range of motion
      Flexion _____ Extension _____
      Walk _____ Shallow knee bend _____

**G. Ankles and feet**

   1. Inspect for size, contour _____ Color, swelling _____
      Mass or deformity _____

   2. Palpate for temperature _____ Pain _____
      Swelling or mass _____

   3. Active range of motion
      Dorsiflexion _____ Plantar flexion _____
      Inversion _____ Eversion _____

**H. Spine**
   1. Inspect for straight spinous processes. _____
      Equal horizontal positions for shoulders, scapulae, iliac crests, gluteal folds _____
      Equal spaces between arms and lateral thorax _____
      Knees and feet align with trunk, point forward _____
      From side, note curvature: cervical, thoracic, lumbar _____
   2. Palpate spinous processes.
   3. Active range of motion
      Flexion _____ Extension _____
      Lateral bending right _____ Left _____
      Rotation right _____ Left _____

**I.  Functional assessment (if indicated)**
   Walk (with shoes on).
   Climb up stairs.
   Walk down stairs.
   Pick up object from floor.
   Rise up from sitting in chair.
   Rise up from lying in bed.

# REGIONAL WRITE-UP—MUSCULOSKELETAL SYSTEM

**Subjective** (reason for seeking care, health history)

**Objective** (physical examination findings)

**Assessment** (assessment of health state or problem, diagnosis)

**Plan** (diagnostic evaluation, follow-up care, patient teaching)

## PURPOSE

This chapter helps you learn the components of the neurologic system, including the cranial nerves, cerebellar system, motor system, sensory system, and reflexes, understand the rationale and methods of examination of the neurologic system, and accurately record the assessment. Together with the mental status assessment presented in Chapter 5, you should be able to perform a complete assessment of the neurologic system at the end of this chapter.

## READING ASSIGNMENT

Jarvis: *Physical Examination and Health Assessment*, 8th ed., Chapter 24, pp. 625-682.

Suggested reading:
Anderson, J. A. (2014). The golden hour: performing an acute ischemic stroke workup. *Nurse Pract, 39* (9), 22-30.

## GLOSSARY

Study the following terms after completing the reading assignment. You should be able to cover the definition on the right and define the term out loud.

**Agnosia** . . . . . . . . . . . . . . . . . . . . loss of ability to recognize importance of sensory impressions

**Agraphia** . . . . . . . . . . . . . . . . . . . loss of ability to express thoughts in writing

**Amnesia** . . . . . . . . . . . . . . . . . . loss of memory

**Analgesia** . . . . . . . . . . . . . . . . . loss of pain sensation

**Aphasia** . . . . . . . . . . . . . . . . . . loss of power of expression by speech, writing, or signs; or loss of comprehension of spoken or written language

**Apraxia** . . . . . . . . . . . . . . . . . . . loss of ability to perform purposeful movements in the absence of sensory or motor damage (e.g., inability to use objects correctly)

**Ataxia** . . . . . . . . . . . . . . . . . . . . inability to perform coordinated movements

**Athetosis** . . . . . . . . . . . . . . . . . . bizarre, slow, twisting, writhing movement, resembling a snake or worm

**Chorea** . . . . . . . . . . . . . . . . . . . . sudden, rapid, jerky, purposeless movement involving limbs, trunk, or face

**Clonus** . . . . . . . . . . . . . . . . . . . . rapidly alternating involuntary contraction and relaxation of a muscle in response to sudden stretch

**Coma** . . . . . . . . . . . . . . . . . . . . state of profound unconsciousness from which person cannot be aroused

**Concussion** . . . . . . . . . . . . . . . collision or trauma causes violent shaking of brain, yielding behavioral changes but no changes on radiologic imaging

**Decerebrate rigidity** . . . . . . . . arms stiffly extended, adducted, internally rotated; legs stiffly extended, plantar-flexed

**Decorticate rigidity** . . . . . . . . arms adducted and flexed, wrists and fingers flexed; legs extended, internally rotated, plantar-flexed

**Dysarthria** . . . . . . . . . . . . . . . . imperfect articulation of speech due to problems of muscular control resulting from central or peripheral nervous system damage

**Dysphasia** . . . . . . . . . . . . . . . . impairment in speech consisting of lack of coordination and inability to arrange words in their proper order

**Extinction** . . . . . . . . . . . . . . . . disappearance of conditioned response

**Fasciculation** . . . . . . . . . . . . . . rapid continuous twitching of resting muscle without movement of limb

**Flaccidity** . . . . . . . . . . . . . . . . . loss of muscle tone, limp

**Graphesthesia** . . . . . . . . . . . . . ability to "read" a number by having it traced on the skin

**Hemiplegia** . . . . . . . . . . . . . . . loss of motor power (paralysis) on one side of the body, usually caused by a stroke; paralysis occurs on side opposite the lesion

**Lower motor neuron** . . . . . . . . motor neuron in the peripheral nervous system with its nerve fiber extending out to the muscle and only its cell body in the central nervous system

**Myoclonus** . . . . . . . . . . . . . . . . rapid sudden jerk of a muscle

**Nuchal rigidity** . . . . . . . . . . . . stiffness in cervical neck area

**Nystagmus** . . . . . . . . . . . . . . . . back and forth oscillation of the eyes

**Opisthotonos** . . . . . . . . . . . . . . prolonged arching of back, with head and heels bent backward, and meningeal irritation

**Paralysis** . . . . . . . . . . . . . . . . . decreased or loss of motor function due to problem with motor nerve or muscle fibers

**Paraplegia** . . . . . . . . . . . . . . . . impairment or loss of motor and/or sensory function in the lower half of the body

**Paresthesia** . . . . . . . . . . . . . . . abnormal sensation (e.g., burning, numbness, tingling, prickling, crawling skin sensation)

**Point localization** . . . . . . . . . . ability of the person to discriminate exactly where on the body the skin has been touched

**Proprioception** . . . . . . . . . . . . sensory information concerning body movements and position of the body in space

**Spasticity** . . . . . . . . . . . . . . . . continuous resistance to stretching by a muscle due to abnormally increased tension with increased deep tendon reflexes

**Stereognosis** . . . . . . . . . . . . . . ability to recognize objects by feeling their form, size, and weight while the eyes are closed

**Tic** . . . . . . . . . . . . . . . . . . . . . . . repetitive twitching of a muscle group at inappropriate times (e.g., wink, grimace)

**Tremor** . . . . . . . . . . . . . . . . . . . involuntary contraction of opposing muscle groups resulting in rhythmic movement of one or more joints

**Two-point discrimination** . . . . ability to distinguish the separation of two simultaneous pinpricks on the skin

**Upper motor neuron** . . . . . . . . nerve located entirely within the central nervous system

## STUDY GUIDE

After completing the reading assignment and the media assignment, write or draw the answers in the spaces provided.

1. List the major function(s) of the following components of the central nervous system:

   Cerebral cortex—frontal lobe _____

   Cerebral cortex—parietal lobe _____

   Cerebral cortex—temporal lobe _____

   Cerebral cortex—Wernicke's area _____

   Cerebral cortex—Broca's area _____

   Basal ganglia _____

   _____

   Thalamus _____

   Hypothalamus _____

   _____

   Cerebellum _____

   Midbrain _____

   Pons _____

   Medulla _____

   Spinal cord _____

2. List the primary sensations mediated by the 2 major sensory pathways of the CNS.

3. Describe 3 major motor pathways in the CNS, including the type of movements mediated by each.

4. Differentiate an upper motor neuron from a lower motor neuron.

5. List the 5 components of a deep tendon reflex arc.

6. List the major symptom areas to assess when collecting a health history for the neurologic system.

7. List and describe 3 tests of cerebellar function.

8. Describe the method of testing the sensory system for pain, temperature, touch, vibration, and position.

9. Define the 4-point grading scale for deep tendon reflexes.

10. Which vertebral level is assessed when eliciting each of these reflexes?

    Biceps reflex _____          Quadriceps reflex _____

    Triceps reflex _____          Achilles reflex _____

    Brachioradialis reflex _____

11. List the components of the neurologic recheck examination that are performed routinely on hospitalized persons being monitored for neurologic deficit.

12. List the 3 areas of assessment on the Glasgow Coma Scale.

Fill in the labels indicated on the following illustrations.

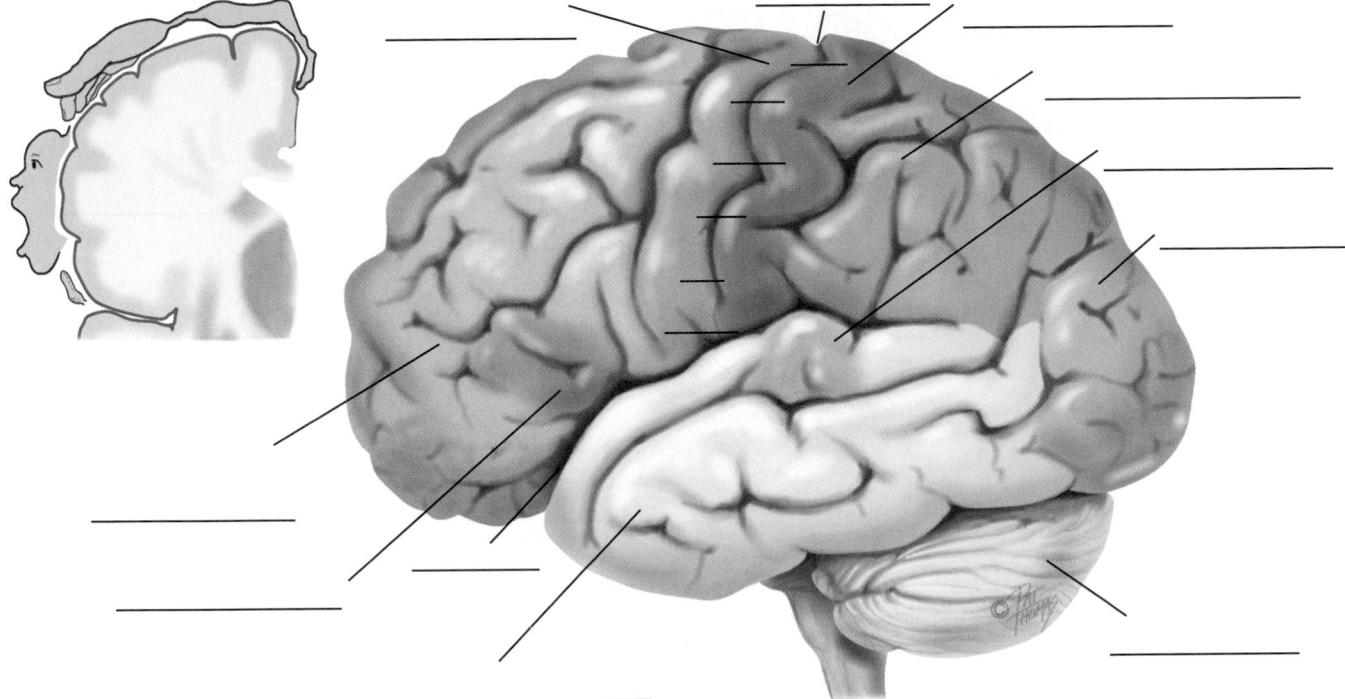

(© Pat Thomas, 2006.)

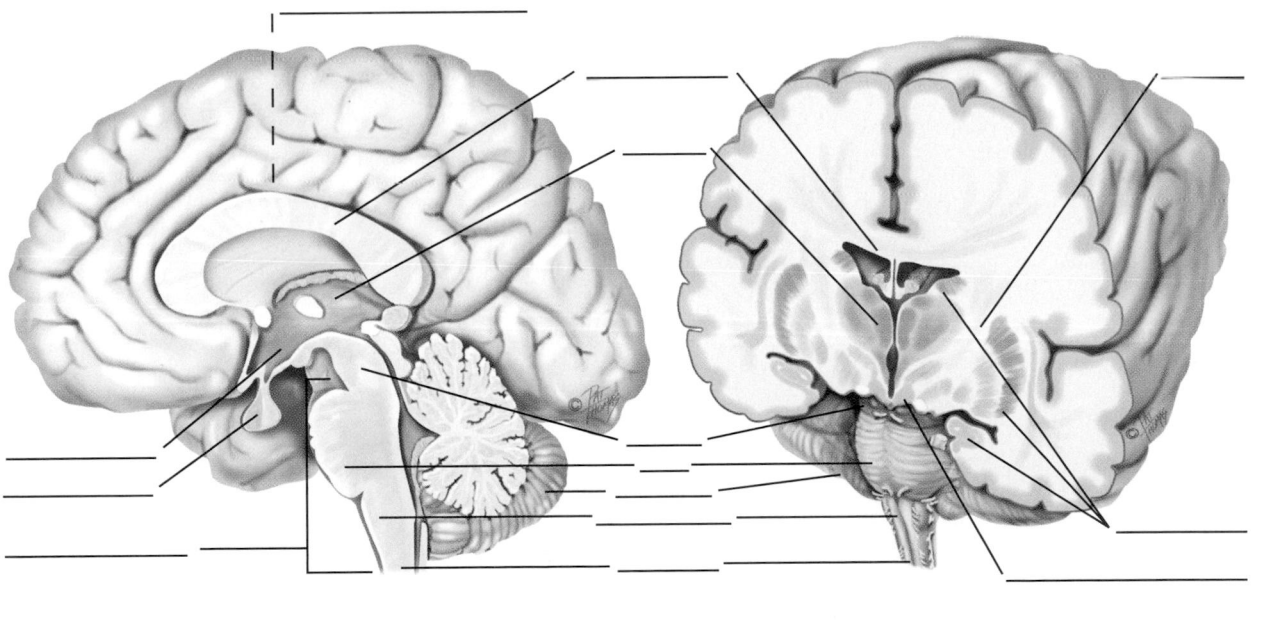

(© Pat Thomas, 2006.)

Fill in the name of each cranial nerve, and then write S (sensory), M (motor), or MX (mixed).

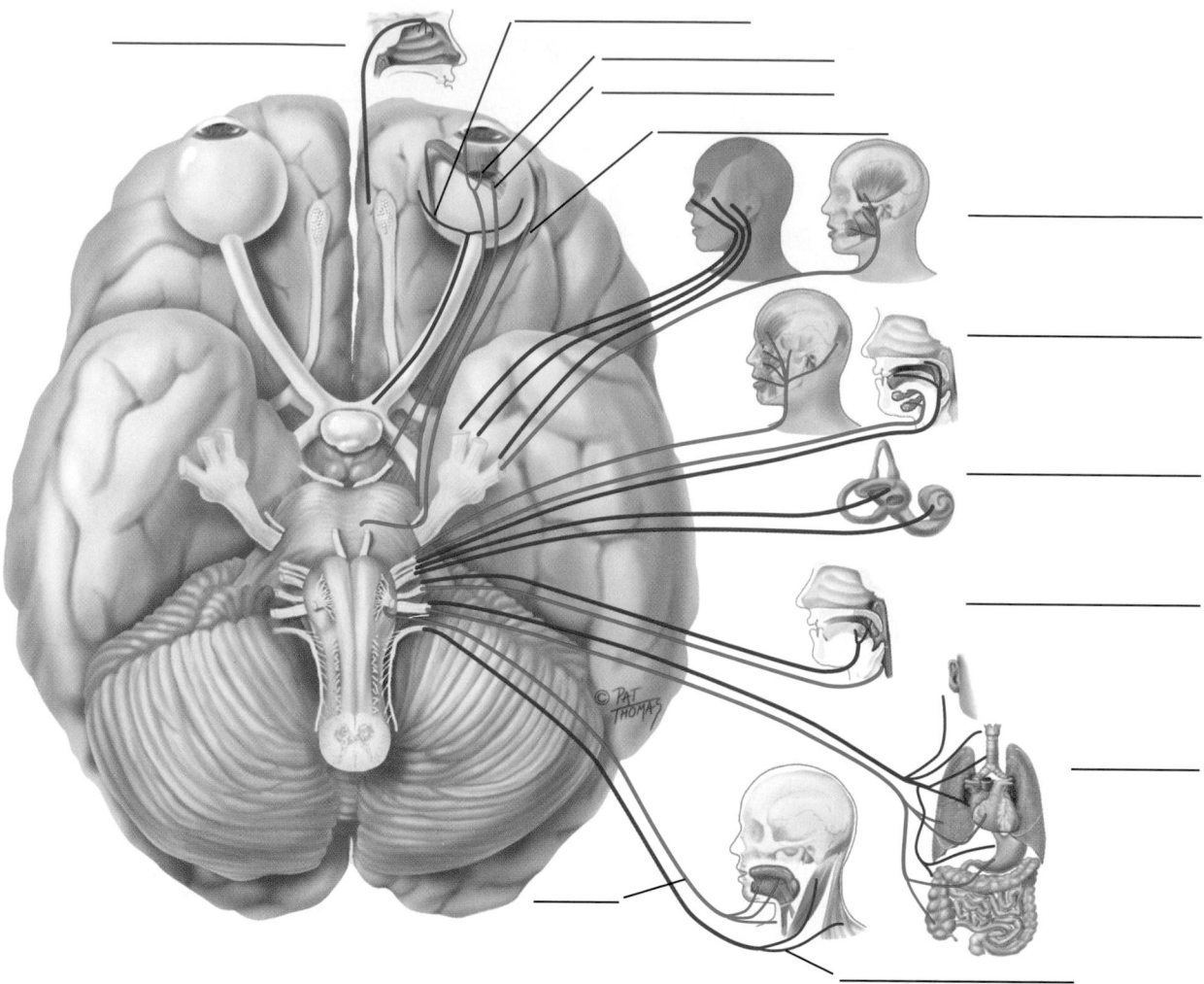

(© Pat Thomas, 2006.)

## REVIEW QUESTIONS

This test is for you to check your own mastery of the content. The answers are provided in Appendix A.

1. The medical record indicates that a person has an injury to Broca's area. When meeting this person, you expect:

    a. Difficulty speaking
    b. Receptive aphasia
    c. Visual disturbances
    d. Emotional lability

2. The control of body temperature is located in:

    a. Wernicke's area.
    b. The thalamus.
    c. The cerebellum.
    d. The hypothalamus.

3. To test for stereognosis, you would:

    a. Have the person close his or her eyes and then raise the person's arm and ask the person to describe its location.
    b. Touch the person with a tuning fork.
    c. Place a coin in the person's hand and ask him or her to identify it.
    d. Touch the person with a cold object.

4. During the examination of an infant, use a cotton-tipped applicator to stimulate the anal sphincter. The absence of a response suggests a lesion of:

    a. L2.
    b. T12.
    c. S2.
    d. C5.

5. During a neurologic examination, the tendon reflex fails to appear. Before striking the tendon again, you use the technique of:

    a. Two-point discrimination.
    b. Reinforcement.
    c. Vibration.
    d. Graphesthesia.

6. Cerebellar function is assessed by which of the following:

    a. Muscle size and strength assessment
    b. Cranial nerve examination
    c. Coordination—hopping on one foot
    d. Spinothalamic test

7. To elicit the Babinski reflex:

    a. Gently tap the Achilles tendon.
    b. Stroke the lateral aspect of the sole of the foot from heel to across the ball.
    c. Present a noxious odor to the person.
    d. Observe the person walking heel to toe.

8. A positive Babinski sign is:

    a. Dorsiflexion of the big toe and fanning of all toes.
    b. Plantar flexion of the big toe with a fanning of all toes.
    c. The expected response in healthy adults.
    d. Withdrawal of the stimulated extremity from the stimulus.

9. Senile tremors may resemble parkinsonism, except that senile tremors do not include:

    a. Nodding the head as if responding yes or no.
    b. Rigidity and weakness of voluntary movement.
    c. Tremor of the hands.
    d. Tongue protrusion.

10. Patients who have Parkinson disease usually have which of the following characteristic styles of speech?

    a. A garbled manner
    b. Loud, urgent
    c. Slow, monotonous
    d. Word confusion

11. The Glasgow Coma Scale (GCS) is divided into three areas. They include:

   a. Pupillary response, a reflex test, and assessing pain.
   b. Eye opening, motor response to stimuli, and verbal response.
   c. Response to fine touch, stereognosis, and sense of position.
   d. Orientation, rapid alternating movements, and the Romberg test.

12. The Landau reflex in the infant is seen when:

   a. The head is held and then flops forward as the baby is pulled to a sitting position by holding her or his wrists.
   b. The infant's toes curl down tightly in response to touch on the ball of his or her foot.
   c. The infant attempts to place his or her foot on the table while being held with the top of the foot touching the underside of the table.
   d. The baby raises her or his head and arches the back, as in a swan dive.

13. A 65-year-old man has noticed a change in his personality and his ability to understand. He also cries and becomes angry very easily. The cerebral lobe responsible for these behaviors is the _____ lobe.

   a. Frontal
   b. Parietal
   c. Occipital
   d. Temporal

Match column A to column B.

**Column A: Cranial Nerve**

14. _____ Olfactory
15. _____ Optic
16. _____ Oculomotor
17. _____ Trochlear
18. _____ Trigeminal
19. _____ Abducens
20. _____ Facial
21. _____ Acoustic
22. _____ Glossopharyngeal
23. _____ Vagus
24. _____ Spinal
25. _____ Hypoglossal

**Column B: Function**

a. Movement of the tongue
b. Vision
c. Lateral movement of the eyes
d. Hearing and equilibrium
e. Talking, swallowing, and sensory information from pharynx and carotid sinus
f. Smell
g. Extraocular movement, pupil constriction, down and inward movement of the eye
h. Mastication and sensation of face, scalp, cornea
i. Phonation, swallowing, tasting on the posterior third of tongue
j. Movement of trapezius and sternomastoid muscles
k. Down and inward movement of the eye
l. Tasting on the anterior two thirds of tongue, closing eyes

## CRITICAL THINKING EXERCISE

Take the Stroke Risk Quiz for yourself (http://www.strokeassociation.org/STROKEORG/AboutStroke/Stroke-Risk-Quiz_UCM_462514_SubHomePage.jsp). Then take it considering an older person in your family or among your acquaintances. Then take on the role of the health care provider and formulate a teaching plan that addresses how the person can reduce her or his risk of stroke.

## SKILLS LABORATORY/CLINICAL SETTING

The purpose of the clinical component is to practice the neurologic regional examination on a peer in the skills laboratory or a patient in the clinical setting and to achieve the following.

### Clinical Objectives

1. Demonstrate knowledge of the neurologic symptoms by obtaining a regional health history from a peer or patient.

2. Demonstrate examination of the neurologic system by assessing the cranial nerves, cerebellar function, sensory system, motor system, and deep tendon reflexes.

3. Record the history and physical examination findings accurately, reach an assessment of the health state, and develop a plan of care.

### Instructions

Gather all equipment for a complete neurologic examination. Wash your hands. Practice the steps of the examination on a peer or on a patient in the clinical setting, giving appropriate instructions as you proceed. Record your findings using the regional write-up sheet that follows. The first section is intended as a worksheet; the last page is intended for your narrative summary recording using the SOAP format.

**NOTES**

# REGIONAL WRITE-UP—NEUROLOGIC SYSTEM

Date _____

Examiner _____

Patient _____ Age _____ Gender _____

Reason for visit _____

## I. Health History

|  | No | Yes, explain |
|---|---|---|
| 1. Any unusually frequent or unusually severe **headaches**? | _____ | _____ |
| 2. Ever had any **head injury**? | _____ | _____ |
| 3. Ever feel **dizziness**? | _____ | _____ |
| 4. Ever had any **siezures**? | _____ | _____ |
| 5. Any **tremors** in hands or face? | _____ | _____ |
| 6. Any **weakness** in any body part? | _____ | _____ |
| 7. Any problem with **coordination**? | _____ | _____ |
| 8. Any **numbness or tingling**? | _____ | _____ |
| 9. Any problem **swallowing**? | _____ | _____ |
| 10. Any problem **speaking**? | _____ | _____ |
| 11. **Past history** of stroke, spinal cord injury, meningitis, congenital defect, alcoholism? | _____ | _____ |
| 12. Any environmental or occupational **hazards** (e.g., insecticides)? | | |

## II. Physical Examination

### A. Cranial nerves

II  _____

III, IV, VI  _____

V  _____

VII  _____

VIII  _____

IX, X  _____

XI  _____

XII  _____

**B. Motor system**
  1. Muscles
     Size, strength, tone _____
     Involuntary movements _____
  2. Cerebellar function
     Rapid alternative movements _____
     Finger-Nose-Finger test _____
     Heel to shin test _____
     Gait _____
     Romberg test _____

**C. Sensory system**
  1. Anterolateral tract
     Sharp or dull _____
     Light touch _____
  2. Posterior column tract
     Vibration _____
     Position (kinesthesia) _____
     Tactile discrimination
        Stereognosis _____
        Graphesthesia _____

**D. Reflexes**

|   | Bi | Tri | BR | P | A | PL (↑/↓) | Abd | Cre | Bab |
|---|----|-----|----|----|----|----------|-----|-----|-----|
| R |    |     |    |    |    |          |     |     |     |
| L |    |     |    |    |    |          |     |     |     |

0 = absent, 1+ = hypoactive, 2+ = normal, 3+ = hyperactive, 4+ = hyperactive with clonus,
↑ = dorsiflexion, ↓ = plantar flexion.

# REGIONAL WRITE-UP—NEUROLOGIC SYSTEM

Summarize your findings using the SOAP format.

**Subjective** (reason for seeking care, health history)

**Objective** (physical examination findings)

Record reflexes on diagram below.

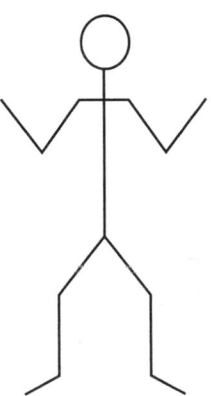

**Assessment** (assessment of health state or problem, diagnosis)

**Plan** (diagnostic evaluation, follow-up care, patient teaching)

**NOTES**

# CHAPTER 25

# Male Genitourinary System

## PURPOSE

This chapter helps you learn the structure and function of the male genitalia, learn the methods of inspection and palpation of these structures, and record the assessment accurately.

## READING ASSIGNMENT

Jarvis: *Physical Examination and Health Assessment*, 8th ed., Chapter 25, pp. 683-712.

Suggested reading:
Thornton, C. P. (2016). Best practice in teaching male adolescents and young men to perform testicular self-examinations. *J Pediatr Health Care, 30*(6), 518-527.

## GLOSSARY

Study the following terms after completing the reading assignment. You should be able to cover the definition on the right and define the term out loud.

**Chancre** . . . . . . . . . . . . . . . . . . . red, round, superficial ulcer with a yellowish serous discharge that is a sign of syphilis

**Condylomata acuminata** . . . . . soft, pointed, fleshy papules that occur on the genitalia and are caused by the human papillomavirus (HPV)

**Cryptorchidism** . . . . . . . . . . . . . undescended testes

**Cystitis** . . . . . . . . . . . . . . . . . . . . inflammation of the urinary bladder

**Epididymis** . . . . . . . . . . . . . . . . . structures composed of coiled ducts located over the superior and posterior surface of the testes, which store sperm

**Epispadias** . . . . . . . . . . . . . . . . . congenital defect in which the urethra opens on the dorsal (upper) side of penis instead of at the tip

**Hernia** . . . . . . . . . . . . . . . . . . . . weak spot in abdominal muscle wall (usually in area of inguinal canal or femoral canal) through which a loop of bowel may protrude

**Herpes genitalis** . . . . . . . . . . . . a sexually transmitted infection characterized by clusters of small painful vesicles, caused by a virus

**Heterosexism** . . . . . . . . . . . . . . an unscientific expectation that heterosexuality is the expected norm and that individuals who are lesbian, gay, bisexual, or transgender are somehow abnormal

**Homophobia** . . . . . . . . . . . . . . an irrational fear of homosexuals, resulting in negative feelings toward them

**Hydrocele** . . . . . . . . . . . . . . . . cystic fluid in tunica vaginalis surrounding the testis

**Hypospadias** . . . . . . . . . . . . . . congenital defect in which urethra opens on the ventral (under) side of penis rather than at the tip

**Orchitis** . . . . . . . . . . . . . . . . . . acute inflammation of testis, usually associated with mumps

**Paraphimosis** . . . . . . . . . . . . . foreskin retracted and fixed behind the glans penis

**Peyronie disease** . . . . . . . . . . . nontender hard plaques on the surface of penis, associated with painful bending of penis during erection

**Phimosis** . . . . . . . . . . . . . . . . . foreskin is advanced and tightly fixed over the glans penis

**Prepuce** . . . . . . . . . . . . . . . . . . foreskin; the hood or flap of skin over the glans penis that often is surgically removed after birth by circumcision

**Priapism** . . . . . . . . . . . . . . . . . prolonged, painful erection of penis without sexual desire

**Spermatic cord** . . . . . . . . . . . . collection of vas deferens, blood vessels, lymphatics, and nerves that ascends along the testis and through the inguinal canal into the abdomen

**Spermatocele** . . . . . . . . . . . . . . retention cyst in epididymis filled with milky fluid that contains sperm

**Torsion** . . . . . . . . . . . . . . . . . . . sudden twisting of spermatic cord; a surgical emergency

**Varicocele** . . . . . . . . . . . . . . . . dilated tortuous varicose veins in the spermatic cord

**Vas deferens** . . . . . . . . . . . . . . duct carrying sperm from the epididymis through the abdomen and then into the urethra

## STUDY GUIDE

After completing the reading assignment and the media assignment, you should be able to answer the following questions in the spaces provided.

1. Identify the structures that provide transport of sperm.

2. Describe the significance of the inguinal canal and the femoral canal.

3. List the pros and cons of circumcision of the male newborn.

4. Discuss ways of creating an environment that will provide psychological comfort for the man and the examiner during examination of the male genitalia.

5. List teaching points to include with the teaching of testicular self-examination.

6. List laboratory tests to assess urinary function.

7. Discuss the rationale for making certain that the testes have descended in the male infant.

8. Contrast phimosis with paraphimosis and hypospadias with epispadias.

9. Describe the following lesions of the penis and genital area:

   Tinea cruris

   Herpes simplex type 2

   Syphilitic chancre

   Penile warts (condylomata acuminata, HPV)

10. Contrast the physical appearance and clinical significance of these scrotal lumps:

Epididymitis

Varicocele

Spermatocele

Testicular tumor

Hydrocele

11. Contrast the anatomic course and clinical significance of these hernias:

Indirect inguinal

Direct inguinal

Femoral

Fill in the labels indicated on the following illustrations.

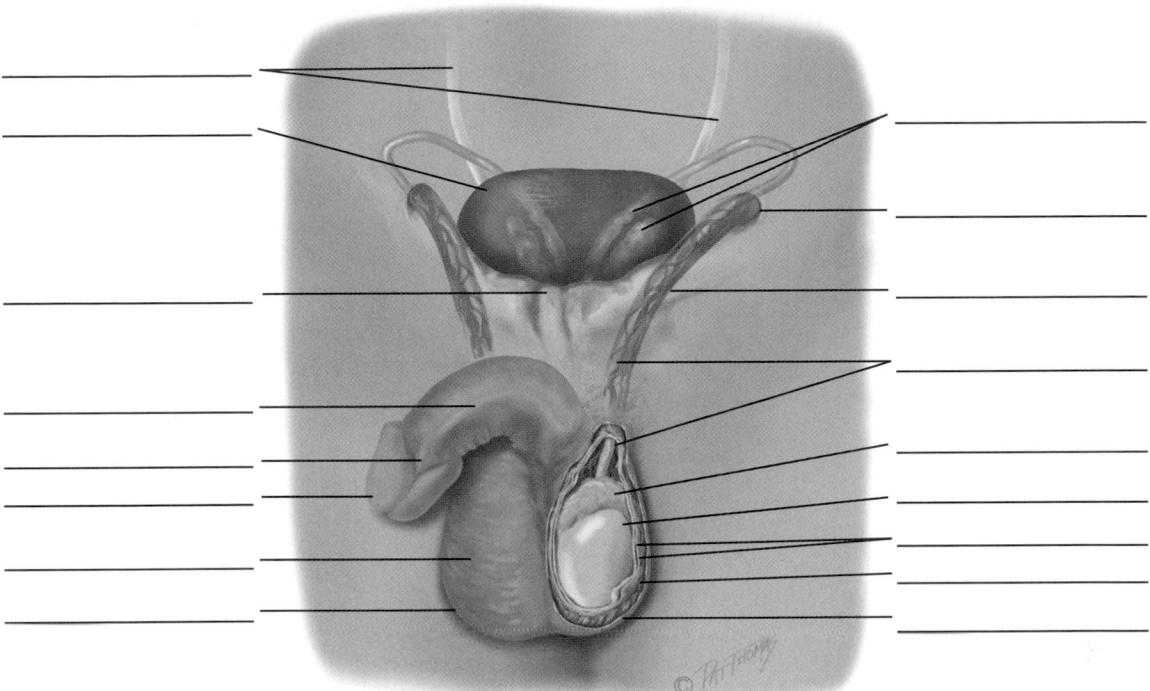

(© Pat Thomas, 2010.)

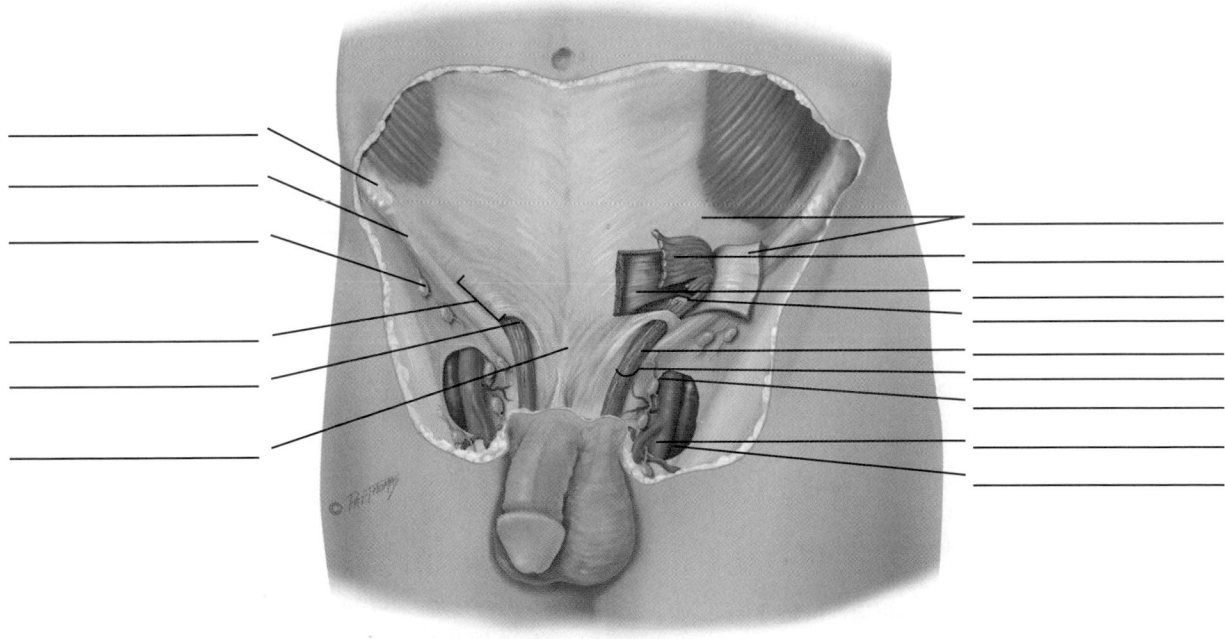

(© Pat Thomas, 2010.)

## REVIEW QUESTIONS

This test is for you to check your own mastery of the content. Answers are provided in Appendix A.

1. The examiner is going to inspect and palpate for a hernia. During this examination, the man is instructed to:

   a. Hold his breath during palpation.
   b. Cough after the examiner has gently inserted the examination finger into the rectum.
   c. Bear down when the examiner's finger is at the inguinal canal.
   d. Relax in a supine position while the examination finger is inserted into the canal.

2. During examination of the scrotum, a normal finding would be that:

   a. The left testicle is firmer to palpation than the right.
   b. The left testicle is larger than the right.
   c. The left testicle hangs lower than the right.
   d. The left testicle is more tender to palpation than the right.

3. H.T. has come to the clinic for a follow-up visit. Six months ago, he was started on a new medication that may cause erectile dysfunction as a side effect; therefore medication classes explored by the nurse are:

   a. Antipyretics.
   b. Bronchodilators.
   c. Corticosteroids.
   d. Antihypertensives.

4. Prostatic hypertrophy occurs frequently in older men. The symptoms that may indicate this problem are:

   a. Polyuria and urgency.
   b. Dysuria and oliguria.
   c. Straining, loss of force, and sense of residual urine.
   d. Foul-smelling urine and dysuria.

5. A 74-year-old man has come for a health examination. A normal age-related change in the scrotum would be:

   a. Testicular atrophy.
   b. Testicular hypertrophy.
   c. Pendulous scrotum.
   d. Increase in scrotal rugae.

6. During palpation of the testes, the normal finding would be:

   a. Firm to hard and rough.
   b. Nodular.
   c. 2 to 3 cm long × 2 cm wide and firm.
   d. Firm, rubbery, and smooth.

7. A 20-year-old man has indicated that he does not perform a testicular self-examination. One of the facts that should be shared with him is that testicular cancer, although rare, does occur in men:

   a. Younger than 15 years.
   b. 15 to 34 years of age.
   c. 35 to 55 years of age.
   d. 55 years and older.

8. During the examination of a full-term male newborn, a finding requiring investigation would be:

   a. An absent testes.
   b. A meatus centered at the tip of the penis.
   c. A wrinkled scrotum.
   d. A penis 2 to 3 cm in length.

9. During transillumination of a scrotum, you note a nontender mass that transilluminates with a red glow. This finding is suggestive of:

   a. Scrotal hernia.
   b. Scrotal edema.
   c. Orchitis.
   d. Hydrocele.

10. Which of the following would be a normal sensitivity to pressure for the testes?

    a. Somewhat
    b. Not at all
    c. Left more sensitive than right
    d. Only when inflammation is present

11. The congenital displacement of the urethral meatus to the inferior surface of the penis is:

    a. Hypospadias.
    b. Epispadias.
    c. Hypoesthesia.
    d. Hypophysis.

12. An adhesion of the prepuce to the head of the penis, making it impossible to retract, is:

    a. Paraphimosis.
    b. Phimosis.
    c. Smegma.
    d. Dyschezia.

13. You are assessing an adolescent boy. The first physical sign of puberty is:

    a. Height spurt.
    b. Penis lengthening.
    c. Sperm production.
    d. Pubic hair development.
    e. Testes enlargement.

14. An older man asks if he is able to father children. In the aging male, when does infertility occur?

    a. At age 60, with the sudden decline in sperm production
    b. At approximately age 55 to 60, when testosterone levels are lower
    c. When the male is no longer able to achieve an erection
    d. There is no specific age; men may be fertile into their 80s and 90s.

15. A patient has soft, moist, fleshy, painless papules around the anus. The examiner suspects this condition is:

    a. HSV-2.
    b. HPV.
    c. Gonorrhea.
    d. Peyronie disease.

## CRITICAL THINKING EXERCISE

Prepare a script for the teaching of testicular self-exam (TSE) to an adolescent or young man. Use the content on the benefits and risks of TSE in the suggested reading article on p. 227. Make your script non-judgmental and free of medical jargon. Practice your delivery on a peer in your lab setting.

## SKILLS LABORATORY AND CLINICAL SETTING

Because of the need to maintain personal privacy, it is likely that you will <u>not</u> practice the male genitalia examination on a classmate. Your practice likely will be with a teaching mannequin in the skills laboratory or with a male patient in the clinical setting. Before you proceed, discuss the feelings that may be experienced by the man and the examiner and methods to increase the comfort of both. Make sure you have discussed the steps of the examination with your instructor before examining a patient.

### Clinical Objectives

1.  Demonstrate knowledge of the signs and symptoms related to the male genitalia by obtaining a pertinent health history.

2.  Inspect and palpate the penis and scrotum.

3.  Palpate the inguinal region for hernia.

4.  Teach testicular self-examination.

5.  Record the history and physical examination findings accurately, reach an assessment of the health state, and develop a plan of care.

### Instructions

Prepare the examination setting, and gather your equipment. Wash your hands; wear gloves during the examination. Practice the steps of the examination on a male patient in the clinical setting, giving appropriate instructions as you proceed. Record your findings using the regional write-up sheet that follows. The front of the page is intended as a worksheet; the back of the page is intended for your narrative summary recording using the SOAP format.

# REGIONAL WRITE-UP—MALE GENITOURINARY SYSTEM

Date _____

Examiner _____

Patient _____ Age _____ Gender _____

Reason for visit _____

## I. Health History

| | No | Yes, explain |
|---|---|---|
| 1. Any urinary **frequency, urgency,** or awakening during night to urinate? | _____ | _____ |
| 2. Any **pain** or **burning** with urinating? | _____ | _____ |
| 3. Any **trouble starting urine stream?** | _____ | _____ |
| 4. Urine **color cloudy** or **foul-smelling?** **Red-tinged** or **bloody?** | _____ | _____ |
| 5. Any **problem controlling your urine?** | _____ | _____ |
| 6. Any **pain** or **sores** on penis? | _____ | _____ |
| 7. Any **lump** in testicles or scrotum? Do you perform testicular self-examination? | _____ | _____ |
| 8. In a relationship now involving intercourse? Use a contraceptive? Which one? | _____ _____ | _____ |
| 9. Any contact with partner who has sexually transmitted infection? Was this treated with antibiotics? | _____ | _____ |

## II. Physical Examination

**A. Inspect and palpate penis.**

Skin condition _____

Glans _____

Urethral meatus _____

Shaft _____

**B. Inspect and palpate scrotum.**

Skin condition _____

Testes _____

Spermatic cord _____

Transillumination (if indicated) _____

**C. Inspect and palpate for hernia.**

Inguinal canal _____

Femoral area _____

**D. Palpate inguinal lymph nodes.** _____

**E. Teach testicular self-examination.** _____

# REGIONAL WRITE-UP—MALE GENITOURINARY SYSTEM

Summarize your findings using the SOAP format.

**Subjective** (reason for seeking care, health history)

**Objective** (physical examination findings)

**Assessment** (assessment of health state or problem, diagnosis)

**Plan** (diagnostic evaluation, follow-up care, patient teaching)

# Anus, Rectum, and Prostate

## PURPOSE

This chapter presents the structure and function of the anus and rectum and the male prostate gland, the methods of inspection and palpation of these structures, and how to record the assessment accurately.

## READING ASSIGNMENT

Jarvis: *Physical Examination and Health Assessment,* 8th ed., Chapter 26, pp. 713-728.

Suggested reading:
Sommers, T., Corban, C., Sengupta, N., et al. (2015). Emergency department burden of constipation in the United States from 2006 to 2011. *Am J Gastroenterol, 110*(4), 572-579, doi:10.1038/ajg.2015.64.

## GLOSSARY

Study the following terms after completing the reading assignment. You should be able to cover the definition on the right and define the term out loud.

**Constipation**. . . . . . . . . . . . . . . decrease in stool frequency, with difficult passing of very hard, dry stools

**Fissure** . . . . . . . . . . . . . . . . . . . . painful longitudinal tear in tissue (e.g., in the superficial mucosa at the anal margin)

**Hemorrhoid** . . . . . . . . . . . . . . . flabby papules of skin or mucous membrane in the anal region caused by a varicose vein of the hemorrhoidal plexus

**Human papillomavirus (HPV)**. . . . . . . . . . . . . . . . . . . a double-stranded DNA virus that enters the nuclei of the squamous and basal cells in oral, nasal, genital, and anal regions; transmitted through vaginal, anal, and oral intercourse

**Melena** . . . . . . . . . . . . . . . . . . . . blood in the stool

**Pruritus**. . . . . . . . . . . . . . . . . . . itching or burning sensation in the skin

**Steatorrhea** . . . . . . . . . . . . . . . . excessive fat in the stool, as in gastrointestinal malabsorption of fat

**Valves of Houston** . . . . . . . . . . set of three semilunar transverse folds that cross half the circumference of the rectal lumen

## STUDY GUIDE

After completing the reading assignment and the media assignment, answer the following questions in the spaces provided.

1. State the length of the anal canal and the rectum in the adult, and describe the location of these structures in the lower abdomen.

2. Describe the size, shape, and location of the male prostate gland.

3. List a few examples of high-fiber foods of the soluble type and of the insoluble type. What advantages do these foods have for the body?

4. List screening measures that are recommended for early detection of colon-rectal cancer and of prostate cancer.

5. State the method of promoting anal sphincter relaxation to aid palpation of the anus and rectum.

6. Describe the normal physical characteristics of the prostate gland that would be assessed by palpation:

   Size

   Shape

   Surface

   Consistency

   Mobility

   Sensitivity

7. Define the condition *benign prostatic hypertrophy,* list the usual symptoms that the man experiences with this condition, and describe the physical characteristics.

Fill in the labels indicated on the following illustrations.

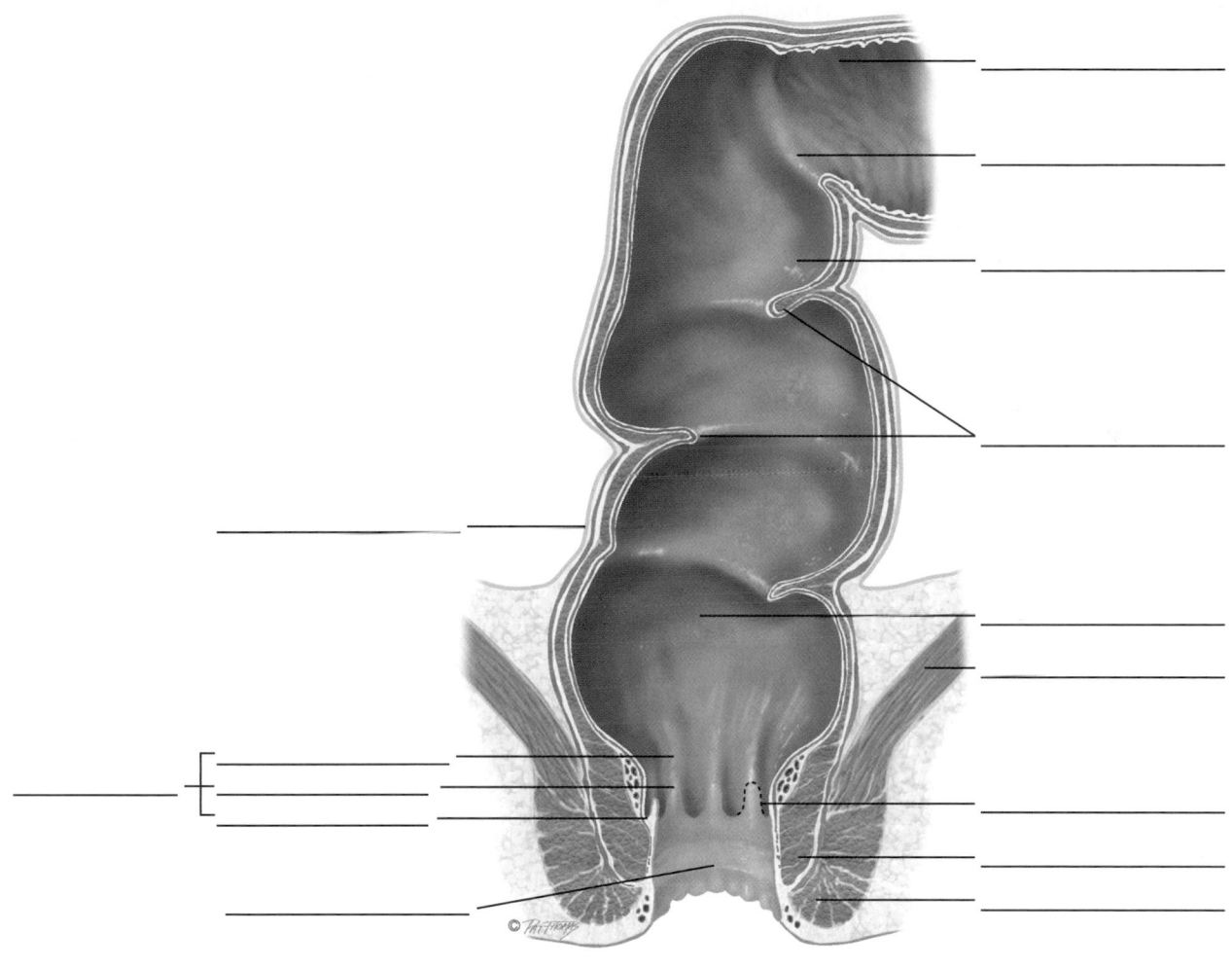

(© Pat Thomas, 2010.)

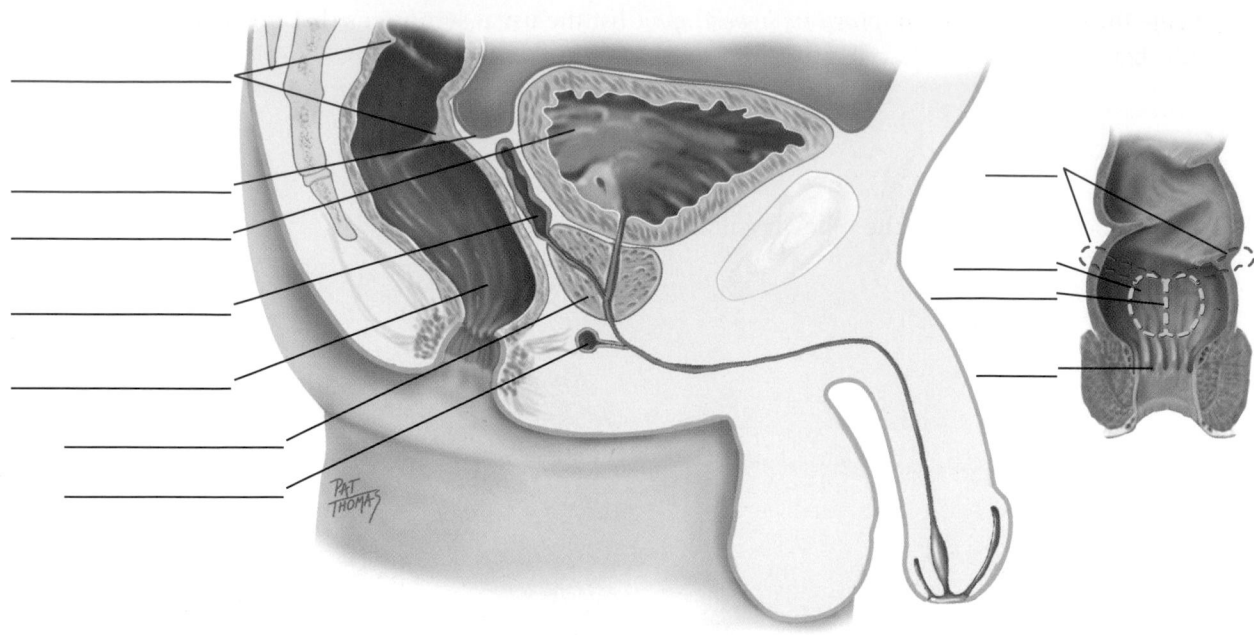

## REVIEW QUESTIONS

This test is for you to check your own mastery of the content. Answers are provided in Appendix A.

1. The gastrocolic reflex is:

   a. A peristaltic wave.
   b. The passage of meconium in the newborn.
   c. Another term for borborygmi.
   d. Reverse peristalsis.

2. Which population has the highest incidence of benign prostatic hypertrophy (BPH)?

   a. European Americans
   b. African Americans
   c. Hispanics
   d. Asians

3. Select the best description of the anal canal.

   a. 12-cm-long portion of the large intestine
   b. Involuntary control of the parasympathetic nervous system
   c. 3.8-cm-long outlet of the gastrointestinal tract
   d. S-shaped portion of the colon

4. Foods that may be beneficial to reduce the risk for colon cancer include:

   a. Foods high in fiber.
   b. Foods low in fat.
   c. Foods high in protein.
   d. Foods high in carbohydrates.

5. Which finding in the prostate gland suggests prostate cancer?

   a. Symmetric smooth enlargement
   b. Extreme tenderness to palpation
   c. Boggy soft enlargement
   d. Diffuse hardness

6. Which is true regarding the bulbourethral gland?

   a. It can be palpated during an examination of a female patient.
   b. It can be palpated during an examination of both male and female patients.
   c. It can be palpated during an examination of a male patient.
   d. It cannot be assessed with a rectal examination.

7. Normal stool is described as:

   a. Black in color and tarry in consistency.
   b. Brown in color and soft in consistency.
   c. Clay-colored and dry in consistency.
   d. Varies depending on the individual's diet.

8. Which symptoms suggest benign prostatic hypertrophy?

   a. Weight loss and bone pain
   b. Fever, chills, urinary frequency, and urgency
   c. Difficulty initiating urination and weak stream
   d. Dark, tarry stools

9. A patient states that he is frequently constipated, and when he has a bowel movement he has rectal bleeding and pain. He does not feel any mass at his anal opening. "Do I have hemorrhoids, or is there something else wrong with me?" The examiner completes a rectal examination and explains that:

   a. There is an indication of rectal prolapse.
   b. It appears to be a pilonidal cyst.
   c. The symptoms are consistent with internal hemorrhoids.
   d. The problem is probably encopresis.

10. A patient states that he has frothy, foul-smelling stools that float on the surface of the water in the toilet bowl. What type of stool is this patient describing?

    a. Steatorrhea
    b. Melena
    c. Dyschezia
    d. A parasitic infection

11. Which of these is the correct technique to assess patency of the anal sphincter?

    a. Inspect the anus and ask the patient to strain.
    b. Palpate the anus with a gloved finger to elicit sphincter control.
    c. Percuss above the anal canal for dull resonance.
    d. There are no sensory nerves in the anal canal or rectum.

12. Which is a structure that secretes a thin, milky alkaline fluid to enhance the viability of sperm?

    a. Cowper gland
    b. Prostate gland
    c. Median sulcus
    d. Bulbourethral gland

13. A newborn infant has a dark green stool 2 days after birth. How should you interpret this?

    a. This type of stool would indicate anal patency.
    b. The dark green color could indicate occult blood in the stool.
    c. Meconium stool can be reflective of distress in the newborn.
    d. The newborn should have passed the first stool within 12 hours after birth.

## CRITICAL THINKING EXERCISE 1

Communication is a crucial component of every patient encounter. Read the suggested article on p. 237 by Sommers et al. (2015). In a small discussion group during your laboratory, address these topics in the article:
- What did you learn about the various causes of constipation?
- What economic and social factors would prompt a person to seek care at an emergency department rather than an outpatient office for the concern of constipation?
- What impact do the ED visits for constipation have on governmental health care policy and insurance coverage?
- Many older persons experience constipation. Some discuss it freely; others do not discuss it unless pressed. Think about the older adults with whom you have had experience—how did you react to their discussions of constipation?

## CRITICAL THINKING EXERCISE 2

Colon cancer is the second cause of cancer death in the United States, but many cases are preventable with screening measures. Search the website at http://www.cdc.gov/cancer/colorectal/sfl.
- Choose materials that are most helpful to you in patient teaching, considering health literacy.
- Choose a family member or family friend older than 50 years, and practice patient teaching with this person.
- Bring your results back to laboratory for group discussion.

## SKILLS LABORATORY AND CLINICAL SETTING

This regional examination usually is combined with examination of the male genitalia or female genitalia.

### Clinical Objectives

1. Demonstrate knowledge of the signs and symptoms related to the rectal area by obtaining a pertinent health history.

2. Inspect and palpate the perianal region.

3. Test any stool specimen for occult blood.

4. Record the history and physical examination findings accurately.

### Instructions

Prepare the examination setting, and gather your equipment. Wash your hands, wear gloves during the examination, and wash hands again after removing gloves. Practice the steps of the examination on a patient in the clinical setting, giving appropriate instructions as you proceed. Record your findings using the regional write-up sheet that follows. Note that only the worksheet is included in this chapter. Your narrative summary recording using the SOAP format can be included with the narrative summary of the genitalia.

# REGIONAL WRITE-UP—ANUS, RECTUM, AND PROSTATE GLAND

Date _____

Examiner _____

Patient _____ Age _____ Gender _____

Reason for visit _____

## I. Health History

| | No | Yes, explain |
|---|---|---|
| 1. Bowels move **regularly**? How often? Usual color? Hard or soft? | | |
| 2. Any **change** in usual bowel habits? Constipation, diarrhea | | |
| 3. Ever had **black or bloody stool**? | | |
| 4. Take any medications? | | |
| 5. Any **rectal itching, pain, or hemorrhoids**? | | |
| 6. Any family history of **colon-rectal polyps or cancer**? | | |
| 7. Describe usual amount of high-fiber foods in diet. | | |

## II. Physical Examination

### A. Inspect the perianal area.

Skin condition _____

Sacrococcygeal area _____

Note skin integrity while patient bears down. _____

### B. Palpate anus and rectum.

Anal sphincter _____

Anal canal _____

Rectal wall _____

Prostate gland (for males)

   Size _____

   Shape _____

   Surface _____

   Consistency _____

   Mobility _____

   Any tenderness _____

Cervix (for females) _____

### C. Examine the stool.

Visual inspection _____

Test for occult blood _____

# REGIONAL WRITE-UP—ANUS, RECTUM, PROSTATE

Summarize your findings using the SOAP format.

**Subjective** (reason for seeking care, health history)

**Objective** (physical examination findings)

**Assessment** (assessment of health state or problem, diagnosis)

**Plan** (diagnostic evaluation, follow-up care, teaching)

# Female Genitourinary System

## PURPOSE

This chapter helps you learn the structure and function of the female genitalia, the methods of inspection and palpation of the internal and external structures, the procedures for collection of cytologic specimens, and how to record the assessment accurately.

## READING ASSIGNMENT

Jarvis: *Physical Examination and Health Assessment*, 8th ed., Chapter 27, pp. 729-766.

Suggested reading:
Wiesenfeld, C. H. (2017). Screening for *Chlamydia trachomatis* infections in women. *New Engl J Med*, *376*(8), 765-773.

## GLOSSARY

Study the following terms after completing the reading assignment. You should be able to cover the definition on the right and define the term out loud.

**Adnexa** . . . . . . . . . . . . . . . . . . . accessory organs of the uterus (i.e., ovaries and fallopian tubes)

**Amenorrhea** . . . . . . . . . . . . . . . absence of menstruation; termed *secondary amenorrhea* when menstruation has begun and then ceases; most common cause is pregnancy

**Bartholin glands** . . . . . . . . . . . vestibular glands, located on either side of the vaginal orifice, that secrete a clear lubricating mucus during intercourse

**Bloody show** . . . . . . . . . . . . . . . dislodging of thick cervical mucus plug at end of pregnancy, which is a sign of beginning of labor

**Caruncle** . . . . . . . . . . . . . . . . . . small, deep red mass protruding from urethral meatus, usually due to urethritis

**Chadwick sign** . . . . . . . . . . . . . bluish discoloration of cervix that occurs normally in pregnancy at 6 to 8 weeks' gestation

**Chancre** . . . . . . . . . . . . . . . . . . red, round, superficial ulcer with a yellowish serous discharge that is a sign of syphilis

**Clitoris** . . . . . . . . . . . . . . . . . . . small, elongated erectile tissue in the female, located at anterior juncture of labia minora

**Cystocele** . . . . . . . . . . . . . . . . . prolapse of urinary bladder and its vaginal mucosa into the vagina with straining or standing

**Dysmenorrhea** . . . . . . . . . . . . . . abdominal cramping and pain associated with menstruation

**Dyspareunia** . . . . . . . . . . . . . . . painful intercourse

**Dysuria** . . . . . . . . . . . . . . . . . . painful urination

**Endometriosis** . . . . . . . . . . . . . aberrant growths of endometrial tissue scattered throughout pelvis

**Fibroid** . . . . . . . . . . . . . . . . . . . (myoma) hard, painless nodule in uterine wall that cause uterine enlargement

**Gonorrhea** . . . . . . . . . . . . . . . . . sexually transmitted infection characterized by purulent vaginal discharge or may have no symptoms

**Hegar sign** . . . . . . . . . . . . . . . . . softening of cervix that is a sign of pregnancy, occurring at 10 to 12 weeks' gestation

**Hematuria** . . . . . . . . . . . . . . . . . red-tinged or bloody urine

**Hymen** . . . . . . . . . . . . . . . . . . . membranous fold of tissue partly closing vaginal orifice

**Leukorrhea** . . . . . . . . . . . . . . . . . whitish or yellowish discharge from vaginal orifice

**Menarche** . . . . . . . . . . . . . . . . . . onset of first menstruation, usually between 11 and 13 years of age

**Menopause** . . . . . . . . . . . . . . . . cessation of menses, usually occurring around 48 to 51 years of age

**Menorrhagia** . . . . . . . . . . . . . . . excessively heavy menstrual flow

**Multipara** . . . . . . . . . . . . . . . . . condition of having two or more pregnancies

**Nullipara** . . . . . . . . . . . . . . . . . . condition of first pregnancy

**Papanicolaou test** . . . . . . . . . . . (Pap test) painless test used to detect cervical cancer

**Polyp** . . . . . . . . . . . . . . . . . . . . . cervical polyp is bright red, soft, pedunculated growth emerging from os

**Rectocele** . . . . . . . . . . . . . . . . . . prolapse of rectum and its vaginal mucosa into vagina with straining or standing

**Rectouterine pouch** . . . . . . . . . (cul-de-sac of Douglas) deep recess formed by the peritoneum between the rectum and cervix

**Salpingitis** . . . . . . . . . . . . . . . . . inflammation of fallopian tubes

**Skene glands** . . . . . . . . . . . . . . . paraurethral glands

**Vaginitis** . . . . . . . . . . . . . . . . . . inflammation of vagina

**Vulva** . . . . . . . . . . . . . . . . . . . . . external genitalia of female

## STUDY GUIDE

After completing the reading assignment and the media assignment, answer the following questions in the spaces provided.

1. Discuss ways of creating an environment that will provide psychological comfort for both the woman and practitioner during the female genitalia examination.

2. Discuss selection, preparation, and insertion of the vaginal speculum.

3. Describe the appearance or sketch these normal variations of the cervix and os:

   Nulliparous

   Parous

   Stellate lacerations

   Cervical eversion

   Nabothian cysts

4. List the steps in the procedure of obtaining these specimens:

   Vaginal pool

   Cervical scrape using spatula

   Endocervical specimen using cytobrush

5. Discuss the procedure and rationale for bimanual examination and list normal findings for the cervix, uterus, and adnexa.

6. Describe the appearance or sketch the appearance of the following abnormalities of the cervix:

Chadwick sign

Erosion

Polyp

Carcinoma

7. List the characteristics of vaginal discharge associated with the following conditions of vaginitis:

Candidiasis (yeast infection)

Trichomoniasis

Bacterial vaginosis

Chlamydia

Gonorrhea

8. List the changes observed during the perimenopausal period.

9. Differentiate the signs and symptoms of these conditions of adnexal enlargement:

Ectopic pregnancy

Ovarian cyst

Fill in the labels indicated on the following illustrations.

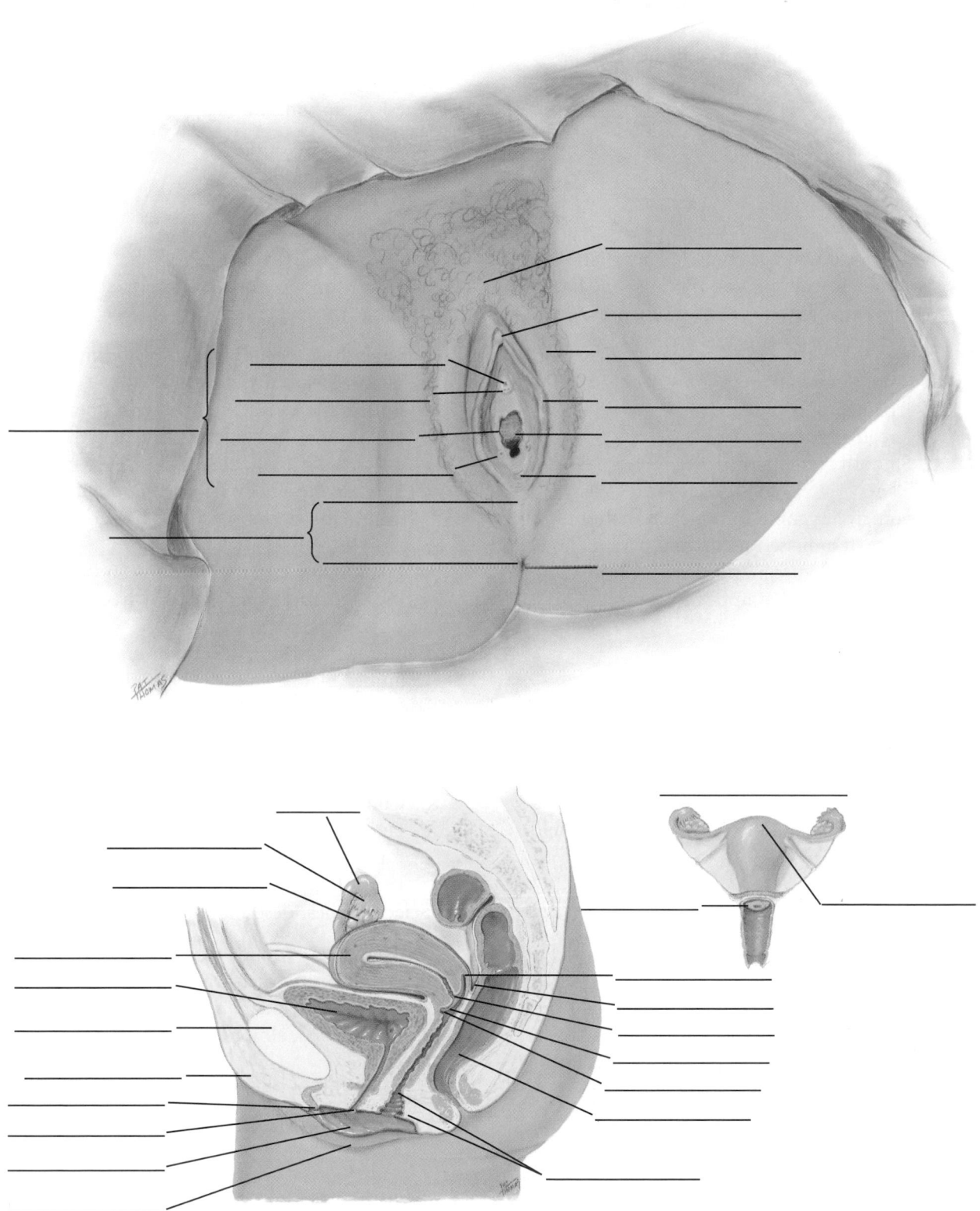

## REVIEW QUESTIONS

This test is for you to check your own mastery of the content. Answers are provided in Appendix A.

1. Vaginal lubrication is provided during intercourse by:

   a. Labia minora.
   b. Sebaceous follicles.
   c. Skene glands.
   d. Bartholin glands.

2. A young woman has come for her first gynecologic examination. Because she has not had any children, the examiner expects the cervical os to appear:

   a. Smooth and circular.
   b. Irregular and slitlike.
   c. Irregular and circular.
   d. Smooth and enlarged.

3. A woman has come for an examination because of a missed menstrual period and a positive home pregnancy test. Examination reveals a cervix that appears cyanotic. This is referred to as the:

   a. Goodell sign.
   b. Hegar sign.
   c. Tanner sign.
   d. Chadwick sign.

4. During the examination of the genitalia of a 70-year-old woman, a normal finding would be:

   a. Hypertrophy of the mons pubis.
   b. Increase in vaginal secretions.
   c. Thin and sparse pubic hair.
   d. Bladder prolapse.

5. For a woman, history of her mother's health during pregnancy is important. A medication that requires frequent follow-up is:

   a. Corticosteroid.
   b. Theophylline.
   c. Diethylstilbestrol.
   d. Aminoglycoside.

6. A woman has come for health care reporting a thick white discharge with intense itching. These symptoms are suggestive of:

   a. Atrophic vaginitis.
   b. Trichomoniasis.
   c. Chlamydia.
   d. Candidiasis.

7. To insert the speculum as comfortably as possible, the examiner:

   a. Opens the speculum slightly and inserts it in an upward direction.
   b. Presses the introitus down with one hand and inserts the blades obliquely with the other.
   c. Spreads the labia with one hand and inserts the closed speculum horizontally with the other.
   d. Pushes down on the introitus and inserts the speculum in an upward direction.

8. Before withdrawing the speculum, the examiner may swab the cervix with a swab soaked in acetic acid. This examination is done to assess for:

   a. Herpes simplex virus.
   b. Contact dermatitis.
   c. Human papillomavirus.
   d. Carcinoma.

9. Select the best description of the uterus.

   a. Anteverted, round, asymmetric organ
   b. Pear-shaped, thick-walled organ flattened anteroposteriorly
   c. Retroverted, almond-shaped, asymmetric organ
   d. Midposition, thick-walled, oval organ

10. In placing a finger on either side of the cervix and moving it side to side, you are assessing:

    a. The diameter of the fallopian tube.
    b. Cervical motion tenderness.
    c. The ovaries.
    d. The uterus.

11. Which of the following is (are) normal, common finding(s) on inspection and palpation of the vulva and perineum?

    a. Labia majora that are wide apart and gaping
    b. Palpable Bartholin glands
    c. Clear, thin discharge from paraurethral glands
    d. Bulging at introitus during Valsalva maneuver

12. Which is the most common bacterial sexually transmitted infection in the United States?

    a. Chlamydia
    b. Gonorrhea
    c. Trichomoniasis
    d. Syphilis
    e. Bacterial vaginosis

13. What does the notation in a health record indicating the patient is a "G2 P3 Ab0" mean?

    a. The woman has delivered 3 children, 2 of whom are living; her blood type is Ab0.
    b. The woman has been pregnant twice with 3 children (twins and another child), and all her children are living.
    c. The woman has been pregnant 3 times, has delivered 2 children, and has had no abortions.
    d. The woman has been pregnant 3 times, has 2 living children, and has had no spontaneous abortions.

14. What problems are associated with smoking and the use of oral contraceptives?

    a. Increased risk for alcoholism and cirrhosis of the liver
    b. Thrombophlebitis and pulmonary emboli
    c. Infertility and weight gain
    d. Urinary tract infections and skin cancer

## CRITICAL THINKING EXERCISE

Read and study the Wiesenfeld article listed on p. 245 concerning a 19-year-old woman's readiness for sexual intercourse and the health needs this situation raises. Answer these questions:
1. Describe how common chlamydia is as a sexually transmitted infection and who is at risk.
2. Chlamydia may or may not have vaginal symptoms. If it is not treated, what are the complications?
3. When a woman has a chlamydial infection, some providers give expedited treatment. That is, the provider gives an extra prescription or extra medications for the woman to give to her partner. This means the woman does not have to name her partner to the clinic. How do you feel about this practice?
4. The article described chlamydial screening by having the woman collect her own vaginal swab and bring it in for testing. What are the advantages of this intervention?

## SKILLS LABORATORY AND CLINICAL SETTING

Because of the need to maintain personal privacy, it is likely you will <u>not</u> practice the female genitalia examination on a peer. Your practice likely will be with a teaching mannequin in the skills laboratory or with a woman in the clinical setting under the guidance of a preceptor. Before you proceed, discuss the feelings that may be experienced by the woman and examiner and methods to increase the comfort of both. With your instructor, discuss methods of positioning the woman, steps in using the vaginal speculum, steps in procuring specimens, and methods of infection control precautions.

### Clinical Objectives

1. Demonstrate knowledge of the signs and symptoms related to the female genitalia by obtaining a pertinent health history.

2. Demonstrate measures to increase the woman's comfort before and during the examination.

3. Demonstrate knowledge of infection control precautions before, during, and after the examination.

4. Inspect and palpate the external genitalia.

5. Using the vaginal speculum, gather materials for cytologic study.

6. Inspect and palpate the internal genitalia.

7. Record the history and physical examination findings accurately, reach an assessment of the health state, and develop a plan of care.

### Instructions

Prepare the examination setting, and gather your equipment. Collect the health history before the woman disrobes for the examination. Wash your hands, wear gloves during the examination, and wash hands again after removing gloves. Practice the steps of the examination on a woman in the clinical setting, giving appropriate instructions as you proceed. Record your findings using the regional write-up sheet that follows. The first section is intended as a worksheet; the last page is intended for your narrative summary recording using the SOAP format. Collection of data for the rectal examination is usually combined with the examination of female genitalia; see Chapter 25 for the regional write-up sheet for the rectal examination.

# REGIONAL WRITE-UP—FEMALE GENITOURINARY SYSTEM

Date _____

Examiner _____

Patient _____ Age _____

Reason for visit _____

## I. Health History

| | No | Yes, explain |
|---|---|---|
| 1. Date of **last menstrual period?** Age at first period? Usual cycle? Duration? Usual amount of flow? Any pain or cramps with period? | | |
| 2. Ever been **pregnant**? How many times? Describe pregnancy(ies). Any complications? | | |
| 3. Periods slowed down or **stopped**? | | |
| 4. How often are **gynecologic checkups**? Date of last Pap test? Results? | | |
| 5. Any problems with **urinating**? | | |
| 6. Any unusual **vaginal discharge**? | | |
| 7. **Sores or lesions** in genitals? | | |
| 8. In a relationship now involving intercourse? | | |
| 9. Use a contraceptive? Which one? | | |
| 10. Any contact with partner who has a sexually transmitted infection? | | |
| 11. Any precautions to reduce risk for STIs? | | |
| 12. Taking any medications? Any hormone therapy? | | |

## II. Physical Examination
### A. Inspect external genitalia.
Skin color and mucous membranes _____

Hair distribution _____ Structures symmetric? _____

Clitoris _____ Labia _____

Urethral opening _____ Vaginal opening _____

Perineum _____

Any lesions? _____

B. **Palpate external genitalia.**
   Bartholin glands _____
   Perineum _____
   Assess for vaginal wall bulging or urinary incontinence. _____
   Discharge, color, odor, consistency _____

C. **Speculum examination**
   Inspect cervix and os.
       Color _____ Position _____
       Size _____ _____Surface _____
       Discharge, color, odor, consistency _____
       Nabothian cysts? _____ IUD string, if present _____
   Obtain cervical smears and cultures.
   Vaginal pool _____ Cervical scrape _____ Endocervical specimen _____
   Other (if indicated) _____
   Complete acetic acid wash _____
   Inspect vaginal wall as speculum is removed. _____

D. **Bimanual examination**
   Cervix
       Consistency _____ Mobility _____
       Tenderness with motion _____
   Uterus
       Size and shape _____ Consistency _____
       Position _____ Mobility _____
       Tenderness _____
   Adnexa
       Able to palpate? (Be honest.) _____
       Size and shape of ovaries _____
       Tenderness _____ Masses _____
   Rectovaginal examination _____

# REGIONAL WRITE-UP—FEMALE GENITOURINARY SYSTEM

Summarize your findings using the SOAP format.

**Subjective** (reason for seeking care, health history)

**Objective** (physical examination findings)                     Record findings on diagram below.

**Assessment** (assessment of health state or problem, diagnosis)

**Plan** (diagnostic evaluation, follow-up care, patient teaching)

**NOTES**

CHAPTER
# 28

# The Complete Health Assessment: Adult

## PURPOSE

This chapter helps you learn the methods of integrating the regional examinations so that you will be able to conduct a complete physical examination on a well young adult.

## READING ASSIGNMENT

Jarvis: *Physical Examination and Health Assessment,* 8th ed., Chapter 28, pp. 767-782.

## CLINICAL OBJECTIVES

1. Demonstrate skills of inspection, percussion, palpation, and auscultation.

2. Demonstrate correct use of instruments, including assembly, manipulation of component parts, and positioning of patient.

3. Use appropriate terminology and correctly pronounce medical terminology with clinical instructor and adapt terms for patient.

4. Choreograph the complete examination in a systematic manner, including integration of certain regional assessments throughout the examination (e.g., skin, musculoskeletal system).

5. Coordinate procedures to limit position changes for examiner and patient.

6. Describe accurately the findings of the examination, including normal and abnormal findings.

7. Demonstrate appropriate infection control measures.

8. Recognize and maintain the privacy and dignity of the patient.
   a. Adequately explain what is being done while limiting small talk.
   b. Consider patient's anxiety and fears.
   c. Consider your own facial expression and comments.
   d. Demonstrate confidence, empathy, and gentle manner.
   e. Acknowledge and apologize for any discomfort caused.
   f. Provide for privacy and warmth at all times.
   g. Determine comfort level, pausing if patient becomes tired.
   h. Wash hands and don gloves appropriately.
   i. Allow adequate time for each step.
   j. Briefly summarize findings to patient, and thank patient for his or her time.

## INSTRUCTIONS

The key to success in this venture is **practice;** you should conduct at least **three** complete physical examination practices in your preparation for this final examination proficiency. You will be assigned a peer "patient" for the examination. You should prepare your own note card "outline" for the examination. You may refer to this minimally during the examination, but overdependence on your notes will constitute failure. You will have 45 minutes in which to conduct the examination (not including setup). Genitalia examination is omitted. If you practice three times, you will have no difficulty completing the examination in the allotted time.

Prepare the examination setting. Arrange for proper lighting. If you are using a hospital bed instead of an examination table, make sure to adjust the bed height during the examination to allow for your own visualization of the patient and for the patient's ease in getting into and out of the bed. Arrange adequate patient gown, bath blankets, and drapes.

Gather your equipment. The following items are needed for a complete physical examination, including female genitalia. Check with your clinical instructor for any items that you may omit for your own examination proficiency.

| | |
|---|---|
| Platform scale with height attachment | Flexible tape measure and ruler marked in |
| Sphygmomanometer with appropriate-size cuff | centimeters |
| Stethoscope with bell and diaphragm endpieces | Reflex hammer |
| Alcohol wipes for cleaning equipment | Sharp object (split tongue blade) |
| Thermometer | Cotton balls |
| Flashlight or penlight | Bivalve vaginal speculum |
| Otoscope, ophthalmoscope | Disposable gloves |
| Tuning fork | Materials for cytologic study |
| Nasal speculum | Lubricant |
| Tongue depressor | Fecal occult blood test materials |
| Pocket vision screener | Hand sanitizer |

Record your findings using the write-up sheets that follow. Your clinical instructor may ask you to write your findings in narrative format. Remember to use appropriate medical terminology and concise phrases.

Following the examination worksheet, a sample form used in an ambulatory care setting has been included. You may use it for your write up.

## COMPLETE PHYSICAL EXAMINATION

Date _____

Examiner _____

Patient _____ Gender _____ Age _____

Occupation _____ Reason for visit _____

### General Survey of Patient

1. Appears stated age _____
2. Level of consciousness _____
3. Skin color _____
4. Nutritional status _____
5. Posture and position _____
6. Obvious physical deformities _____
7. Mobility: gait, use of assistive devices, ROM of joints, no involuntary movement _____
8. Facial expression _____
9. Mood and affect _____
10. Speech: articulation, pattern, content appropriate, native language _____
11. Hearing _____
12. Personal hygiene _____

### Measurement and Vital Signs

1. Weight _____
2. Height _____
3. Waist circumference _____
4. Body mass index _____
5. Vision using Snellen eye chart
   Right eye _____ Left eye _____ Correction? _____
6. Radial pulse, rate, and rhythm _____
7. Respirations, rate, depth _____
8. Blood pressure
   Right arm _____ (sitting or lying?)
   Left arm _____ (sitting or lying?)
9. Temperature (if indicated) _____
10. Pain assessment _____

## Stand in Front of Patient, Patient Sitting

### Skin

1. Hands and nails _____
2. (For remainder of examination, examine skin with corresponding region.)
   Color and pigmentation _____
   Temperature _____
   Moisture _____
   Texture _____
   Turgor _____
   Any lesions _____

## Head and Face

1. Scalp, hair, cranium _____
2. Face (cranial nerve VII) _____
3. Temporal artery, temporomandibular joint _____
4. Maxillary sinuses, frontal sinuses _____

## Eyes

1. Visual fields (cranial nerve II) _____
2. Extraocular muscles, corneal light reflex _____
   Cardinal positions of gaze (cranial nerves III, IV, VI) _____
3. External structures _____
4. Conjunctivae _____
   Sclerae _____
   Corneas _____
   Irides _____
5. Pupils _____
6. Ophthalmoscope, red reflex _____
   Disc _____
   Vessels _____
   Retinal background _____

## Ears

1. External ear _____
2. Any tenderness _____
3. Otoscope, ear canal _____
   Tympanic membrane _____
4. Hearing (cranial nerve VIII), whispered voice test _____

## Nose

1. External nose _____
2. Patency of nostrils _____
3. Speculum, nasal mucosa _____
   Septum _____
   Turbinates _____

## Mouth and Throat

1. Lips and buccal mucosa _____
   Teeth and gums _____
   Tongue _____
   Hard and soft palate _____
2. Tonsils _____
3. Uvula (cranial nerves IX, X) _____
4. Tongue (cranial nerve XII) _____

## Neck

1. Symmetry, lumps, pulsations _____
2. Cervical lymph nodes _____
3. Carotid pulse (bruits if indicated) _____
4. Trachea _____
5. ROM and muscle strength (cranial nerve XI) _____
6. Palpate thyroid gland _____

## Move to Back of Patient, Patient Sitting

### Chest and Lungs, Posterior and Lateral

1. Thoracic cage configuration _____
   Skin characteristics _____
   Symmetry _____
2. Symmetric expansion _____
   Tactile fremitus _____
   Lumps or tenderness _____
3. Spinous processes _____
4. Percussion over lung fields _____
5. CVA tenderness _____
6. Breath sounds _____
7. Adventitious sounds _____

## Move to Front of Patient

### Chest and Lungs, Anterior

1. Respirations and skin characteristics _____
2. Tactile fremitus, lumps, tenderness _____
3. Percuss lung fields _____
4. Breath sounds _____

### Upper Extremities

1. ROM and muscle strength, shoulder _____
   Elbow _____
   Wrist and hand _____
2. Epitrochlear nodes _____

### Breasts

1. Symmetry, mobility, dimpling _____
2. Supraclavicular and infraclavicular areas _____

## Patient Supine, Stand at Patient's Right

### Breasts

1. Breast palpation _____
2. Nipple _____
3. Axillae and regional nodes _____
4. Teach breast self-examination _____

### Neck Vessels

1. Jugular venous pulse _____
2. Jugular venous pressure, if indicated _____

### Heart

1. Precordium: pulsations and heave _____
2. Apical impulse _____
3. Precordium, thrills _____

　4. Apical rate and rhythm _____
　5. Heart sounds _____

**Abdomen**
　1. Contour, symmetry _____
　　 Skin characteristics _____
　　 Umbilicus and pulsations _____
　2. Bowel sounds _____
　3. Vascular sounds _____
　4. Percussion _____
　5. Light and deep palpation _____
　6. Palpation of liver, spleen, kidneys, aorta _____
　7. Abdominal reflexes, if indicated _____

**Inguinal Area**
　1. Femoral pulse _____
　2. Inguinal nodes _____

**Lower Extremities**
　1. Symmetry _____
　　 Skin characteristics, hair distribution _____
　2. Pulses, popliteal _____
　　 Posterior tibial _____
　　 Dorsalis pedis _____
　3. Temperature, pretibial edema _____
　4. Toes _____
　5. ROM and muscle strength, hips _____

## Patient Sitting Up

**Lower Extremities**
　1. ROM and muscle strength, knees _____
　　 Ankles and feet _____

**Neurologic**
　1. Sensation, face _____
　　 Arms and hands _____
　　 Legs and feet _____
　2. Position sense _____
　3. Stereognosis or graphesthesia _____
　4. Cerebellar function, finger to nose _____
　5. Cerebellar function, heel to shin _____
　6. Deep tendon reflexes
　　 Biceps _____ Triceps _____
　　 Brachioradialis _____ Patellar _____
　　 Achilles _____
　7. Babinski reflex _____

## Patient Standing Up

### Musculoskeletal
1. Walk across room _____
   Walk, heel to toe _____
2. Walk on tiptoes, and then walk on heels _____
3. Romberg sign _____
4. Shallow knee bend _____
5. Touch toes _____
6. ROM of spine _____

### Male Genitalia
1. Penis and scrotum _____
2. Testes and spermatic cord _____
3. Inguinal hernia _____
4. Teach testicular self-examination _____

### Male Rectum
1. Perianal area _____
2. Rectal walls and prostate gland _____
3. Stool for occult blood _____

## Female Patient in Lithotomy Position

### Female Genitalia and Rectum
1. Perineal and perianal areas _____
2. Vaginal speculum: cervix and vaginal walls _____
3. Procure specimens _____
4. Bimanual: cervix, uterus, and adnexa _____
   _____
5. Rectovaginal _____
6. Stool for occult blood _____

### Closure
1. Help patient sit up.
2. Thank patient for time, and depart from patient.

# NOTES

## Comprehensive Adult History and Physical*

Date of Visit: _____

Patient Name: _____

Medical Record #: _____

Address: _____

Telephone: (home)_____ (business) _____    Informant/Relationship: _____

Date of Birth: _____ Age: ____ Gender: Male  Female    Language _____ Interpreter present: ☐ Yes ☐ No

Provider: _____    Reliability: ☐ Adequate   ☐ Inadequate

### History of Present Illness

### Past Medical History

☐ HTN       ☐ Asthma/COPD ☐ Seizure Disorder ☐ Breast Disease
☐ DM        ☐ GERD        ☐ Renal Disease    ☐ Anemia
☐ CVD/CAD   ☐ Hepatitis   ☐ Thyroid Disorder ☐ Transfusions
☐ CVA       ☐ Osteoporosis ☐ Bleeding Disorder ☐ Psychiatric
☐ CA        ☐ Arthritis   ☐ Infectious Disease ☐ Childhood
Other/Details of Above:                          Illnesses

### Past Surgical History/Trauma/Hospitalization

☐ T & A:            Other/Details:
☐ Appendectomy:
☐ Cholecystectomy:
☐ Hernia repair:
☐ Hysterectomy:
☐ Laparotomy:
☐ Cesarean section:
☐ Biopsy: _____ ☐ ORIF: _____

### Medications

☐ OTC
☐ Vitamins
☐ Supplements/Herbals

### Allergies

☐ Drugs
☐ Environment
☐ Foods ☐ Latex
☐ IV Contrast

### Reproductive History

Menstrual: _____ Age at menarche _____ LMP _____

Interval _____ Duration _____ Flow _____
☐ Reg ☐ Irreg ☐ Cramping ☐ Intermenstrual Bleeding ☐ PMS
Obstetrical: G _____ T _____ P _____ A _____ L _____
Complications: _____
Menopause: Age _____ Abnl Bleeding: _____
Symptoms: _____
Hormones: ☐ ERT ☐ HRT ☐ topical _____

Contraceptives: _____
Sexual Activity:
☐ same sex          ☐ opposite sex        ☐ abstinent
☐ single partner    ☐ multiple partners   ☐ >4 lifetime partners
STD hx:_____
Concerns:

*From Loretz L. (2005). Primary care tools for clinicians. St. Louis: Elsevier.

## Comprehensive Adult History and Physical - 2*

Patient Name: _____

Date of Birth: _____ Date of Exam: _____

### Social History

**Marital Status:** ☐ Single ☐ Married ☐ Domestic Partner
☐ Divorced ☐ Widowed

**Cohabitants:** _____

**Children:** _____

**Education:** _____

**Occupation:** _____

**Interests/Activities:** _____

**Exercise:** ☐ Aerobic ☐ Weights _____

**Diet:** ☐ Balanced ☐ Calcium _____

**Sleep/Rest:** _____ **Caffeine:** ☐ No ☐ Yes cups/day _____

**Tobacco:** ☐ No ☐ Yes PPD _____ # Years _____ Quit Year _____

Smoking in home: ☐ Yes ☐ No _____

**ETOH:** ☐ Yes ☐ No ☐ Daily ☐ Weekly ☐ Monthly # drinks_____

**Recreational Drugs:** _____

**Support Systems/Coping Skills:** ☐ Adequate ☐ Inadequate

### Family History

☐ **Family History Unknown**

**Father:** _____

**Mother:** _____

**Siblings:** _____

_____

**MGF:** _____

**MGM:** _____

**PGF:** _____

**PGM:** _____

**Other:** _____

_____

**Cultural/Religious Influences:** _____

_____

### Health Maintenance History

| Exam | Last Date | Results | N/A | Refused | Exam | Last Date | Results | N/A | Refused |
|------|-----------|---------|-----|---------|------|-----------|---------|-----|---------|
| Pap test | | | | | Dental | | | | |
| Mammogram | | | | | Vision | | | | |
| SBE/TSE | | | | | Hearing | | | | |
| Stool guaiac | | | | | Lipid Profile | | | | |
| Flex sig/Colonoscopy | | | | | FBS | | | | |
| CXR | | | | | PSA | | | | |
| ECG | | | | | PPD | | | | |

| Immunizations (dates): | | | | Safety: | | | |
|------------------------|--|--|--|---------|--|--|--|
| Td | MMR/titers | Hep B | Polio | ☐ Seatbelt Use | ☐ Cycling Helmet | ☐ Sunscreen | ☐ Occupational |
| Varicella vaccine/chickenpox | Influenza | Pneumovax | | ☐ Smoke Detectors | ☐ Housing | ☐ Dom. Violence | ☐ Firearms |

### Review of Systems (Check box at left if all systems negative.)

Comments/Details:

☐ **General:** ☐ fever ☐ chills ☐ night sweats ☐ fatigue ☐ unexplained weight loss ☐ weight gain

☐ **Skin:** ☐ pruritus ☐ rash ☐ hair loss ☐ worrisome lesion ☐ pigment change ☐ moles ☐ sweating ☐ dry skin ☐ nail change

☐ **HEENT:** ☐ headache ☐ dizziness ☐ earache ☐ hearing loss ☐ tinnitus ☐ vision change ☐ eye pain/sensitivity
☐ excessive tearing ☐ eyeglasses/contact use ☐ glaucoma ☐ rhinorrhea ☐ nasal congestion ☐ postnasal drip ☐ sinus pain
☐ nosebleeds ☐ hay fever ☐ sore throat ☐ mouth sores ☐ hoarseness ☐ toothache ☐ bleeding gums ☐ dentures

☐ **Breast:** ☐ pain ☐ lumps ☐ discharge ☐ history of breast disease ☐ implants

☐ **Pulmonary:** ☐ cough ☐ sputum ☐ hemoptysis ☐ SOB ☐ pain with respiration ☐ wheezing ☐ cyanosis

☐ **CV:** ☐ chest pain ☐ palpitations ☐ DOE ☐ orthopnea ☐ PND ☐ diaphoresis ☐ syncope ☐ heart murmur ☐ leg edema

☐ **PVD:** ☐ claudication ☐ varicose veins ☐ phlebitis ☐ coldness of hands/feet ☐ leg ulcers

☐ **GI:** ☐ dysphagia ☐ heartburn ☐ change in appetite ☐ food intol ☐ nausea ☐ vomiting ☐ hematemesis ☐ abdominal pain ☐ bloating
☐ flatulence ☐ diarrhea ☐ constipation ☐ melena ☐ jaundice ☐ dark urine ☐ BRBPR ☐ change in BM ☐ hemorrhoids ☐ hernia

☐ **GU:** ☐ dysuria ☐ urgency ☐ frequency ☐ hematuria ☐ nocturia ☐ polyuria ☐ suprapubic pain ☐ flank pain ☐ incontinence ☐ lesions
♂ ☐ hesitancy ☐ dribbling ☐ decreased force stream ☐ testicular pain ☐ testicular mass/swelling ☐ penile discharge ☐ erectile dysfunction
♀ ☐ vaginal itch ☐ abnl vaginal discharge ☐ vaginal dryness ☐ dyspareunia ☐ sexual dysfunction ☐ abnl vaginal bleeding

☐ **Endocrine:** ☐ polyuria ☐ polydipsia ☐ polyphagia ☐ heat/cold intol ☐ tremor ☐ lump in throat ☐ unexplained wt change ☐ hair changes

☐ **Heme:** ☐ anemia ☐ easy bruising ☐ swollen glands ☐ bleeding of skin/mucous membranes ☐ freq infections ☐ allergies ☐ delayed healing

☐ **MSK:** ☐ joint pain (location _____) ☐ stiffness ☐ restriction of motion ☐ swelling ☐ erythema
☐ bony deformity ☐ myalgia ☐ muscle cramps ☐ weakness ☐ antalgic gait ☐ back pain

☐ **Neuro:** ☐ focal weakness ☐ paralysis ☐ numbness ☐ tremor ☐ seizure ☐ syncope ☐ gait disturbance ☐ memory loss ☐ aphasia

☐ **Psych:** ☐ anxiety ☐ panic attacks ☐ depression ☐ mood changes ☐ irritability ☐ nervousness ☐ decreased libido
☐ eating disorder ☐ sleep disturbance ☐ suicidal thoughts ☐ impaired judgment ☐ hallucinations ☐ confusion

*From Loretz L. (2005). *Primary care tools for clinicians.* St. Louis: Elsevier.

## Comprehensive Adult History and Physical - 3*

Patient Name: _____

Date of Birth: _____ Date of Exam: _____

### Physical Exam

| N = Normal   A = Abnormal   (Check appropriate box) | N | A |
|---|---|---|
| **1. General Appearance:** age • LOC • nutrition • development • mobility • affect • speech • hygiene | | |
| **2. Skin:** hydration • color • texture • hair • nails • lesions | | |
| **3. Head:** shape • size • symmetry • scalp • TMJ • lesions | | |
| **4. Eyes:** lids • conjunctiva • sclera | | |
| Extraocular Muscles | | |
| Visual fields | | |
| Pupils: size, reaction to light and accommodation | | |
| Fundi | | |
| **5. Ears:** pinna • canals • TMs • hearing | | |
| **6. Nose:** patency • nares • sinuses • nasal mucosa • septum • turbinates | | |
| **7. Mouth:** lips • gums • teeth • mucosa • palate • tongue | | |
| **8. Throat:** pharynx • tonsils • uvula | | |
| **9. Neck:** ROM • symmetry • palpation • thyroid • trachea • carotids • jugular veins • lymph nodes | | |
| **10. Breasts:** size • symmetry • skin • nipples • palpation • nodes | | |
| **11. Chest/Lungs:** excursion • palpation • percussion • auscultation | | |
| **12. Cardiac:** PMI • palpation • rate • rhythm • S1 • S2 • murmurs • gallops • bruits • extra sounds | | |
| **13. Abdomen:** appearance • bowel sounds • bruits • percussion • palpation • liver • spleen • flank • suprapubic • hernia | | |
| **14. Anorectal:** perianal | | |
| digital rectal | | |
| stool guaiac | | |
| prostate exam | | |
| **15. Female Genitalia:** perineum • labia • urethral meatus • introitus | | |
| Internal: vaginal mucosal • cervix | | |
| Bimanual: vagina • cervix • uterus • adnexa | | |
| **16. Male Genitalia:** penis • scrotum • testes • hernia | | |
| **17. Lymph Nodes:** cervical • subclavian • axillary • inguinal • other | | |
| **18. Musculoskeletal:** Back/Spine: ROM • palpation | | |
| Upper Extremity: ROM • strength • palpation | | |
| Lower Extremity: ROM • strength • palpation | | |
| **19. Peripheral Vascular:** Upper extremity: pulses • appearance • temp | | |
| Lower extremity: pulses • appearance • temp | | |
| **20. Neurologic:** cranial nerves • motor • sensory • cerebellar • reflexes • gait • mental status | | |

### Vitals

Ht _____ Wt _____ Temp _____ Resp _____ Pulse _____

BP (upright) _____ (supine) _____ Staff Initials _____

### Visual Acuity

Right        /                Left        /
Corrective lenses     ☐ Yes     ☐ No

### Document Abnormals (by number)/Comments

### Lab/Studies

### Assessment and Plan

*From Loretz L. (2005). *Primary care tools for clinicians*. St. Louis: Elsevier.

## Comprehensive Adult History and Physical - 4*

*Patient Name:* _____

*Date of Birth:* _____ *Date of Exam:* _____

### Assessment and Plan (continued)

### Periodic Health Screening Plan

| Exam | Performed | Scheduled | N/A | Refused |
|---|---|---|---|---|
| Breast Exam | | | | |
| Mammogram | | | | |
| Pap Test | | | | |
| Prostate exam | | | | |
| Testicular exam | | | | |
| Digital rectal with stool guaiac | | | | |
| Flexible Sigmoidoscopy/Colonoscopy | | | | |
| Bone Density | | | | |
| PPD | | | | |

### Health Counseling (check if discussed, describe any intervention)

☐ Smoking cessation _____
☐ Alcohol/Drug Use _____
☐ Diet/Weight _____
☐ Vitamins/Calcium _____
☐ Periodic Dental/Vision care _____
☐ Exercise/Sleep _____
☐ Sun exposure _____
☐ Seatbelts/Helmets _____
☐ Stress/Family issues _____
☐ Safety: Weapons/ Domestic Violence _____
☐ BSE/TSE _____
☐ Sexual issues/risks _____
☐ Contraception _____
☐ Living Will/Power of atty/DNR _____

*From Loretz L. (2005). *Primary care tools for clinicians*. St. Louis: Elsevier.

### Immunizations

Immunizations current: ☐ Yes  ☐ No

| Vaccine | Given | Planned | Refused |
|---|---|---|---|
| Td | | | |
| Hepatitis B | | | |
| Influenza | | | |
| Pneumonia | | | |
| Other: | | | |

### Lab/Studies Ordered

☐ CXR   ☐ Lipids   ☐ Creat/BUN   ☐ $HbA_1C$
☐ ECG   ☐ CBC/diff   ☐ LFTs   ☐ TSH
        ☐ Electrolytes   ☐ FBS   ☐ UA/UC
☐ Other:

**Provider's Signature** _____ Date
☐ Note dictated/written

# The Complete Physical Assessment: Infant, Young Child, and Adolescent

## PURPOSE

This chapter helps you learn the methods of integrating the health history and physical examination on those of varying ages. You will note specific developmental and behavioral items to address.

## READING ASSIGNMENT

Jarvis: *Physical Examination and Health Assessment*, 8th ed., Chapter 29, pp. 783-792.

## CLINICAL OBJECTIVES

1. Demonstrate skills of inspection, percussion, palpation, and auscultation.

2. Demonstrate correct use of instruments, including assembly, manipulation of component parts, and positioning with patient.

3. Use appropriate terminology and correctly pronounce medical terminology with clinical instructor and adapt for patient, parent, or caregiver.

4. Choreograph the complete examination in a systematic manner, including integration of certain regional assessments throughout the examination (e.g., skin, musculoskeletal).

5. Coordinate procedures to limit position changes for examiner and patient.

6. Describe accurately the findings of the examination, including normal and abnormal findings.

7. Demonstrate appropriate infection control measures.

8. Recognize and maintain the privacy and dignity of the patient.
   a. Adequately explain what is being done while limiting small talk, appropriate to child's age.
   b. Consider patient's and caregiver's anxiety and fears.
   c. Consider your own facial expression and comments.
   d. Demonstrate confidence, empathy, and gentle manner.
   e. Acknowledge and apologize for any discomfort caused.
   f. Provide for privacy and warmth at all times.
   g. Determine comfort level, pausing if patient becomes tired.
   h. Wash hands and don gloves appropriately.
   i. Allow adequate time for each step.
   j. Briefly summarize findings to patient and parent, and thank patient and parent for his or her time.

## INSTRUCTIONS

If your clinical instructor has arranged for you to perform a complete health assessment on an infant or young child, please review the instructions on p. 258 of the preceding chapter. Please review the age appropriate considerations found in Chapters 8 and 28 of Jarvis: *Physical Examination and Health Assessment*, 8th ed.

Following you will find age-appropriate forms for assessment findings: Pediatric Initial Health Questionnaire to be completed with the parent or caregiver; 0- to 1-month Well-Child Visit; 5-Year Well-Child Visit; and 15- to 17-Year Well Visit. For each form, note the age-specific points for Daily Activities, Health History, Development, and Anticipatory Guidance, in addition to the examination findings. If you do not perform these examinations, find a partner in your laboratory group and discuss these points thoroughly. State the rationale for including each point.

## Pediatric Initial Health Questionnaire*

Date of Visit: _____

Your Name: _____

Child's Name:_____

Relationship to Child:_____

**THIS FORM IS FOR MEDICAL RECORD USE ONLY AND WILL REMAIN CONFIDENTIAL. PLEASE ANSWER EACH QUESTION TO THE BEST OF YOUR ABILITY.**

### Vital Information

**Child's Birth date** _____  ☐ Boy  ☐ Girl

**Birthplace:**  City/State_____

   Hospital _____  Other_____

**Mother's Name** _____  Birth date: _____

   Occupation _____  Ht _____  Wt _____

**Father's Name** _____  Birth date:_____

   Occupation _____  Ht _____  Wt _____

**Names of living brothers and sisters**        Birth dates

_____

_____

_____

_____

**Was child adopted?**  ☐ Yes  ☐ No   At what age? _____

   If adopted, country of origin _____

**Religious Preference**_____

### Pregnancy

Number of pregnancies before this one: _____

How long was this pregnancy? _____ weeks

How many months pregnant when prenatal care was begun? _____

Were there any of the following illnesses or problems?

   ☐ Rubella (measles)     ☐ Accident/injury     ☐ Bleeding

   ☐ High blood pressure   ☐ Swelling            ☐ Sugar in urine

   ☐ Excessive weight gain ☐ Other infections

Explain: _____

Medicines or drugs used during pregnancy:

_____

_____

Smoking while pregnant:  ☐ None  ☐ Moderate  ☐ Heavy

Alcohol while pregnant:  ☐ None  ☐ <1 per week  ☐ >1 per week

### Birth

How long was labor? _____  Was labor induced? _____

**At delivery (check all that apply):**

☐ Breech (feet or bottom first)     ☐ Cesarean section  ☐ VBAC

☐ Breathed and cried immediately    ☐ Resuscitated      ☐ In oxygen

**Did baby require:**

☐ special nursery  ☐ blood transfusion  ☐ antibiotics  ☐ lights

**Did baby have:**

☐ breathing problems  ☐ yellow jaundice  ☐ other _____

**At birth:**

Weight: _____  Length: _____  Apgar score_____

Discharge weight: _____  Length of hospital stay: _____

**Describe any problems:**_____

_____

_____

### Family Background

**Ethnic origin/Race:**  Mother: _____  Father: _____

☐ Married  ☐ Living together  ☐ Separated  ☐ Divorced  ☐ Single

**Child lives with:**

☐ Both parents  ☐ Mother  ☐ Father  ☐ Guardian

**Other members of household:**_____

Age of home or apartment: _____  Any pets? _____

Has any parent, brother, or sister died? _____  Who? _____

Cause of death _____  Age _____

| Please check the box of your child's blood relatives who have ever had any of the following conditions; circle examples in parentheses or write in name of disease, if known: | Father | Mother | Father's side | Mother's side | Siblings |
|---|---|---|---|---|---|
| Headaches (migraine, cluster, tension)........... | | | | | |
| Eye Disease (blindness, tumor, glaucoma)........ | | | | | |
| Ear Disease (deafness, infections, defects)........ | | | | | |
| Allergies (eczema, hay fever, sinus, hives) ........ | | | | | |
| Lung Disease (asthma, cystic fibrosis, bronchitis).. | | | | | |
| Tuberculosis..................................... | | | | | |
| High Blood Pressure............................. | | | | | |
| High Cholesterol................................ | | | | | |
| Heart Attack (age _____)..................... | | | | | |
| Heart Disease................................... | | | | | |
| Anemia (Sickle Cell, Mediterranean, other)........ | | | | | |
| Bleeding Disorders (hemophilia) ................. | | | | | |
| Stomach or Duodenal Ulcers ..................... | | | | | |
| Liver or Gallbladder Disease (hepatitis) .......... | | | | | |
| Intestinal Disease (colitis, polyps) ............... | | | | | |
| Kidney Disease (nephritis, cysts, stones) ......... | | | | | |
| Diabetes ....................................... | | | | | |
| Thyroid Problems (goiter, nodules, hyper-, hypo-).. | | | | | |
| Bone or Joint Disease (arthritis, osteoporosis)..... | | | | | |
| Muscle Weakness or Dystrophy ................... | | | | | |
| Seizure Disorder (epilepsy)....................... | | | | | |
| Neurologic Disorder ............................. | | | | | |
| Learning Disability .............................. | | | | | |
| Mental Retardation (Down syndrome, other)...... | | | | | |
| Mental Illness (depression, anxiety, other)........ | | | | | |
| Alcoholism or Drug Abuse ....................... | | | | | |
| Birth Defects (cleft lip, other deformity) .......... | | | | | |
| Obesity........................................ | | | | | |
| Cancer: Breast, Cervix, Uterine, or Ovarian........ | | | | | |
| Lung, Thyroid, Pancreas, or Kidney....... | | | | | |
| Bladder, Prostate, or Testicular .......... | | | | | |
| Colon, Stomach, or Oral Cavity .......... | | | | | |
| Leukemia, Myeloma, or Lymphoma....... | | | | | |
| Skin, Brain, or Bone................... | | | | | |
| Other _____ ... | | | | | |

*From Loretz L. (2005). *Primary care tools for clinicians.* St. Louis: Elsevier.

## Pediatric Initial Health Questionnaire - 2*

### Nutrition in Infancy

**Feeding:** Breast ☐     Duration _____ months/weeks

Formula ☐     Type _____

☐ Vitamins     ☐ Fluoride     ☐ Iron     ☐ Uses pacifier

**Problems:** ☐ Vomiting   ☐ Colic   ☐ Diarrhea   ☐ Allergies

**Solid foods:** Age when started _____   Intolerances _____

### Growth and Development

**At what age did your child:**

Sit alone _____   Walk alone _____   Feed self _____

Talk (2-3-word sentences) _____   Dress self _____

Toilet trained:  Day _____   Night _____

**School-age child:** Current grade _____   Days missed this year _____

**School problems:** ☐ reading, writing  ☐ behavior  ☐ special needs

**Are there any behavior problems at home?** _____

Please describe: _____

_____

_____

### Medical History

**Please check the diseases that your child has had and give age:**

☐ Measles, Rubella _____   ☐ Anemia _____

☐ Mumps _____   ☐ Heart Disease _____

☐ Chickenpox _____   ☐ Allergies/Hay fever _____

☐ Whooping cough _____   ☐ Eczema _____

☐ Scarlet fever _____   ☐ Asthma _____

☐ Rheumatic fever _____   ☐ Pneumonia _____

☐ Convulsions/Seizures _____   ☐ Hepatitis _____

☐ Strep throat _____   ☐ Ear Infection _____

☐ Other illnesses _____

Has your child ever been injured? _____   Age _____

Injury _____

Any fractures? _____   Which bone(s)? _____

Any loss of consciousness or concussion? _____

Any accidental poisoning? _____   Age _____   Substance _____

Has your child ever had surgery? _____   Age _____

Type of operation _____

Has your child ever been hospitalized other than for the above? _____

Describe: _____

Has your child ever had a blood transfusion? _____   Age _____

Does your child take any medications regularly? _____

Please list: _____

_____

_____

**Does your child take any of the following:**

☐ Vitamins   ☐ Fluoride   ☐ Food supplements _____

**Has your child worn:**

☐ Glasses   ☐ Contact lenses   ☐ Dental braces   ☐ Leg braces

☐ Corrective shoes   ☐ Orthotics in shoes   ☐ Other braces

*From Loretz L. (2005). *Primary care tools for clinicians.* St. Louis: Elsevier.

**Does your child have allergies to any of the following?**

☐ Penicillin   ☐ Sulfa   ☐ Other medicines _____

☐ Pollen   Foods _____   ☐ Animals _____

Type of allergic reaction to above: _____

**Please check if your child has had:**

☐ Frequent headaches          ☐ Crossed eyes

☐ Pinkeye                      ☐ More than two earaches a year

☐ Trouble hearing             ☐ Frequent nosebleeds

☐ Stuffy nose most of time    ☐ More than 6 colds a year

☐ Chronic cough               ☐ Shortness of breath with exercise

☐ Heart murmur                ☐ Constant or frequent fatigue

☐ Frequent stomachaches       ☐ Frequent diarrhea or constipation

☐ Poor appetite               ☐ Frequent urination or accidents

☐ Bloody, red, or brown urine ☐ Frequent bed-wetting after age 5

☐ Joint pains or swelling     ☐ Dizziness or fainting spells

☐ Inability to get to sleep   ☐ Frequent nightmares or sleepwalking

☐ Excessive thirst            ☐ Excessive weight gain

☐ Signs of sexual development before age 9

**Other concerns:** _____

_____

_____

### Immunizations & Screenings

**Please give approximate dates for each immunization, if known:**

| Series | #1 | #2 | #3 | #4 | #5 |
|---|---|---|---|---|---|
| DtaP/DT | | | | | |
| Tetanus booster | | | | | |
| Polio IPV/OPV | | | | | |
| MMR | | | | | |
| Hib | | | | | |
| Hepatitis B | | | | | |
| Pneumococcal | | | | | |
| Varicella | | | | | |
| Meningococcal | | | | | |
| Influenza | | | | | |

**Please give approximate dates for the following, if done:**

| Test | No | Yes | Date(s) | Result |
|---|---|---|---|---|
| Lead blood test | | | | |
| TB skin test | | | | |
| Vision exam | | | | |
| Hearing test | | | | |
| Hemoglobin blood test | | | | |
| Urine test | | | | |

## 0- to 1-Month Well-Child Visit*

Date of Visit: _____

Medical Record Number: _____

Child's Name: _____

Address: _____

Telephone: _____

Date of Birth: _____   Age: ____   Gender:   Male   Female

Provider: _____

Informant: _____   Interpreter present:   ☐ Yes   ☐ No

Relationship to child:_____   Language _____

### Measurements

Ht _____ _____ %  Wt _____ _____ %  OFC _____ _____ %  Staff

Temp _____  Pulse _____  Resp _____   Initials ____

### Birth Data

Ht _____  Wt _____  OFC _____  Gest Age _____  Wks

| | | |
|---|---|---|
| L&D record on baby's chart? | ☐ Yes | ☐ No |
| Significant prenatal history on baby's chart? | ☐ Yes | ☐ No |
| Hepatitis B vaccine given in nursery? | ☐ Yes | ☐ No |

**Newborn Metabolic Screening**

☐ Normal   ☐ Abnormal (specify):

### Vision/Hearing

**Newborn Hearing Screening**

☐ Normal   ☐ Not screened   ☐ Abnormal (specify):

*Vision concerns*   ☐ No   ☐ Yes (explain)_____

*Hearing concerns*   ☐ No   ☐ Yes (explain)_____

### Child Health History

*Family/social history (refer to chart)*   ☐ Completed   ☐ Updated

*Parental concerns:*_____

_____

*Recent injury/illness/surgery/hospitalizations:*

*Allergies:* _____

*Medications:* _____

### Review of Systems

| | N | AB |
|---|---|---|
| **HEENT** (eye discharge, thrush) | | |
| **Skin** (rashes) | | |
| **CV** (color) | | |
| **Resp** (wheezing) | | |
| **GI** (projectile vomiting/stools) | | |
| **GU** (pain/stream/frequency) | | |
| **Neuromuscular** (moves all extremities equally) | | |

Remainder of review of systems (unlisted) negative ☐

### Daily Activities

**Nutrition/Elimination**

☐ Breast frequency _____   # feedings/day _____

☐ Formula _____   # feedings/amount _____

☐ Iron/vitamins   # stools/day _____   # voids/day _____

**Sleep** (arrangements/patterns) _____

**Hygiene** (cord/circ care)_____

**Caregivers**   ☐ Mother   ☐ Father   ☐ Other relative

Caregiver working/in school   ☐ Yes   ☐ No

Who cares for baby during day or other time?   ☐ Parent/other relative
                                               ☐ Day care

**Stresses for Caregivers** _____

**Environmental Risks**—*Check if assessed*

☐ Lead risk            ☐ Guns in house/bldg       ☐ TB exposure

☐ Alcohol use in house/bldg  ☐ Housing inadequate   ☐ Domestic violence

☐ Smokers in house/bldg   ☐ Drug use in house/bldg  ☐ Other

☐ Identified risks _____

**Active community supports/resources:**

_____

**Mental Health/Behavior Risks:**

☐ No concerns

☐ Concerns (explain) _____

**Observation of parent/child interaction:**

☐ Appropriate

☐ Not appropriate (explain)_____

**Other:**

### Development

| Personal/Social/Cognitive | N | AB | |
|---|---|---|---|
| • Regards face | | | |
| • Smiles responsively | | | |
| **Fine motor/adaptive** | | | ☐ Development screening tool, if used: |
| • Follows to midline | | | Name of tool _____ |
| **Language** | | | |
| • Vocalizes | | | |
| • Responds to sound | | | Staff initials _____ |
| • "Ooo/aah" | | | |
| **Gross motor** | | | ☐ By observation/exam/ parent report. No tool used. |
| • Lifts head 45° | | | |
| **Breastfeeding** | | | |
| • Latch-on/positioning | | | |
| • Quality of suck | | | |

*From Loretz L. (2005). *Primary care tools for clinicians.* St. Louis: Elsevier.

## 0- to 1-Month Well-Child Visit - 2*

*Child's Name:* _____    *Medical Record Number:* _____

### Physical Exam

| N = normal    Ab = abnormal (check appropriate box) | N | AB |
|---|---|---|
| **1. General appearance:** | | |
| **2. Skin:** color • character • birthmarks • jaundice | | |
| **3. Nodes:** cervical • axillary • inguinal | | |
| **4. Head:** shape • AF size • PF size • sutures • scalp | | |
| **5. Eyes:** tear ducts • EOM • red reflex • corneal light reflex • PERL • lids | | |
| **6. Vision:** follows light, movement | | |
| **7. Ears:** pinna • canals • TMs | | |
| **8. Hearing:** responds to loud sound | | |
| **9. Nose:** patency • nares | | |
| **10. Mouth:** gums • tongue • frenulum • palate • mucosa • throat | | |
| **11. Neck:** position • ROM • thyroid | | |
| **12. Chest:** shape • symmetry • lungs • respiration rate • clavicles | | |
| **13. CV:** rate • rhythm • $S_1$ • $S_2$ • murmur • femoral pulses | | |
| **14. ABD:** contour • umbilicus • liver • spleen • masses • anus • bowel sounds | | |
| **15. GU:** ♀ labia • vaginal mucosa • discharge ♂ circ • penis • testes • hydrocele • hernia | | |
| **16. MS:** ROM • Ortolani • spine | | |
| **17. Neuro:** jitteriness • head control • posture • tone • DTRs • clonus • Babinski • Moro • TNR • suck • root • grasp • stepping crossed • extension • positive supporting | | |

*Document Abnormals (by number):*

### Anticipatory Guidance

✔ *Topics discussed*

**Nutrition**

| | |
|---|---|
| No solids | Spitting up/vomiting |
| Always hold to feed Never prop bottle | Encourage continuation of breastfeeding (if appropriate) on demand |
| No honey before one year | |

**Safety**

| | |
|---|---|
| Car seat | Supervise sibling and pet interaction |
| Never leave unattended | Safe crib/sleep on back or side |
| Support head and neck | No strings |
| Care with talc | Smoke detectors |
| Sun protection | No smoking around baby |
| Hot water temp < 125° F | |

**Parenting**

| | |
|---|---|
| Show affection to baby | Diarrhea care |
| Interact by responding to cry | Thermometer use |
| Never punish, jerk, or shake | When to call office |
| Day care concerns | Bulb syringe for congestion |
| Fever care | Infection risk reduction |
| Skin care | |

*Other:*

### Laboratory Tests (none routinely required at this age)

### Additional Plan

### Assessment

☐ Child well
☐ Additional diagnoses (specify):

### Plan
#### Immunizations

*Are immunizations on schedule?*  ☐ Yes  ☐ No  (Update Record Card)
*If not, catch-up plan?* _____
*Previous reaction?*  ☐ Yes    ☐ No

*Comments:* _____
*Immunizations ordered/given:*  ☐ Hepatitis B  ☐ PCV
☐ DTaP  ☐ IPV  ☐ Hib  ☐ Other _____
*If immunization(s) due but not given, explain:*

**Referrals**
☐ *Smoking cessation class*
☐ *Breastfeeding class/support group*
☐ *Other:*

☐ *Encouraged smoking cessation*
☐ *Need for financial assistance*
☐ *Social services*
☐ *Requires additional health education*
☐ *Schedule 2-month visit*

**Provider signature**
☐ Note dictated

*From Loretz L. (2005). *Primary care tools for clinicians.* St. Louis: Elsevier.

## 5-Year Well-Child Visit*

Date of Visit: _____

Medical Record Number: _____

Child's Name: _____

Address: _____

Telephone: _____

Date of Birth: _____ Age: ____ Gender:  Male   Female

Provider: _____

Informant: _____     Interpreter present:  ☐ Yes   ☐ No

Relationship to Child:_____     Language _____

### Measurements

Ht _____ _____ %   Wt _____ _____ %   BP _____     Staff

Temp _____   Pulse _____   Resp _____     Initials ____

### Vision/Hearing

| Hearing | | | | | | | | Vision | | |
|---|---|---|---|---|---|---|---|---|---|---|
| Right Ear | | | | Left Ear | | | | Glasses  ☐ Yes  ☐ No | | |
| 500 | 1000 | 2000 | 4000 | 500 | 1000 | 2000 | 4000 | Right eye      / | | |
| | | | | | | | | Left eye      / | | |
| ☐ Normal ☐ Abnormal ☐ Question validity/retest | | | | | | | | ☐ Normal | | |
| Comments:              Staff Initials _____ | | | | | | | | ☐ Refer to eye clinic | | |
| | | | | | | | | ☐ Question validity/ retest | | |

Vision concerns      ☐ No    ☐ Yes (explain) _____

Hearing concerns    ☐ No    ☐ Yes (explain) _____

### Child Health History

Family/social history (refer to chart)    ☐ Completed    ☐ Updated

Parental concerns:_____

_____

Recent injury/illness/surgery/hospitalizations:

Allergies: _____

Medications: _____

### Review of Systems

| | N | AB |
|---|---|---|
| HEENT | | |
| Skin (rashes) | | |
| CV (activity level) | | |
| Resp (wheezing) | | |
| GI (vomiting/stools) | | |
| GU (pain on voiding/stream/bedwetting) | | |
| Neuromuscular (headaches, limb pain) | | |

Remainder of review of systems (unlisted) negative  ☐

### Daily Activities

Nutrition: (variety/misses meals/wt concern)_____

Milk: (whole, 2%, 1%, skim)_____

Sleep: bedtime _____   awakes _____

*From Loretz L. (2005). Primary care tools for clinicians. St. Louis: Elsevier.

### Child Health History (continued)

Dental: (brushing) _____

Exercise: _____

Recreation/Hobbies/TV: _____

Environmental Risks—Check if assessed

☐ Lead risk                    ☐ Guns in house/bldg          ☐ TB exposure

☐ Alcohol use in house/bldg    ☐ Housing inadequate          ☐ Domestic violence

☐ Smokers in house/bldg        ☐ Drug use in house/bldg      ☐ Other

☐ Identified risks _____

Active community supports/resources:

_____

Mental Health/Behavior Risks:

☐ No concerns

☐ Concerns (explain)_____

Observation of parent/child interaction:

☐ Appropriate

☐ Not appropriate (explain) _____

Other:

### Development

| Personal/social/cognitive | N | AB |
|---|---|---|
| • Dresses without help | | |
| • Plays make believe | | |
| • Plays board games | | |
| Language | | |
| • Names 4 colors | | |
| • Counts 5 blocks | | |
| • Understands 4 prepositions | | |
| • Able to define 5 words | | |
| • Speech all understandable | | |
| Gross motor | | |
| • Balances each foot 5 sec | | |
| • Heel-to-toe walk | | |
| Fine motor/adaptive | | |
| • Copies square demonstrated | | |
| • Copies + | | |
| • Recognizes some letters | | |
| • Draws a person with 6 parts | | |

☐ Developmental screening tool, if used:

Name of tool _____

_____

Staff initials _____

☐ By observation/exam/ parent report. No tool used.

## 5-Year Well-Child Visit - 2*

Child's Name: _____     Medical Record Number: _____

### Physical Exam

| N = normal     Ab = abnormal (check appropriate box) | N | AB |
|---|---|---|
| 1. General appearance: | | |
| 2. Skin: color • character • birthmarks | | |
| 3. Nodes: cervical • axillary • inguinal | | |
| 4. Head: shape • hair | | |
| 5. Eyes: EOM • red reflex • corneal light reflex • PERL • cross cover accommodation • fundi • lids | | |
| 6. Ears: pinna • canals • TMs | | |
| 7. Nose: patency • nares • turbinates | | |
| 8. Mouth: mucosa • tonsils • teeth • throat | | |
| 9. Neck: ROM • thyroid | | |
| 10. Chest: shape • symmetry • lungs • respiration rate | | |
| 11. CV: rate • rhythm • $S_1$ • $S_2$ • murmur • femoral pulses | | |
| 12. Abd: contour • liver • spleen • masses • anus • bowel sounds | | |
| 13. GU: ♀ labia • vaginal mucosa • urethra       ♂ penis • testes • hernia | | |
| 14. MS: ROM • gait • spine | | |
| 15. Neuro: DTRs • clonus • motor strength • sensory | | |

Document Abnormals (by number): _____

### Assessment

☐ Child well
☐ Additional diagnoses (specify):

### Plan

#### Immunizations

Are immunizations on schedule?  ☐ Yes ☐ No  (update record card)

If not, catch-up plan? _____

Previous reaction?  ☐ Yes     ☐ No

Comments: _____

Immunizations ordered/given:  ☐ Hepatitis B   ☐ DTaP   ☐ IPV
☐ Hib       ☐ MMR       ☐ Varicella

If immunization(s) due but not given, explain:

☐ Has had chickenpox infection
☐ Other _____

*From Loretz L. (2005). Primary care tools for clinicians. St. Louis: Elsevier.

### Anticipatory Guidance

✔ Topics discussed

#### Healthy Habits

| Limit TV | Food choices (friuts, vegetables, grains) |
|---|---|
| Safety: matches/poisons/guns | Safe after school environment |
| Safety: water/playground/stranger | Adequate sleep/physical activity |
| Safety: car seat/seat belt/ bike helmet | Curiosity about sex |
| | Infection risk reduction |
| Dental sealants | Eliminate lead risk |

#### Social Competence

| School readiness | Family rules, respect, right from wrong |
|---|---|
| Praise, encourage | |
| Knows address and phone number | Anger control/conflict resolution |

#### Family Relationships

| Affection | Know child's friends/families |
|---|---|
| Sibling relationships | Ethical role model |

Other:

### Laboratory Tests

☐ Blood lead (if never tested)          ☐ UA (optional)
☐ Other

### Dental

☐ Verbal referral for preventive dental visit

### Additional Plan

| Referrals |
|---|
| ☐ Smoking cessation class |
| ☐ Other: |

☐ Encouraged smoking cessation
☐ Need for financial assistance/social services
☐ Requires additional health education
☐ Dental resource information given
☐ Schedule 6-year preventive visit

Provider Signature
☐ Note dictated

## 15- to 17-Year Well Visit*

Date of Visit: _____

Medical Record Number: _____

Child's Name: _____

Address: _____

Telephone: _____

Date of Birth: _____    Age: _____    Gender:  Male    Female

Provider: _____

Informant: _____     Interpreter present:   ☐ Yes     ☐ No

Relationship to Child:_____     Language _____

### Measurements

Ht _____ _____ %  Wt _____ _____ %  BP _____     Staff

Temp _____   Pulse _____   Resp _____   Initials _____

### Vision/Hearing

| Hearing | | | | | | | | Vision |
|---|---|---|---|---|---|---|---|---|
| Right Ear | | | | Left Ear | | | | Glasses  ☐ Yes ☐ No |
| 500 | 1000 | 2000 | 4000 | 500 | 1000 | 2000 | 4000 | Right eye        / |
|  |  |  |  |  |  |  |  | Left eye         / |

☐ Normal ☐ Abnormal ☐ Question validity/retest
Comments:                  Staff Initials _____

Vision box:
- ☐ Normal
- ☐ Refer to eye clinic
- ☐ Question validity/retest

Vision concerns        ☐ No   ☐ Yes (explain) _____

Hearing concerns      ☐ No   ☐ Yes (explain)_____

### Health History

Family/social history (refer to chart)   ☐ Completed   ☐ Updated

Adolescent/parental concerns: _____
_____

Recent injury/illness/surgery/hospitalizations:

Allergies: _____

Medications: _____

### Review of Systems

|  | N | AB |
|---|---|---|
| HEENT |  |  |
| Skin (rashes/acne) |  |  |
| CV (dizziness, chest pain) |  |  |
| Resp (wheezing) |  |  |
| GI (vomiting/stools) |  |  |
| GU (pain/stream) |  |  |
| Neuromuscular (headaches) |  |  |

Remainder of review of systems (unlisted) negative ☐

### Daily Activities

Nutrition: (variety/misses meals/wt concern) _____

Milk: (whole, 2%, 1%, skim) _____

Sleep: bedtime _____   awakes _____

### Health History (continued)

Dental: _____

Exercise: _____

Recreation/Hobbies/TV: _____

Tobacco/Alcohol/Drugs/Driving: _____

Menstrual Hx (female):

   Menarche _____   LMP _____   Regularity _____

Sexual History (activity, partners, birth control, STDs, pregnancy):

_____

Practices self-breast/testicular exam?:   ☐ Yes    ☐ No

Environmental Risks—Check if assessed

☐ Guns in house/bldg        ☐ TB exposure        ☐ Alcohol use in house/bldg

☐ Housing inadequate        ☐ Violence/rape       ☐ Smokers in house/bldg

☐ Drug use in house/bldg    ☐ Other: _____

☐ Identified risks _____

Active community supports/resources:

_____

Mental Health/Behavior Risks:

☐ No concerns

☐ Concerns (explain) _____

Observation of parent/child interaction:

☐ Appropriate

☐ Not appropriate (explain)_____

Other: _____

☐ Adolescent risk assessment tool (if used)

### Development

|  | N | AB | Comments: |
|---|---|---|---|
| School (employment) performance/attendance: |  |  |  |
| Future plans, college, career |  |  |  |
| Family relationships |  |  |  |
| Ability to form/maintain peer relationships |  |  |  |
| Dating/sexual activity |  |  |  |
| Activities or sports involvement |  |  |  |
| Emotional stability |  |  |  |

*From Loretz L. (2005). Primary care tools for clinicians. St. Louis: Elsevier.

## 15- to 17-Year Well Visit - 2*

*Child's Name:* _____    *Medical Record Number:* _____

### Physical Exam

| N = normal    Ab = abnormal (check appropriate box) | N | AB |
|---|---|---|
| *1. General appearance:* | | |
| *2. Skin:* rash • acne | | |
| *3. Nodes:* cervical • axillary • inguinal | | |
| *4. Head:* scalp • hair | | |
| *5. Eyes:* EOM • red reflex • corneal light reflex • PERL • lids | | |
| *6. Ears:* pinna • canals • TMs | | |
| *7. Nose:* patency • nares | | |
| *8. Mouth:* gums • teeth/caries • occlusion • throat | | |
| *9. Neck:* ROM • thyroid | | |
| *10. Chest:* lungs • respiration rate | | |
| ♀ *Female:* Breasts • Tanner Stage: | | |
| ♂ *Male:* Gynecomastia | | |
| *11. CV:* rate • rhythm • S1 • S2 • murmur • femoral pulses | | |
| *12. Abd:* liver • spleen • masses • anus • bowel sounds | | |
| *13. GU:* ♀ labia • vaginal mucosa | | |
| ♂ penis • testes • hernia | | |
| Tanner Stage: _____ | | |
| *Pelvic:* EG _____    Vag _____  BUS _____    CX _____  Uterus _____    Adnexa _____ | | |
| *14. MS:* ROM • spine • gait | | |
| *15. Neuro:* DTRs • coordination • sensory • motor | | |

*Document Abnormals (by number):*

### Assessment

☐ Adolescent well

☐ Additional Diagnoses (specify):

### Plan
### Immunizations

*Are immunizations on schedule?*    ☐ Yes ☐ No  (Update Record Card)

*If not, catch-up plan?* _____

*Previous reaction?*    ☐ Yes    ☐ No

*Comments:* _____

*Immunizations ordered/given:*    ☐ Hepatitis B    ☐ Td    ☐ IPV
☐ MMR    ☐ Varicella    ☐ Meningococcal

*If immunization(s) due but not given, explain:*

☐ Has had chickenpox infection

☐ Other _____

*From Loretz L. (2005). *Primary care tools for clinicians.* St. Louis: Elsevier.

### Anticipatory Guidance

✔ *Topics discussed*

*Healthy Habits*

| Self-protection | Adequate sleep/exercise |
|---|---|
| Weight management/food choices | Athletic conditioning, weight training |
| Sexual feelings | Handle anger/conflict resolution |
| How to say no, abstinence | Weapons |
| Birth control, STDs, safer sex | Seat belts, bike helmets |
| Alcohol/Drugs/Tobacco use | Stress, nervousness, sadness |
| Infection risk reduction | |

*Social Competence*

| Family time | Social activities/groups/sports |
|---|---|
| Peer pressure/peer refusal | Respect parents' limits/consequences |

*Responsibility*

| Respect others | Rules, chores, responsibility |
|---|---|
| Ethical role model | Religious, cultural, volunteer activities |

*School Achievement*

| Attendance, homework | Frustrations, dropping out |
|---|---|
| Future plans, college, career | |

*Other:*

### Laboratory Tests

☐ *Hgb/Hct* (once in adolescence for menstruating females) _____

☐ *Urinalysis* (once in adolescence) _____

☐ *Other* (STD, Pap, TB, cholesterol if at risk) _____

### Dental

☐ *Verbal referral for preventive dental visit*

### Additional Plan

**Referrals**
☐ *Smoking cessation class*
☐ *Other:*

☐ *Encouraged smoking cessation*

☐ *Need for financial assistance/social services*

☐ *Requires additional health education*

☐ *Dental resource information given*

☐ *Schedule visit in 1 to 2 years*

**Provider Signature**
☐ Note dictated

# Bedside Assessment and Electronic Documentation

## PURPOSE

This chapter helps you learn the methods of integrating the regional examinations for the hospital setting. The selection and sequencing of the techniques provide an assessment that is efficient, thorough, and consistent with the assessments performed by other nurses in the course of 24-hour care.

## READING ASSIGNMENT

Jarvis: *Physical Examination and Health Assessment,* 8th ed., Chapter 30, pp. 793-799.

Suggested reading:
Pearce, P. F., Ferguson, L. A., George, G. S., & Langford, C. A. (2016). The essential SOAP note in an EHR age. *Nurse Pract, 41*(2), 29-36.

## CLINICAL OBJECTIVES

1. Demonstrate skills of inspection, palpation, and auscultation.

2. Demonstrate correct use of instruments, including assembly, manipulation of component parts, and positioning with patient.

3. Use appropriate terminology and correctly pronounce medical terminology with clinical instructor and adapt for patient.

4. Choreograph the examination in a systematic manner, including integration of certain regional assessments throughout the examination (e.g., skin, musculoskeletal).

5. Coordinate procedures to limit position changes for examiner and patient.

6. Describe accurately the findings of the examination, including normal and abnormal findings.

7. Demonstrate appropriate infection control measures.

8. Recognize and maintain the privacy and dignity of the patient.
   a. Adequately explain what is being done while limiting small talk.
   b. Consider patient's anxiety and fears.
   c. Consider your own facial expression and comments.
   d. Demonstrate confidence, empathy, and gentle manner.

e. Acknowledge and apologize for any discomfort caused.
f. Provide for privacy and warmth at all times.
g. Determine comfort level, pausing if patient becomes tired.
h. Wash hands and don gloves appropriately.
i. Allow adequate time for each step.
j. Briefly summarize findings to patient, and thank patient for his or her time.

9. Complete all procedures with attention to specifics of technique, which allows clear and consistent replication of the procedures by others assessing the same patient.

## INSTRUCTIONS

As with other assessments, this particular version of the head-to-toe examination requires a great deal of practice before you will feel truly confident. The good news about this sequence is that it is directly applicable in any inpatient clinical sites that you attend. If you are already attending clinicals, use any available time to practice this sequence on real patients.

You are responsible for recruiting a friend or classmate to act as your patient for this examination. You will have 20 minutes for this examination, not including setup. If you have practiced the individual regional assessments thoroughly and can complete this particular sequence three times, you will be able to complete it satisfactorily within the time allotted.

Prepare the examination setting. Arrange the lighting, furniture, and bed to allow for the most efficient and comfortable activity for yourself and your patient. Think carefully about the functions of the patient's hospital bed. It can be useful to raise the bed closer to your eyes and stethoscope, but you cannot expect the patient to get out of bed safely from that height. Position sheets, drapes, and bath blankets strategically to achieve the proper balance of modesty, efficiency, and comfort.

Gather and arrange your equipment before you begin. The following items are needed for this sequence, but your instructor may modify the equipment list slightly for your individual class or exercise:

| | |
|---|---|
| Water (in a cup) | Ruler in millimeters |
| Watch with a second hand | Oxygen equipment (as indicated by your instructor) |
| Stethoscope | Doppler (as indicated by your instructor) |
| Blood pressure cuff | Bladder scanner (as indicated by your instructor) |
| Pulse oximeter | Standardized scales to calculate patient's risk for skin breakdown and falling |
| Penlight | Documentation forms (as included here, or provided by your instructor) |

Verify with your instructor whether you should submit documentation of this particular assessment after your demonstration or documentation that you have prepared to reflect one of your earlier practice sessions.

Good luck!

## COMPLETE INPATIENT REASSESSMENT

Date _____

Examiner _____

Patient _____    Age _____    Gender _____

Occupation _____    Reason for admission _____

### Introduction
1. Check for flags or markers at doorway.
2. Introduce yourself.
3. Perform hand hygiene.
4. Make eye contact.
5. Offer water (if appropriate).
6. Check name band.
7. Ask appropriate interview questions, including current pain.
8. Elevate the bed to appropriate height.

### General Appearance
1. Facial expression  _____
2. Body position  _____
3. Level of consciousness _____
4. Skin color _____
5. Nutritional status _____
6. Speech: articulation, pattern, content appropriate _____
7. Hearing  _____
8. Personal hygiene _____

### Measurement
1. Temperature _____
2. Pulse _____
3. Respiration _____
4. Blood pressure _____
5. Pulse oximetry _____
6. Weight on admission or daily weight if indicated  _____
7. Rate pain level on scale of 0 to 10; note ability to tolerate pain. _____
8. Pain reassessment, if appropriate _____

### Neurologic System
1. Glasgow Coma Scale:
   Eye opening _____
   Motor response _____
   Verbal response _____
2. Pupil size in millimeters and reaction
   a. R _____    b. L _____
3. Upper muscle strength
   a. R _____    b. L _____

4. Lower muscle strength
   a. R _____     b. L _____
5. Any ptosis, facial droop _____
6. Sensation (if indicated) _____
7. Communication _____
8. Ability to swallow _____

## Respiratory

1. Oxygen by mask, nasal cannula; check fitting _____
2. $F_{IO_2}$ _____
3. Respiratory effort _____
4. Auscultate breath sounds:
   Anterior lobes:
       Right upper _____
       Left upper _____
       Right middle _____
       Right lower _____
       Left lower _____
   Posterior lobes:
       Left upper _____
       Right upper _____
       Left lower _____
       Right lower _____
   Cough and deep breathe; any mucus? Check color and amount. _____
   Educate on use of incentive spirometry, if ordered.

## Cardiovascular System

1. Auscultate rhythm at apex: regular, irregular? _____
2. Check apical versus radial pulse
3. Assess heart sounds in all auscultatory areas: first with diaphragm, repeat with bell.
4. Check capillary refill _____
5. Check pretibial edema
   a. R _____     b. L _____
6. Palpate posterior tibial pulse
   a. R _____     b. L _____
7. Palpate dorsalis pedis pulse
   a. R _____     b. L _____
8. Pulses by Doppler, if appropriate _____
9. IV fluid and rate, if present _____

## Skin (may be integrated with rest of assessment)

1. Color _____
2. Temperature _____
3. Skin turgor _____
4. Note any lesions; check any dressings _____
5. Note skin around IV site _____
6. Standardized scale regarding skin breakdown _____
7. Settings and application of specialized surface, if present _____

## Abdomen

1. Contour of abdomen: flat, rounded, protuberant _____
2. Bowel sounds _____
3. Check any tube drainage and site _____
4. Inquire if passing flatus or stool _____
5. Can patient tolerate current diet? Should diet be advanced or changed? _____

## Genitourinary

1. Inquire if voiding regularly _____
2. Urine for color, clarity, quantity _____
3. Bladder scan, if indicated _____

## Activity

1. If on bed rest, check head of bed, risk for skin breakdown _____
2. Any SCDs or TED hose? Must be hooked up/on _____
3. Transfer to chair (if appropriate) _____
4. Note any assistance needed, how movement is tolerated, distance walked to chair, ability to turn
   _____
5. Need for ambulatory aid or equipment _____
6. Standardized fall scale _____

## Closure

1. Return bed to lowest position
2. Verify that brakes are locked
3. Make sure appropriate side rails are up
4. Ensure call light is within reach
5. Verify bed alarm, if indicated
6. Thank the patient for his or her attention and cooperation
7. Initiate or continue appropriate plan of care
8. Complete assessment and document

The SBAR framework (Situation, Background, Assessment, Recommendation) is used in many hospital units to improve verbal communication and reduce medical errors. Practice with the SBAR form on the next page. It will keep your message concise and focused on the patient, yet give your colleague enough information to grasp the current situation and make a decision.

## TELEMETRY UNIT SBAR

<table>
<tr>
<td>S</td>
<td colspan="3">
Patient name　　　　　　　Age<br><br>
Room number　　　　　　　Admit date<br><br>
1 Dx　　　　　　　　　　　2 Dx<br><br>
C/O
</td>
<td>
Allergies<br><br>
Code status<br><br>
Advanced directive on chart?
</td>
<td>
Physician<br>
Attending<br><br>
Consultants<br><br>
Pgr/#
</td>
</tr>
<tr>
<td>B</td>
<td colspan="3">
History<br><br>
Surgery　　　　　　Surgeon<br><br>
Anesthesia　　　　Anesthesiologist　　　EBL
</td>
<td colspan="2">
Isolation　　　Core Measures<br><br>
Restraints　　CHF MI PNA<br><br>
Fall risk　　　Vaccine - PNA Flu
</td>
</tr>
<tr>
<td rowspan="6">A</td>
<td colspan="3">
Cardiac: BP/HR/Peripheral pulses/Edema/Heart sounds<br><br>
Current rhythm<br><br>
Daily wt?<br><br>
DVT prophylaxis
</td>
<td colspan="2">
Pain/sedation<br><br>
Pain scale<br><br>
Location<br><br>
Meds type and last dose
</td>
</tr>
<tr>
<td colspan="2">
Pulmonary: Breath sounds/Secretions/SpO$_2$/UPAs/PIP/ Spontaneous VT & VE
</td>
<td>
Vent/bipap etc<br><br>
settings
</td>
<td colspan="2">
Accu checks　　　　A1C<br><br>
Frequency<br><br>
Last results
</td>
</tr>
<tr>
<td colspan="2">
GI　　　　NG/OGT<br><br>
BS　　　　Last BM
</td>
<td>
Diet　　　　GI Prophylaxis
</td>
<td colspan="2">
Skin<br>
Wounds/drainage<br><br>
Staples<br>
Drains<br><br>
Location<br><br>
Ducub photo on admission
</td>
</tr>
<tr>
<td colspan="3">
GU Foley/void<br><br>
Output
</td>
<td colspan="2"></td>
</tr>
<tr>
<td colspan="3">
IV　　　　　　Date inserted<br><br>
Fluids　　　　Gtts
</td>
<td colspan="2">
Psych social
</td>
</tr>
<tr>
<td colspan="3">
Meds
</td>
<td colspan="2">
Pending orders
</td>
</tr>
<tr>
<td>A</td>
<td colspan="5">

| Na | Cl | BUN | gluc | mg | BNP | Coags<br>INR | | Hct | UA | CT<br>CXR |
|----|----|-----|------|-----|------|------|---|-----|------|------|
| K | Co | Cr | Ca | Phos | D dimer | PTT Next<br>Lab | W | Pl | Cultures | MRI<br>Echo |
| Cardiac enz | | 1 | 2 | 3 | | | | Hgb | | |

</td>
</tr>
<tr>
<td>R</td>
<td colspan="3">
DC Plan. Is pt informed of plan____24 hour orders reviewed____
</td>
<td colspan="2">
Shift goals
</td>
</tr>
</table>

Courtesy of Scrubs Magazine, The Nurses Guide to Good Living, at scrubsmag.com.

# The Pregnant Woman

## PURPOSE

This chapter helps you learn the changes and function of the female genitalia during pregnancy; the methods of inspection and palpation of the internal and external structures and the maternal abdomen; and how to record the assessment accurately.

## READING ASSIGNMENT

Jarvis: *Physical Examination and Health Assessment*, 8th ed., Chapter 31, pp. 801-824.

Suggested reading:
Anderson, C. M. (2017). Preeclampsia: Current approaches to nursing management. *Am J Nurs, 117*(11), 30-40.

## GLOSSARY

Study the following terms after completing the reading assignment. You should be able to cover the definition on the right and define the term out loud.

**Amniocentesis** . . . . . . . . . . . . . the transabdominal perforation of the amniotic sac for the purpose of obtaining a sample of amniotic fluid; helps identify genetic disorders, such as Down syndrome or sickle cell anemia

**Amniotic fluid** . . . . . . . . . . . . . fluid in the sac surrounding the fetus in the mother's uterus

**Anemia**. . . . . . . . . . . . . . . . . . . condition in which the number of red blood cells/mm$^3$ are less than normal

**Antenatal testing** . . . . . . . . . . . consists of monitoring fetal growth, amniotic fluid volume, umbilical cord Doppler blood flow, and fetal monitoring via non-stress or contraction stress testing using a fetal monitor

**Antepartum** . . . . . . . . . . . . . . . the period occurring before childbirth

**Blastocyst** . . . . . . . . . . . . . . . . the fertilized ovum; a specialized layer of cells around the blastocyst that becomes the placenta

**Chadwick sign** . . . . . . . . . . . . . bluish purple discoloration of the cervix during pregnancy due to venous congestion

**Chloasma** . . . . . . . . . . . . . . . . the "mask of pregnancy"; butterfly-shaped pigmentation of the face

**Chorionic villi sampling** . . . . . transabdominal or transvaginal sampling of trophoblastic tissue surrounding the gestational sac

**Colostrum** . . . . . . . . . . . . . . . . the precursor to milk that contains minerals, proteins, and antibodies

**Corpus luteum** . . . . . . . . . . . . . "yellow body"; a structure on the surface of the ovary that is formed by the remaining cells in the follicle; acts as a short-lived endocrine organ that produces progesterone to help maintain the pregnancy in its early stages

**Diastasis recti** . . . . . . . . . . . . . . separation of the abdominal muscles during pregnancy, returning to normal after pregnancy

**Engagement** . . . . . . . . . . . . . . . referes to when the widest diameter of the presenting part has descended into the pelvic inlet

**Fetal lie** . . . . . . . . . . . . . . . . . . orientation of the fetal spine to the maternal spine

**Goodell sign** . . . . . . . . . . . . . . the softening of the cervix due to increased vascularity, congestion, and edema

**Hegar sign** . . . . . . . . . . . . . . . . occurs when the uterus becomes globular in shape, softens, and flexes easily over the cervix

**Leopold maneuver** . . . . . . . . . . external palpation of the maternal abdomen to determine fetal lie, presentation, attitude, and position

**Linea nigra** . . . . . . . . . . . . . . . . a median line of the abdomen that becomes pigmented (darkens) during pregnancy

**Morning sickness** . . . . . . . . . . . nausea and vomiting of pregnancy that usually begins between weeks 4 and 6, peaks between weeks 8 and 12, and resolves between weeks 14 and 16

**Mucus plug** . . . . . . . . . . . . . . . mucus that forms a thick barrier in the cervix that is expelled at various times before or during labor

**Multigravida** . . . . . . . . . . . . . . . a pregnant woman who has previously carried a fetus to the point of viability

**Multipara** . . . . . . . . . . . . . . . . . a woman who has had two or more viable pregnancies and deliveries

**Nägele rule** . . . . . . . . . . . . . . . a rule for calculating the estimated date of delivery; add 7 days to first day of the last menstrual period and subtract 3 months

**Nuchal translucency** . . . . . . . . the amount of fluid behind the neck of the fetus; also known as the *nuchal fold*. Fetuses at risk for Down syndrome tend to have a higher amount of fluid.

**Position** . . . . . . . . . . . . . . . . . . the location of a fetal part to the right or left of the maternal pelvis

**Postpartum** . . . . . . . . . . . . . . . the period occurring after delivery

**Presentation** . . . . . . . . . . . . . . the part of the fetus that is entering the pelvis first

**Primigravida** . . . . . . . . . . . . . . a woman pregnant for the first time

**Primipara** . . . . . . . . . . . . . . . . . a woman who has had one pregnancy and delivery

**Striae gravidarum** . . . . . . . . . . "stretch marks" that may be seen on the abdomen and breasts (in areas of weight gain) during pregnancy

**Ultrasound (US) image**.......the use of sound waves to examine the fetus, amniotic fluid, and placenta in the uterus

**Umbilical cord** .............a ropelike structure containing blood vessels that connect the fetus to the placenta, carrying oxygen and nutrients from the mother and waste products away from the fetus

**VBAC**.....................vaginal birth after cesarean delivery

## STUDY GUIDE

After completing the reading assignment and the media assignment, write or draw the answers in the spaces provided.

1. Describe the function of the placenta.

2. Using Nägele rule, calculate the estimated date of delivery if the LMP is August 22.

3. Give examples of the following signs of pregnancy.

   Presumptive: _____

   Probable: _____

   Positive: _____

4. When can serum hCG be detected in maternal blood? In maternal urine?

5. Describe three physical and physiologic changes that are seen in the:

   First trimester: _____

   Second trimester: _____

   Third trimester: _____

6. Describe the "recommended" weight gain during pregnancy.

7. List the major concerns for teenage pregnancy.

8. List at least 3 risk factors concerning pregnant women of advanced maternal age.

9. Discuss the importance of how culture and genetics play a role in a woman's pregnancy.

10. True or false: Please circle the best answer.

| | | |
|---|---|---|
| True | False | A woman who has had a classic uterine incision is a good candidate for a VBAC. |
| True | False | A woman who is pregnant for the first time is called a *primipara.* |
| True | False | The fetal period begins after the 9th gestational week. |
| True | False | Preeclampsia is seen only in the third trimester of pregnancy. |
| True | False | Vaginal bleeding in pregnancy always indicates a miscarriage. |
| True | False | Cervical incompetence is always accompanied by painful contractions. |

11. What is the importance of fetal movement counting, and when should it be initiated?

12. Describe why it is important to ask a pregnant woman if she feels safe in her relationships and environment.

13. Label, list the order, and describe the purpose of the following maneuvers.

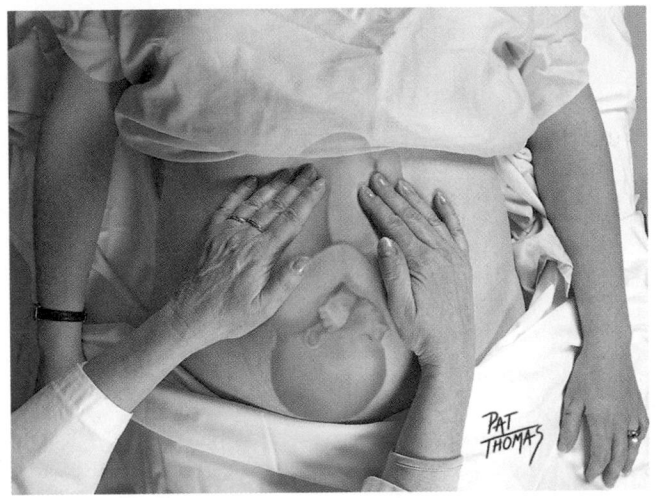

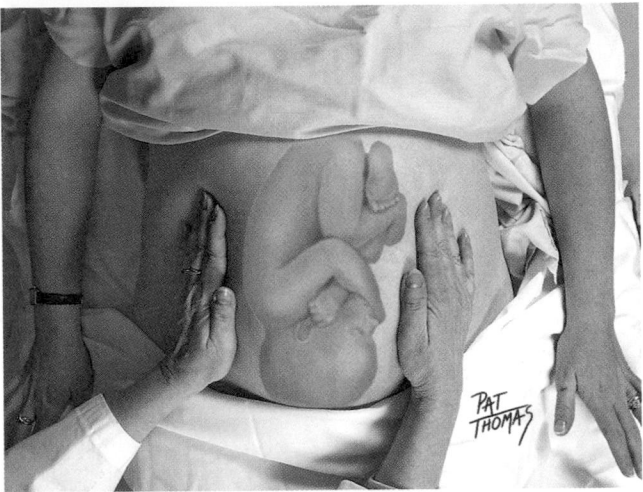

_____

_____

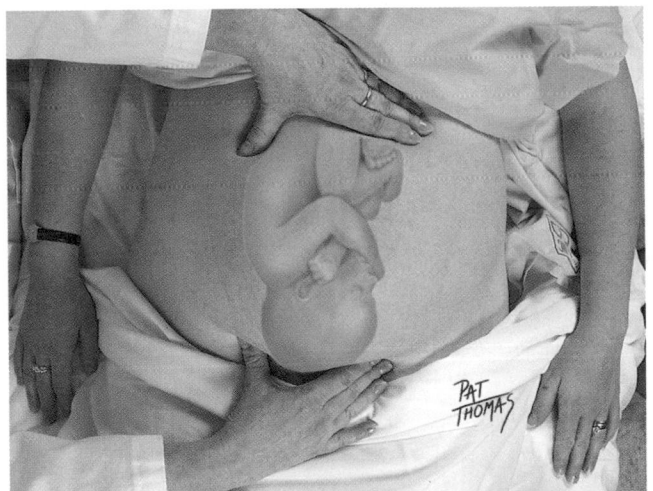

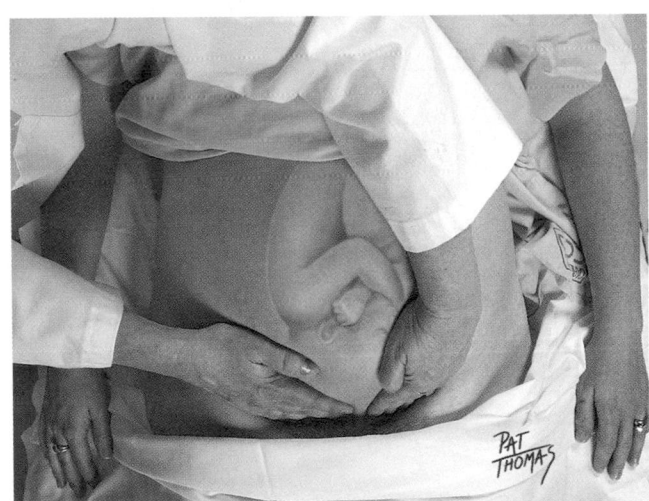

_____

_____

14. Describe the following for this figure.

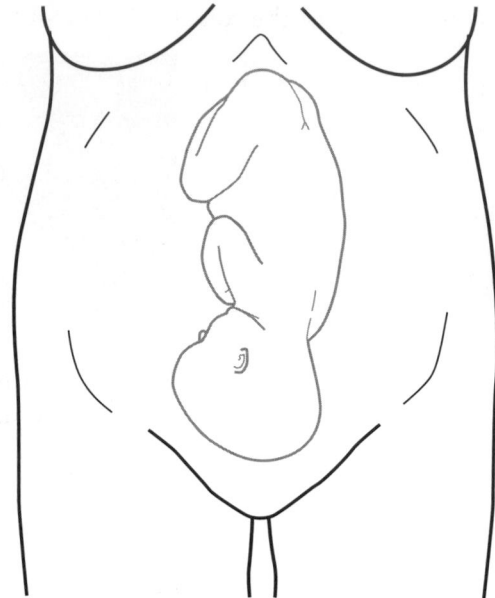

Fetal lie: _____

Fetal presentation: _____

Fetal position: _____

15. List the symptoms of preeclampsia.

16. List at least 2 reasons why fundal height may be small for gestational age.

17. List at least 2 reasons why fundal height may be large for gestational age.

# REVIEW QUESTIONS

This test is for you to check your own mastery of the content. Answers are provided in Appendix A.

1. Using Nägele rule, the estimated date of delivery (EDD) if a woman's last menstrual period started on January 13 is:

   a. 1/13 + 7 = 20, 20 − 3 months, EDD ≈ October 29.
   b. 1/13 + 10 = 23, 23 − 3 months, EDD ≈ October 18.
   c. 1/13 + 14 = 27, 27 − 3 months, EDD ≈ September 30.
   d. 1/13 − 7 = 6, 6 − 3 months, EDD ≈ October 6.

2. A woman reports nausea, fatigue, breast tenderness, urinary frequency, and amenorrhea. These are:

   a. Probable signs of pregnancy.
   b. Positive signs of pregnancy.
   c. Presumptive signs of pregnancy.
   d. Signs of stress.

3. Approximately 2 to 3 weeks before labor, the woman will experience which sign that the baby has "dropped" into the pelvis?

   a. Extreme fatigue
   b. Braxton-Hicks contractions
   c. Lightening
   d. Back pain

4. Cardiac output in a pregnant woman:

   a. Drops dramatically.
   b. Remains the same.
   c. Increases along with stroke volume.
   d. Decreases along with stroke volume.

5. A pregnant adolescent is medically at risk for:

   a. Poor weight gain, preeclampsia, thyroiditis, miscarriage.
   b. Poor weight gain, preeclampsia, prolonged labor.
   c. Stress, abuse, inadequate housing, inadequate education.
   d. Miscarriage, hypothyroidism, poor weight gain.

6. Women older than 35 years who desire a pregnancy are at possible risk for:

   a. Congenital defects.
   b. Infertility.
   c. Diabetes.
   d. Hypertension.
   e. All of the above.

7. Sexually transmitted infections place the pregnant woman at risk for:

   a. Infertility.
   b. Premature rupture of membranes.
   c. Preterm labor.
   d. Postpartum maternal infections.
   e. All of the above.

8. Abdominal pain in the first trimester may be indicative of:

   a. Preterm labor.
   b. Ectopic pregnancy.
   c. Appendicitis.
   d. All of the above.

9. A woman at approximately 20 weeks' gestation reports lower right and/or left quadrant pain. Which of the following may be the cause of this pain?

   a. Appendicitis
   b. Constipation
   c. Urinary tract infection
   d. Stretching of the round ligament

10. You palpate the maternal abdomen at approximately 35 weeks. Your left hand is on the maternal right, and your right hand is on the maternal left. What maneuver is this?

    a. Leopold first maneuver
    b. Leopold second maneuver
    c. Schmidt third maneuver
    d. Schmidt second maneuver

11. Fetal heart tones are best auscultated over the fetus's:

    a. Back.
    b. Abdomen.
    c. Shoulder.
    d. Head.

12. Chadwick sign is:

    a. Softening of the cervix.
    b. Rotation of the cervix to the left.
    c. The fundus of the uterus tipping forward.
    d. A bluish color of the cervix and vaginal walls during early pregnancy.

13. Three of these findings can be assessed with an obstetric ultrasound. Which one cannot?

    a. Thickness of the uterine wall
    b. Fetal position
    c. Placental location
    d. Amniotic fluid volume

# SKILLS LABORATORY AND CLINICAL SETTING

You are now ready for the clinical component of the pregnant female examination. Some clinical settings may arrange for pregnant women to participate, or your practice setting may have available a pregnant teaching mannequin that you may use to practice your skills. If you have a pregnant woman available, discuss with her, in the presence of your instructor, the methods of examination that will be used. Maintain her comfort and adequate positioning to prevent maternal dizziness, nausea, and hypotension and to maintain adequate uterine blood flow.

## Clinical Objectives

1. Demonstrate knowledge of the physical changes related to pregnancy in the first, second, and third trimesters.

2. Demonstrate obtaining a pertinent health history during the first prenatal visit.

3. Demonstrate cultural sensitivity during the examination.

4. Inspect and palpate the maternal abdomen for uterine size and fetal position.

5. Demonstrate obtaining fetal heart tones.

6. Record the history and physical examination findings accurately; reach an assessment of the health state, estimated gestational age, and fetal position (when appropriate); and develop a plan of care.

## Instructions

Prepare the examination setting, and gather your equipment. Collect the health history before the woman disrobes for the examination. Calculate the EDD. Wash your hands. Practice the steps of the examination on a woman in the clinical setting, giving appropriate instructions and explanations as you proceed. Record your findings using the regional write-up sheet that follows. The first section is intended as a worksheet; the last page is intended for your narrative summary recording using the SOAP format. See Chapter 27 for the female genital examination.

**REGIONAL WRITE-UP—PREGNANT FEMALE**

_____

Patient Name                                Date

# PRENATAL HISTORY QUESTIONNAIRE

Having a healthy baby is a special event. Once a baby is born, families take certain precautions to ensure the baby's health and safety. The unborn child deserves similar care.

# QUESTIONNAIRE

The following questions will help in the care of your pregnancy. Please answer these questions as well as you can. All answers will remain private. If you need help answering the questions, please ask your health care provider. The first question relates to your family history. The next 7 questions will be about you, your baby's father, and both your families. When thinking about your families, please include your child (or unborn baby), mother, father, sisters, brothers, grandparents, aunts, uncles, nieces, nephews, and cousins.

Yes    No    1.    Will you be 35 years or older when the baby is due? Age when due: _____ .

Yes    No    2.    Are you and the baby's father related to each other (e.g., cousins)?

Yes    No    3.    Have you had three or more pregnancies that ended in miscarriage?

Yes    No    4.    Have you or the baby's father had a stillborn baby or a baby who died around the time of delivery?

Yes    No    5.    Do either you or the baby's father have a birth defect or genetic condition such as a baby born with an open spine (spina bifida), a heart defect, or Down syndrome?

Yes    No    6.    Does anyone in your family or anyone in the baby's father's family have a birth defect or condition that has been diagnosed as genetic or inherited, such as open spine (spina bifida), a heart defect, or Down syndrome?

Yes    No    7.    Where your ancestors came from may sometimes give us important information about the health of your baby. Are you or the baby's father from any of the following ethnic/racial groups: Jewish, African American, Asian, Mediterranean (Greek, Italian)?

Yes    No    8.    Have you or the baby's father ever been screened to see if you are carriers of the gene for any of the following: Tay-Sachs, sickle cell, thalassemia?

Sometimes, the unborn baby can be exposed to outside factors that can cause birth defects. The next 8 questions will give us important information about possible exposure to the baby.

Yes    No    9.    Have you had any x-rays during this pregnancy?

Yes    No    10.   Have you had any alcohol during this pregnancy?

11.   Prior to your pregnancy, how often did you drink alcoholic beverages?
☐ Every day                              ☐ Less than once a month
☐ At least once a week, not daily        ☐ I do not drink alcoholic beverages.
☐ At least once a month, not weekly

12.   Prior to your pregnancy, about how many alcoholic beverages did you usually have per occasion? (1 = one can of beer, one wine cooler, one glass of wine, or one shot of liquor.)
☐ 3 or more
☐ 1 to 2
☐ I do not drink alcoholic beverages.

Yes    No    13.    Have you taken any over-the-counter, prescription, or "street" drugs during this pregnancy? If yes, list drugs.

_____

_____

Yes    No    14.    Have you ever sought and/or received treatment for alcohol or drug problems? If yes, how long ago?_____

Yes    No    15.    Do you think you are at increased risk for having a baby with a birth defect or genetic disorder?

Yes    No    16.    At any time during the first 2 months of your pregnancy, have you had a rash or a fever of 103° F or greater?

A test for HIV is strongly recommended for all pregnant women, regardless of your responses to the next questions. The test is voluntary. There are two reasons to be tested: [1] New medications are available to reduce the chance of an infected mother passing HIV to her baby; and [2] most women do not know if they are infected with HIV until late in the disease. Sometimes other infections can put you and your baby at risk. The following questions will help your health care provider determine other areas for counseling and evaluation.

Yes    No    Unsure    17.    Have you or your sexual partners ever had a sexually transmitted infection (STI or VD) such as chlamydia, gonorrhea, syphilis, or herpes?

Yes    No    Unsure    18.    Have you ever had a serious pelvic infection or pelvic inflammatory disease (PID)?

Yes    No    Unsure    19.    Do you think any of your male sexual partners have ever had sex with other men?

Yes    No    Unsure    20.    Have you or your sexual partners ever used IV street drugs?

Yes    No    Unsure    21.    Have you had sex with two or more partners in the last 12 months?

Yes    No    Unsure    22.    Do you think any of your sexual partners may have HIV or AIDS?

Yes    No    Unsure    23.    Have you or your sexual partners ever had a blood transfusion?

How safe you feel in your daily living gives us important information about risks to you and your baby.
Please answer these questions as well as you can. All answers will remain private.

24.    Do you feel safe....
Yes    No    -    in your personal relationship?
Yes    No    -    within your home?
Yes    No    -    in your own neighborhood?
Yes    No    -    other (specify)_____

Yes    No    25.    Have you ever had your feelings repeatedly hurt, been repeatedly put down, or experienced other kinds of hurting?

Yes    No    26.    Are you being or have you ever been hit, slapped, kicked, pushed, or otherwise physically hurt? If yes, by whom?
☐ Husband          ☐ Family member
☐ Ex-husband       ☐ Stranger
☐ Partner          ☐ Other (specify)_____

Yes    No    27.    Are you experiencing or have you ever experienced uncomfortable touching or forced sexual contact? If yes, by whom?
☐ Husband          ☐ Family member
☐ Ex-husband       ☐ Stranger
☐ Partner          ☐ Other (specify)_____

RM/603  REV 6/97

# PRENATAL RECORD

| DATE | AGE | RACE | RELIGION | OCCUPATION | YRS. ED. | MARITAL STATUS | FATHER OF BABY | FATHER'S WORK PHONE |
|---|---|---|---|---|---|---|---|---|

| PHONE-HOME | PHONE-WORK | ADDRESS | | REFERRAL-SOURCE | MOTHER'S PRIMARY CARE PROVIDER |
|---|---|---|---|---|---|

## GYNECOLOGICAL HISTORY | MEDICAL HISTORY - CONTINUED

| MENARCHE | YRS | INTERVAL | ☐ REGULAR ☐ IRREGULAR | DURATION | DAYS | | CARDIOVASCULAR |
|---|---|---|---|---|---|---|---|

RESPIRATORY/TB

✔ IF NEGATIVE-DESCRIBE POSITIVE HISTORY

| PAP HISTORY | | GI |
| INFERTILITY | | GU |
| GYN DISORDER | | METABOLIC |
| GYN SURGERY | | NEURO |
| DES EXPOSURE | | PSYCH-EMOTIONAL |
| PRIOR CONTRACEPTION | | HEPATITIS |
| BCP W/IN 90 DAYS CONCEP | | MUSCULOSKELETAL |
| BREASTS | | SKIN DISORDERS |
| OTHER GYN HX | | OTHER DISEASE/DX |
| GONORRHEA | | OPERATIONS |
| SYPHILIS | | TRANSFUSIONS |
| CHLAMYDIA | | ALLERGIES |
| HERPES-SELF/PARTNER | |
| OTHER STI/HIV | |

### FAMILY HISTORY - NOTE IF FATHER OF BABY
| DIABETES |
| HYPERTENSION |
| TWINS |
| CONGENITAL ANOM |
| OTHER FAMILY HX |

## MEDICAL HISTORY
✔ IF NEGATIVE-DESCRIBE POSITIVE HISTORY
| HEENT |

## PREVIOUS PREGNANCIES

| NO. | DATE | LENGTH (WKS) | LABOR (HRS) | TYPE DELIVERY | ANES. | SEX | WEIGHT | WHERE DELIVERED | COMPLICATIONS-AP, IP, PP, NEONATAL | OUTCOME/ NAME |
|---|---|---|---|---|---|---|---|---|---|---|

## PRESENT PREGNANCY HISTORY | PHYSICAL EXAMINATION | DATE

| LMP | LNMP | EDC | + PG TEST  TYPE  DATE |
|---|---|---|---|
☐ NORM ☐ ABNORM

PLANNED PREGNANCY/OK? | FATHER SUPPORTIVE?

✔ IF NEGATIVE-DESCRIBE POSITIVE FINDINGS

✔ IF NEGATIVE-DESCRIBE POSITIVE HISTORY

| NAUSEA/VOMITING | | HEIGHT |
| BLEEDING | | WEIGHT |
| URINARY SX | | B.P. |
| VAGINAL DISCHARGE | | HEENT |
| INFECTION | | NECK |
| FEVER/RASH | | LUNGS |
| TOBACCO/SMOKING | | BREASTS |
| ETOH | | HEART |
| PHYSICAL/SEXUAL ABUSE | | ABDOMEN |
| | | NEURO |
| | | EXTREMITIES/SKIN |

PATIENT NO.

### PELVIC EXAMINATION | DATE
| EXT. GENITALIA |
| VAGINA/CERVIX |
| UTERUS-SIZE |
| PELVIS |
| ADNEXA |
| BONY PELVIS/ADEQUATE? |
| HEMORRHOIDS |

PATIENT NAME

D.O.B.

PROVIDER SIGNATURE

| FIRST TRIMESTER | DATE | WEEKS | EDC/RANGE | DATE | PROBLEMS AND RISK FACTORS |
|---|---|---|---|---|---|
| LMP | | | | | |
| LNMP | | | | | |
| OVU/CONCEP | | | | | |
| FIRST EXAM | | | | | |
| + HCG URINE | | | | | |
| + HCG SERUM | | | | | |
| FHT DOPPLER | | | | | |
| FHT FETOSCOPE | | | | | |
| FM | | | | | |
| ULTRASOUND | | | | | |
| ULTRASOUND | | | | | |
| ULTRASOUND | | | | | |
| | | | | | |

## ANTICIPATORY GUIDANCE

| FIRST TRIMESTER | SECOND TRIMESTER | THIRD TRIMESTER |
|---|---|---|
| CLINIC PROCEDURES/OUTLINE PRENATAL CARE<br>HIV COUNSELING/TESTING<br>NUTRITION<br>VITAMINS/MINERALS<br>DENTAL/VISION CARE<br>WEIGHT GAIN<br>SEAT BELTS<br>EXERCISE<br>PRENATAL DIAGNOSIS<br>HAZARDS: SMOKING, ETOH, DRUGS, OVERHEATING, CATS,<br>RAW MEAT, UNPASTEURIZED MILK<br>DISCOMFORTS/RELIEF MEASURES<br>WARNING SIGNS: BLEEDING, CRAMPS, ABDOMINAL<br>PAINS, DYSURIA, ETC.<br>BROCHURES | FETAL DEVELOPMENT/QUICKENING<br>FAMILY/FATHER/SIBLINGS<br>HOSPITAL PRE-ADMISSION/TOUR?<br>FEEDING PLANS (BREAST/BOTTLE)<br>EXERCISES/BODY MECHANICS<br>WARNING SIGNS: SROM, BLEEDING, PRE-TERM LABOR<br>BABY'S CARE PROVIDER _____<br>NEWBORN CARE/ROOMING-IN<br>CIRCUMCISION<br>BROCHURES<br>PRENATAL CLASSES<br>SUPPORT PERSON _____<br>BIRTH PLANS/OPTIONS<br>SEXUALITY | DISCOMFORTS/RELIEF MEASURES<br>WARNING SIGNS<br>FETAL ACTIVITY MONITORING<br>LABOR SIGNS: WHEN AND HOW TO CALL<br>TRAVEL RESTRICTIONS<br>LABOR & DELIVERY ROUTINE<br>ELECTRONIC FETAL MONITORING<br>ANESTHESIA/ANALGESIA<br>EPISIOTOMY/PERINEAL INTEGRITY<br>LABOR & DELIVERY COMPLICATIONS/OPERATIVE DELIVERY<br>BREAST CARE<br>CAR SEAT<br>DISCUSS POST-TERM MANAGEMENT<br>EARLY DISCHARGE/HELP AT HOME |

| DATE | MEDICATIONS | POSTPARTUM CONTRACEPTIVE PLANS |
|---|---|---|
| | RHOGAM | ☐ ORAL CONTRACEPTION    ☐ LONG-ACTING CONTRACEPTION |
| | | ☐ STERILIZATION - DATE TUBAL FORM SIGNED _____ |
| | | ☐ BARRIER    ☐ OTHER |
| | | |
| | | |
| | | |
| | | |
| | | |
| | | |
| | | |
| DRUG ALLERGIES/REACTIONS    ☐ NKA | | |
| | | |
| PATIENT NAME | | |
| | | |

## LABORATORY DATA

| TYPE RH | RUBELLA | SEROLOGY | HBsAg | HIV | URINE | | DIABETIC SCREEN ___ @ ___ WKS | SICKLE PREP | PPD/TINE |
|---|---|---|---|---|---|---|---|---|---|

| ANTIBODY SCREEN ___ @ ___ WKS ___ @ ___ WKS | HCT ___ @ ___ WKS ___ @ ___ WKS | HSV SEROLOGY I ____ II ____ MSAFP / MOM PAP      DATE | CERVICAL CULTURES DATE CHLAMYDIA GC HSV STREP | GTT @ ___ WKS FBS 1 HR ___ 2 HR ___ 3 HR ___ | OTHER COPY SENT ___ COPY SENT ___ |
|---|---|---|---|---|---|

| EDC | REVISED EDC | REVISED EDC | AGE | GRAVIDA | PARA | | ABORTIONS | | | DEATHS | | LIVING CHILDREN |
|---|---|---|---|---|---|---|---|---|---|---|---|---|
| | | | | | TERM | PRETERM | SPONT | ELEC | ECTOPIC | FETAL | NEONATAL | |

## WEIGHT AND FUNDAL HEIGHT GRAPH

DATE

WEEKS GESTATION: 6 8 10 12 14 16 18 20 22 24 26 28 30 32 33 34 35 36 37 38 39 40 41 42 43

## PRENATAL VISITS

WEIGHT NON PG ___
BLOOD PRESSURE
BLOOD PRESSURE RE-CHECK
URINE PROTEIN/GLUCOSE
FHR D-DOPPLER F-FETOSCOPE
PRESENTATION
ESTIMATE UTERINE SIZE
FETAL ACTIVITY

WEEKS GESTATION: 6 8 10 12 14 16 18 20 22 24 26 28 30 32 33 34 35 36 37 38 39 40 41 42 43

FUTURE PARAMETERS TO CHECK — M S A F P OR TRIPLE SCREEN — HCT DIABETIC SCREEN RhNEG - ANTIBODY SCREEN ? RHOGAM — FETAL SURVEILLANCE

SEE NOTE (✔)
RETURN WEEKS
INITIALS

PATIENT NO.                    HOSPITAL
PATIENT NAME
D.O.B.

| RISK FACTOR GUIDELINES | PROGRESS NOTES |
|---|---|

**PATIENT PROFILE**
AGE > 34 OR PREGNANCY WITHIN 2 YEARS OF MENARCHE
OCCUPATION AND AVOCATION
DRUG ABUSE OR ADDICTION
   ALCOHOL
   SMOKING
   COCAINE
   MARIJUANA
   NARCOTICS
   SEDATIVES/HYPNOTICS
   SALICYLATES AND OTHER PGSI'S
   OTHER
LOW SOCIO-ECONOMIC STATUS
   WELFARE
   EDUCATION < 9TH GRADE
   CROWDED LIVING CONDITIONS
   OTHER
BODY HABITUS
   SMALL STATURE (< 5 FEET TALL)
   OBESE ( > 50# OVER IDEAL WEIGHT FOR HEIGHT)
   UNDERWEIGHT ( > 20# UNDER IDEAL WEIGHT FOR HEIGHT)
   MATERNAL BIRTHWEIGHT (LOW BIRTHWEIGHT OR LARGE FOR DATES)
PARTNER
   MEDICAL OR SURGICAL DISORDERS
   DRUG, SMOKING OR ALCOHOL ABUSE
   OCCUPATION, AVOCATION, HOBBIES
   STI'S (HERPES, URETHRITIS)
   HIV RISK FACTORS

**GYNECOLOGICAL HISTORY**
UTERINE AND CERVICAL ABNORMALITIES
   PAST UTERINE SURGERY (NON-CESAREAN)
   UTERINE ANOMALIES (CONGENITAL ANOMALIES, DES STIGMATA, MYOMATA)
   CERVICAL LACERATIONS OR CONIZATIONS
MENSTRUAL HISTORY AND GESTATIONAL DATING
   IRREGULAR MENSES OR OLIGOMENORRHEA
   ORAL CONTRACEPTIVE USE PRIOR TO CONCEPTION

**MEDICAL HISTORY**
   ANEMIA (HGB < 9.5 OR HCT < 30)
   HEART DISEASE (SYMPTOMATIC OR ASYMPTOMATIC)
   THROMBOEMBOLISM (DURING PREVIOUS PREGNANCY OR PRIOR TO
      CURRENT PREGNANCY)
   ANTICOAGULANT USE
   CHRONIC HYPERTENSION (BP > 140/90 AT FIRST PRENATAL VISIT)
   ASTHMA OR OTHER CHRONIC LUNG DISEASE
   SEIZURE DISORDER (WITH OR WITHOUT ANTICONVULSANT USE)
   DIABETES MELLITUS (GESTATIONAL OR PREGESTATIONAL)
   HEPATITIS
   HIV RISK FACTORS
   CHRONIC RENAL DISEASE (BUN > 20, CREATININE > 1.2 AT FIRST PRENATAL
      VISIT)
   PYELONEPHRITIS

**OBSTETRICAL FACTORS**
PARITY
   PRIMIGRAVIDA
   GRAND MULTIPARA (> 4)
PAST PREGNANCIES
   HABITUAL ABORTION (> 3)
   PREMATURE BIRTH (< 37 WEEKS)
   PREMATURE RUPTURE OF MEMBRANES
   LOW BIRTH WEIGHT INFANT (BIRTHWEIGHT < 10TH PERCENTILE FOR DATES)
   LARGE FOR DATES INFANT (BIRTHWEIGHT > 90TH PERCENTILE FOR DATES)
   FETAL OR NEONATAL DEATH
   CONGENITAL ANOMALIES
   SURVIVING NEUROLOGICALLY IMPAIRED INFANT
   CERVICAL INCOMPETENCY
   MIDFORCEP OR DIFFICULT DELIVERY (E.G., SHOULDER DYSTOCIA)
   ABNORMAL LABOR (ARREST OR PROTRACTION DISORDER OF FIRST OR
      SECOND STAGE)
   ANTEPARTUM HEMORRHAGE (PLACENTAL ABRUPTION, PLACENTA PREVIA)
   BLEEDING PRIOR TO 20 WEEKS
   RH ISOIMMUNIZATION
   PREGNANCY-INDUCED HYPERTENSION
   CESAREAN DELIVERY (LOW TRANSVERSE, LOW VERTICAL, CLASSIC,
      UNKNOWN)
   INTERVAL FROM LAST DELIVERY < 12 MONTHS
   ANESTHESIA INTOLERANCE OR REACTIONS

**PRESENT PREGNANCY**
   EMOTIONAL STRESS
   POOR COMPLIANCE
   LATE REGISTRATION FOR CARE
   UNCERTAIN DATES
   FAILURE TO GAIN WEIGHT (< 1/2 # PER WEEK AFTER 12 WEEKS)
   EXCESSIVE WEIGHT GAIN (> 2 # PER WEEK AFTER 12 WEEKS)
   BLEEDING PRIOR TO 20 WEEKS
   LACK OF PREGNANCY NAUSEA AND VOMITING (MORNING SICKNESS)
   PLACENTAL ABRUPTION
   PLACENTA PREVIA
   OTHER VAGINAL BLEEDING
   PREMATURE RUPTURE OF MEMBRANES
   POLYHYDRAMNIOS OR OLIGOHYDRAMNIOS
   THREATENED PREMATURE LABOR

PATIENT NAME

RM 612  REV 5/97

# Functional Assessment of the Older Adult

## PURPOSE

This chapter describes the functional assessment of the older adult using a systems perspective, including the normal changes of aging and ongoing chronic geriatric syndromes. Tools that may be used as part of the functional assessment of the older adult are described.

## READING ASSIGNMENT

Jarvis: *Physical Examination and Health Assessment,* 8th ed., Chapter 32, pp. 825-835.

Suggested readings:
Phillips Burkhart, K. (2016). Frailty syndrome: A weakly addressed problem. *Am Nurse Today, 11*(7), 7-9.

## GLOSSARY

Study the following terms after completing the reading assignment. You should be able to cover the definition on the right and define the term out loud.

**Activities of daily living** . . . . . . tasks that are necessary for self-care, such as eating/feeding, bathing, grooming, toileting, walking, and transferring

**Advanced activities of daily living** . . . . . . . . . . . . . activities that an older adult performs as a family member or as a member of society or community, including occupational and recreational activities

**Caregiver assessment** . . . . . . . . assessment of the health and well-being of an individual's caregiver

**Caregiver burden** . . . . . . . . . . . the perceived strain by the person who cares for an older, chronically ill, or disabled person

**Domains of cognition** . . . . . . . . domains included in mental status assessments, such as attention, memory, orientation, language, visuospatial skills, and higher cognitive functions

**Environmental** . . . . . . . . . . . . . assessment of an individual's home environment and community system, including hazards in the home

**Functional ability** . . . . . . . . . . the ability of a person to perform activities necessary to live in modern society; may include driving, using the telephone, or performing personal tasks such as bathing and toileting

**Functional assessment** . . . . . . . a systematic assessment that includes assessment of an individual's activities of daily living, instrumental activities of daily living, and mobility

**Functional status** . . . . . . . . . . . . a person's actual performance of activities and tasks associated with current life roles (as defined by Richmond et al., 2004)

**Geriatric assessment** . . . . . . . . multidimensional assessment: physical examination and assessments of mental status, functional status, social and economic status, pain, and physical environment for safety

**Home care** . . . . . . . . . . . . . . . . . supportive services provided in the home: skilled nursing care, primary care, therapy (physical, occupational, speech), social work, nutrition, case management, ADL assistance, durable medical equipment

**Instrumental activities**
**of daily living** . . . . . . . . . . . . . . functional abilities necessary for independent community living, such as shopping, meal preparation, housekeeping, laundry, managing finances, taking medications, and using transportation

**Katz Index of Independence**
**in Activities of Daily Living** . . . an instrument used to measure physical function in older adults and the chronically ill

**Lawton Instrumental**
**Activities of Daily Living** . . . . . an instrument used to measure an individual's ability to perform instrumental activities of daily living; may assist in assessing one's ability to live independently

**Physical performance**
**measures** . . . . . . . . . . . . . . . . . . tests that measure balance, gait, motor coordination, and endurance

**Social domain** . . . . . . . . . . . . . . the domain that focuses on an individual's relationships within family, social groups, and the community

**Social networks** . . . . . . . . . . . . informal supports accessed by older adults, such as family members and close friends, neighbors, church societies, neighborhood groups, and senior centers

**Spiritual assessment** . . . . . . . . assessment of an individual's spiritual health

# STUDY GUIDE

After completing the reading and media assignment, you should be able to answer the following questions in the spaces provided.

1. Differentiate the following, and provide 2 examples of each:

   Activities of daily living (ADLs)

   Instrumental activities of daily living (IADLs)

   Advanced activities of daily living (AADLs)

2. Discuss at least 2 disorders that may alter an older adult's cognition.

3. What are some indications of possible caregiver burnout?

4. Describe a method of assessing an older adult for depression.

5. Describe 3 contexts of care of an older adult.

6. How do falls affect older adults? Name some interventions.

7. List 4 ways in which driving cessation negatively affects the older adult.

8. Define an environmental assessment and list at least 4 common environmental hazards that may be found in an individual's home.

9. State the priority when assessing an older adult who is in pain.

10. Describe 4 nonpharmacologic interventions to improve sleep.

## CRITICAL THINKING EXERCISE

Consider the importance of home safety, especially as it relates to fall risk in older adults. Go online and review home safety checklists from the AARP and the National Safety Council. Use the checklists to determine the safety of your home. As you walk around your home, make note of anything that may be a trip hazard or anything that could be considered unsafe. Use the same checklists to assess the safety of an older adult's home. Were there any differences between the assessments? Did you notice anything within the older adult's home that should be changed to assure safety and prevent falls? Did you assess the older adult's home differently than you did your own home?

## REVIEW QUESTIONS

This test is for you to check your own mastery of the content. Answers are provided in Appendix A.

1. An appropriate tool to assess an individual's instrumental activities of daily living is a tool by:

   a. Katz.
   b. Lawton.
   c. Tinetti.
   d. Norbeck.

2. Which statement is true regarding an individual's functional status?

   a. Functional status refers to one's ability to care for another person.
   b. An older adult's functional status is usually static over time.
   c. An older adult's functional status may vary from independence to disability.
   d. Dementia is an example of functional status.

3. An older person is experiencing an acute change in cognition. You recognize that this disorder is:

   a. Alzheimer dementia.
   b. Attention deficit disorder.
   c. Depression.
   d. Delirium.

4. Assessment of the social domain includes:

   a. Family relationships.
   b. Ability to cook meals.
   c. Ability to balance the checkbook and pay bills.
   d. Hazards found in the home.

5. You will use which technique when assessing an older individual who has cognitive impairment?

   a. Ask open-ended questions.
   b. Complete the entire assessment in one session.
   c. Ask the family members for information instead of the older individual.
   d. Ask simple questions that have "yes" or "no" answers.

6. An older person needs to be assessed before going home as to whether he or she is able to go outside alone safely. Which test is best for this assessment?

   a. Timed Up and Go Test
   b. Performance of Activities of Daily Living test
   c. Older Americans Resources and Services Multidimensional Functional Assessment Questionnaire
   d. Lawton IADL instrument

7. An older adult has had surgery for a fractured hip and has a history of dementia. You should keep in mind that older adults with mild cognitive impairment:

   a. Experience less pain.
   b. Can provide a self-report of pain.
   c. Cannot be relied on to self-report pain.
   d. Will not express pain sensations.

8. An appropriate use of the Caregiver Strain Index would be which situation?

   a. A daughter who is taking her older father home to live with her
   b. An older patient who lives alone
   c. A wife who has cared for her husband for the past 4 years at home
   d. A son whose parents live in an assisted living facility

9. Which is an example of an informal social support network for the aging adult?

   a. A neighbor who drops by with newspapers and magazines on a regular basis
   b. An area church that offers a weekly activity and luncheon for seniors in the neighborhood
   c. A home health care agency that provides weekly blood pressure screenings at the church luncheon
   d. A senior citizen chess club whose members hold classes at the local Boys' Club

10. When completing a spiritual assessment, you should:

    a. Use "yes" and "no" questions as the foundation for future dialogue.
    b. Use open-ended questions to help the patient understand potential coping mechanisms.
    c. Try to complete this assessment as soon as possible after meeting the patient.
    d. Wait until a member of the clergy can be involved in the assessment.

11. When you perform a functional assessment of an older patient, which is most appropriate?

    a. Observe the patient's ability to perform the tasks.
    b. Ask the patient's partner how he or she does when performing tasks.
    c. Review the medical record for information on the patient's abilities.
    d. Ask the patient's physician for information on the patient's abilities.

12. The Lawton IADL instrument is described by which of the following?

    a. The nurse uses direct observation to implement this tool.
    b. It is designed as a self-report measure of performance rather than ability.
    c. It is not useful in the acute hospital setting.
    d. It is best used for those residing in an institutional setting.

13. An older adult's advanced activities of daily living would include:

    a. Recreational activities.
    b. Meal preparation.
    c. Balancing the checkbook.
    d. Self-grooming activities.

14. When using the various instruments to assess an older person's activities of daily living (ADLs), remember that a disadvantage of these instruments includes:

    a. The reliability of the tools.
    b. Self or proxy report of functional activities.
    c. Lack of confidentiality during the assessment.
    d. Insufficient detail about the deficiencies identified.

## SKILLS LABORATORY AND CLINICAL SETTING

The purpose of this component is to practice a functional assessment of an older adult. If possible, complete at least two assessments in different settings (e.g., acute care, ambulatory clinic, assisted living, home setting), noting the differences between settings and how you adapted the assessment based on the context of care.

### Clinical Objectives

1. Correctly administer the Timed Up and Go Test to an older adult.
2. Demonstrate the ability to assess ADLs and IADLs in an older adult.
3. Analyze differences between functional assessment findings (either between 2 or more assessments you completed or with a partner who assessed a different person).
4. Identify potential causes of decreased functional ability in an older adult.
5. Measure caregiver strain in an adult caregiver of an older dependent adult.

### Instructions

#### Functional Assessment of an Older Adult

Using the instructions and checklists below, complete a functional assessment of at least 1 older adult. If possible, assess at least 2 older adults in different settings (e.g., acute care hospital, ambulatory clinic, assisted living, home environment). Compare the results of each assessment. Did you identify areas of dependence? Were you able to observe each area, or was self-reporting used? What medical conditions, if any, lead to a decrease in independence for the older person? If only one assessment was completed, discuss your findings with a partner who assessed a different older adult. Note similarities and differences in your findings. Did context of care shape the results?

- **Timed Up and Go Test**
  - Equipment: arm chair, tape measure, tape, stopwatch.
  - Place a piece of tape 10 feet (3 meters) away from the chair so that it is easily seen by the subject.
  - Instructions to the subject: "When I say go, you will stand up, walk to the line on the floor, turn around, walk back to the chair, and sit down. Please walk at your regular pace."
  - The subject should wear normal footwear and use any assistive device typically used during ambulation. You will begin timing when you say go and end when the subject has returned to a seated position. The subject should begin the test completely seated with hips all the way to the back of the seat. Give the subject a practice run that is not timed so that he or she understands the test.
  - Note gait, balance, and the amount of time it takes for the person to complete the test.
  - If the person takes ≥12 seconds to complete the test, he or she is at risk of falling.
- **Katz Index of Independence in Activities of Daily Living and Lawton Instrumental Activities of Daily Living Scale**

  Review the questions on each scale. In the clinical setting, use the Katz ADL form and the Lawton IADL form to assess an older adult.

| **Katz Activities of Daily Living** | | |
|---|---|---|
| **Activities**<br>Points (1 or 0) | **Independence**<br>(1 point)<br>NO supervision, direction,<br>or personal assistance | **Dependence**<br>(0 points)<br>WITH supervision, direction,<br>personal assistance, or total care |
| Bathing<br>Points _____ | (1 point) Bathes self completely or needs help in bathing only a single part of the body such as the back, genital area, or disabled extremity | (0 points) Needs help with bathing more than one part of the body or getting in or out of the tub or shower; requires total bathing |
| Dressing<br>Points _____ | (1 point) Gets clothes from closet and drawers and puts on clothes and outer garments complete with fasteners; may have help tying shoes | (0 points) Needs help with dressing self or needs to be completely dressed |
| Toileting<br>Points _____ | (1 point) Gets to toilet, gets on and off, arranges clothes, cleans genital area without help | (0 points) Needs help transferring to the toilet, cleaning self, or using bedpan or commode |
| Transferring<br>Points _____ | (1 point) Moves in and out of bed or chair unassisted. Mechanical transferring aids are acceptable | (0 points) Needs help in moving from bed to chair or requires a complete transfer |
| Continence<br>Points _____ | e.(1 point) Exercises complete self-control over urination and defecation | (0 points) Is partially or totally incontinent of bowel or bladder |
| Feeding<br>Points _____ | (1 point) Gets food from plate into mouth without help. Preparation of food may be done by another person | (0 points) Needs partial or total help with feeding or requires parenteral feeding |
| Total points = _____ | 6 = High (patient independent) | 0 = Low (patient very dependent) |

Adapted from Gerontological Society of America. Katz, S., Downs, T. D., Cash, H. R., et al. (1970). Progress in the development of the index of ADL. *Gerontologist, 10,* 20-30.

## The Lawton Instrumental Activities of Daily Living Scale

A. Ability to Use Telephone
    1. Operates telephone on own initiative; looks up and dials numbers     1
    2. Dials a few well-known numbers     1
    3. Answers telephone, but does not dial     1
    4. Does not use telephone at all     0

B. Shopping
    1. Takes care of all shopping needs independently     1
    2. Shops independently for small purchases     0
    3. Needs to be accompanied on any shopping trip     0
    4. Completely unable to shop     0

C. Food Preparation
    1. Plans, prepares, and serves adequate meals independently     1
    2. Prepares adequate meals if supplied with ingredients     0
    3. Heats and serves prepared meals or prepares meals, but does not maintain adequate diet     0
    4. Needs to have meals prepared and served     0

D. Housekeeping
    1. Maintains house alone with occasional assistance (heavy work)     1
    2. Performs light daily tasks such as dishwashing, bed making     1
    3. Performs light daily tasks, but cannot maintain acceptable level of cleanliness     1
    4. Needs help with all home maintenance tasks     1
    5. Does not participate in any housekeeping tasks     0

E. Laundry
    1. Does personal laundry completely     1
    2. Launders small items, rinses socks, stockings, etc     1
    3. All laundry must be done by others     0

F. Mode of Transportation
    1. Travels independently on public transportation or drives own car     1
    2. Arranges own travel via taxi, but does not otherwise use public transportation     1
    3. Travels on public transportation when assisted or accompanied by another     1
    4. Travel limited to taxi or automobile with assistance of another     0
    5. Does not travel at all     0

G. Responsibility for Own Medications
    1. Is responsible for taking medication in correct dosages at correct time     1
    2. Takes responsibility if medication is prepared in advance in separate dosages     0
    3. Is not capable of dispensing own medication     0

H. Ability to Handle Finances
    1. Manages financial matters independently (budgets, writes checks, pays rent and bills, goes to bank); collects and keeps track of income     1
    2. Manages day-to-day purchases, but needs help with banking, major purchases, etc     1
    3. Incapable of handling money     0

Scoring: For each category, circle the item description that most closely resembles the client's highest functional level (either 0 or 1).

From Lawton, M.P., & Brody, E.M. (1969). Assessment of older people: self-maintaining and instrumental activities of daily living. *Gerontologist, 9,* 179-186. © The Gerontological Society of America.

Jarvis, Carolyn: PHYSICAL EXAMINATION AND HEALTH ASSESSMENT: Study Guide and Laboratory Manual, Eighth Edition. Copyright © 2020, 2016, 2012, 2008, 2004, 2000, 1996 by Elsevier Inc. All rights reserved.

## Caregiver Assessment

Too often, health care workers fail to assess the caregivers of older dependent patients. Assessment of the caregiver is an integral part of identifying the needs of the older adult; it helps to assure that the caregiver is not suffering from burnout, depression, or increased stress. After completing your assessment and discussing it with the caregiver, discuss the results with a partner who assessed a different caregiver. Were there any significant differences? If so, what do you think contributed to the differences?

- **Modified Caregiver Strain Index**
  Identify an adult who is the primary caregiver for a dependent older adult. If you are unable to identify an adult caregiver of an older dependent adult, identify a caregiver to a disabled or dependent adult >18 years old. Administer the Modified Caregiver Strain Index. Discuss the results with the caregiver. While no specific cutoff for caregiver strain is identified, the higher the score, the more strain the caregiver is under and the more likely it is that he or she will need assistance.

## Modified Caregiver Strain Index

**Directions:** Here is a list of things that other caregivers have found to be difficult. Please put a checkmark in the columns that apply to you. We have included some examples that are common caregiver experiences to help you think about each item. Your situation may be slightly different, but the item could still apply.

| | Yes, on a regular basis = 2 | Yes, sometimes = 1 | No = 0 |
|---|---|---|---|
| **My sleep is disturbed**<br>(For example, *the person I care for* is in and out of bed or wanders around at night) | | | |
| **Caregiving is inconvenient**<br>(For example, helping takes so much time or it's a long drive over to help) | | | |
| **Caregiving is a physical strain**<br>(For example, lifting in or out of a chair; effort or concentration is required) | | | |
| **Caregiving is confining**<br>(For example, helping restricts free time or *I* cannot go visiting) | | | |
| **There have been family adjustments**<br>(For example, helping has disrupted *my* routine; there has been no privacy) | | | |
| **There have been changes in personal plans**<br>(For example, *I* had to turn down a job; *I* could not go on vacation) | | | |
| **There have been other demands on my time**<br>(For example, other family members *need me*) | | | |
| **There have been emotional adjustments**<br>(For example, severe arguments *about caregiving*) | | | |
| **Some behavior is upsetting**<br>(For example, incontinence; *the person cared for* has trouble remembering things; or *the person I care for* accuses people of taking things) | | | |
| **It is upsetting to find the person I care for has changed so much from his or her former self**<br>(For example, he or she is a different person than he or she used to be) | | | |
| **There have been work adjustments**<br>(For example, *I* have to take time off *for caregiving duties*) | | | |
| **Caregiving is a financial strain** | | | |
| **I feel completely overwhelmed**<br>(For example, *I* worry about *the person I care* for; *I* have concerns about how *I* will manage) | | | |

Total Score =

Words appearing in *italics* represent modifications from Thornton, M., & Travis, S. S. (2003). Analysis of the reliability of the modified caregiver strain index. *The Journals of Gerontology, 58B*(2), S129. © The Gerontological Society of America. Reproduced by permission of the publisher.

# NOTES

# Answers to Review Questions

## Chapter 1: Evidence-Based Assessment

| | | |
|---|---|---|
| 1. c | 6. a | 11. c |
| 2. d | 7. a | 12. c |
| 3. c | 8. c | 13. d |
| 4. b | 9. c | 14. d |
| 5. c | 10. b | 15. c |

## Chapter 2: Cultural Assessment

| | | |
|---|---|---|
| 1. a | 6. a | 11. d |
| 2. c | 7. b | 12. c |
| 3. d | 8. d | 13. d |
| 4. c | 9. b | 14. b |
| 5. c | 10. a | 15. c |

## Chapter 3: The Interview

| | | |
|---|---|---|
| 1. a | 6. b | 11. b |
| 2. a | 7. a | 12. c |
| 3. b | 8. d | 13. a |
| 4. c | 9. b | 14. b |
| 5. d | 10. d | 15. b |

## Chapter 4: The Complete Health History

| | | |
|---|---|---|
| 1. d | 6. c | 11. c |
| 2. a | 7. a | 12. d |
| 3. c | 8. d | 13. d |
| 4. b | 9. b | |
| 5. c | 10. d | |

## Chapter 5: Mental Status Assessment

| | | |
|---|---|---|
| 1. d | 6. c | 11. c |
| 2. a | 7. b | 12. d |
| 3. d | 8. a | 13. c |
| 4. c | 9. b | 14. a |
| 5. b | 10. a | 15. c |

| | | |
|---|---|---|
| 16. i | for season | remote |
| 17. d | and setting. | memory |
| 18. b | Posture | intact. Affect |
| 19. g | is erect, | and verbal |
| 20. f | with no | responses |
| 21. a | involuntary | appropriate. |
| 22. e | body | Perceptions |
| 23. h | movements | and thought |
| 24. Patient is | Oriented to | processes |
| dressed and | time, person, | logical and |
| groomed | and place. | coherent. |
| appropriately | Recent and | |

## Chapter 6: Substance Use Assessment

| | | |
|---|---|---|
| 1. c | 6. b | 11. a |
| 2. b | 7. c | 12. b |
| 3. a | 8. c | 13. c |
| 4. c | 9. a | 14. c |
| 5. b | 10. b | |

## Chapter 7: Domestic and Family Violence Assessment

| | | |
|---|---|---|
| 1. d | 6. e | 11. b |
| 2. a | 7. d | 12. d |
| 3. b | 8. d | 13. b |
| 4. b | 9. b | 14. d |
| 5. a | 10. c | 15. a |

## Chapter 8: Assessment Techniques and Safety in the Clinical Setting

| | | |
|---|---|---|
| 1. d | 5. c | 9. d |
| 2. c | 6. d | 10. b |
| 3. b | 7. c | 11. d |
| 4. a | 8. c | |

## Chapter 9: General Survey and Measurement

| | | |
|---|---|---|
| 1. d | 3. b | 5. c |
| 2. c | 4. c | |

## Chapter 10: Vital Signs

| | | |
|---|---|---|
| 1. a | 5. a | 9. c |
| 2. b | 6. d | 10. b |
| 3. b | 7. c | |
| 4. d | 8. a | |

## Chapter 11: Pain Assessment

| | | |
|---|---|---|
| 1. c | 6. b | 11. d |
| 2. b | 7. c | 12. b |
| 3. c | 8. b | 13. d |
| 4. d | 9. d | 14. d |
| 5. d | 10. c | 15. d |

## Chapter 12: Nutrition Assessment

| | | |
|---|---|---|
| 1. c | 5. b | 9. b |
| 2. d | 6. a | 10. d |
| 3. c | 7. b | 11. c |
| 4. c | 8. c | 12. b |

## Chapter 13: Skin, Hair, and Nails

| | | |
|---|---|---|
| 1. b | 12. c | 23. a |
| 2. a | 13. c | 24. b |
| 3. d | 14. b | 25. d |
| 4. b | 15. a | 26. b |
| 5. d | 16. c | 27. a |
| 6. c | 17. b | 28. g |
| 7. a | 18. c | 29. c |
| 8. a | 19. a | 30. f |
| 9. c | 20. a | 31. d |
| 10. d | 21. b | 32. e |
| 11. c | 22. c | |

## Chapter 14: Head, Face, Neck, and Regional Lymphatics

| | | |
|---|---|---|
| 1. d | 5. d | 9. a |
| 2. c | 6. d | 10. a |
| 3. b | 7. c | 11. a |
| 4. a | 8. d | 12. c |

| | | |
|---|---|---|
| 13. a | 17. f | 21. j |
| 14. b | 18. h | 22. b |
| 15. c | 19. g | 23. d |
| 16. e | 20. i | 24. a |

## Chapter 15: Eyes

| | | |
|---|---|---|
| 1. b | 10. b | d. R—react (to) |
| 2. a | 11. c | |
| 3. b | 12. b | e. L—light (and) |
| 4. d | 13. a | |
| 5. c | 14. b | f. A—accommo-dation |
| 6. a | 15. a. P—pupils | |
| 7. c | b. E—equal | |
| 8. a | c. R—round | 16. c |
| 9. c | | |

## Chapter 16: Ears

| | | |
|---|---|---|
| 1. c | 6. d | 11. b |
| 2. a | 7. b | 12. d |
| 3. d | 8. d | 13. c |
| 4. b | 9. b | 14. b |
| 5. c | 10. a | |

## Chapter 17: Nose, Mouth, and Throat

| | | |
|---|---|---|
| 1. c | 6. b | 11. a |
| 2. d | 7. d | 12. c |
| 3. a | 8. c | 13. a |
| 4. a | 9. a | 14. c |
| 5. b | 10. d | 15. a |

## Chapter 18: Breasts, Axillae, and Regional Lymphatics

| | | |
|---|---|---|
| 1. d | 6. c | 11. c |
| 2. b | 7. c | 12. d |
| 3. a | 8. c | 13. a |
| 4. c | 9. b | 14. b |
| 5. a | 10. d | 15. b |

## Chapter 19: Thorax and Lungs

| | | |
|---|---|---|
| 1. a | 5. b | 9. d |
| 2. b | 6. b | 10. b |
| 3. b | 7. d | 11. c |
| 4. a | 8. c | 12. a |

| | | |
|---|---|---|
| 13. c | 18. d | 23. f |
| 14. a | 19. b | 24. c |
| 15. e | 20. e | 25. b |
| 16. a | 21. a | |
| 17. c | 22. d | |

## Chapter 20: Heart and Neck Vessels

| | | |
|---|---|---|
| 1. c | 16. Fill in the | carotid |
| 2. b | following | artery and |
| 3. c | blanks: | coincides |
| 4. b | $S_1$ is best | with the R |
| 5. d | heard at | wave if the |
| 6. d | the apex of | patient is |
| 7. b | the heart, | on an ECG |
| 8. b | whereas $S_2$ | monitor. |
| 9. a | is loudest | 17. e |
| 10. a | at the base | 18. c |
| 11. a | of the | 19. f |
| 12. b | heart. $S_1$ | 20. a |
| 13. c | coincides | 21. b |
| 14. c | with the | 22. d |
| 15. b | pulse in the | |

## Chapter 21: Peripheral Vascular System and Lymphatic System

| | | |
|---|---|---|
| 1. a | 6. d | 11. a |
| 2. c | 7. a | 12. c |
| 3. c | 8. d | 13. a |
| 4. b | 9. b | 14. b |
| 5. c | 10. d | 15. b |

## Chapter 22: Abdomen

| | | |
|---|---|---|
| 1. c | 6. a | 11. c |
| 2. c | 7. d | 12. b |
| 3. a | 8. d | 13. d |
| 4. d | 9. a | |
| 5. c | 10. a | |

## Chapter 23: Musculoskeletal System

| | | |
|---|---|---|
| 1. d | 6. a | 11. d |
| 2. b | 7. c | 12. d |
| 3. d | 8. b | 13. b |
| 4. c | 9. c | 14. e |
| 5. a | 10. b | 15. g |

| | | |
|---|---|---|
| 16. i | 20. m | 24. h |
| 17. d | 21. k | 25. f |
| 18. a | 22. n | 26. c |
| 19. j | 23. l | |

## Chapter 24: Neurologic System

| | | |
|---|---|---|
| 1. a | 10. c | 19. c |
| 2. d | 11. b | 20. l |
| 3. c | 12. d | 21. d |
| 4. c | 13. a | 22. i |
| 5. b | 14. f | 23. e |
| 6. c | 15. b | 24. j |
| 7. b | 16. g | 25. a |
| 8. a | 17. k | |
| 9. b | 18. h | |

## Chapter 25: Male Genitourinary System

| | | |
|---|---|---|
| 1. c | 6. d | 11. a |
| 2. c | 7. b | 12. b |
| 3. d | 8. a | 13. e |
| 4. c | 9. d | 14. d |
| 5. c | 10. a | 15. b |

## Chapter 26: Anus, Rectum, and Prostate

| | | |
|---|---|---|
| 1. a | 6. c | 11. b |
| 2. b | 7. b | 12. b |
| 3. c | 8. c | 13. a |
| 4. a | 9. c | |
| 5. d | 10. a | |

## Chapter 27: Female Genitourinary System

| | | |
|---|---|---|
| 1. d | 6. d | 11. a |
| 2. a | 7. b | 12. a |
| 3. d | 8. c | 13. b |
| 4. c | 9. b | 14. b |
| 5. c | 10. b | |

## Chapter 31: The Pregnant Woman

| | | |
|---|---|---|
| 1. a | 6. e | 11. a |
| 2. c | 7. e | 12. d |
| 3. c | 8. d | 13. a |
| 4. c | 9. d | |
| 5. b | 10. b | |

## Chapter 32: Functional Assessment of the Older Adult

| | | | | |
|---|---|---|---|---|
| 1. b | 4. a | 7. b | 9. a | 11. a | 13. a |
| 2. c | 5. d | 8. c | 10. b | 12. b | 14. b |
| 3. d | 6. a | | | | |